# BREAST SURGERY

# A Companion to Specialist Surgical Practice

**Series Editors**
O. James Garden
Simon Paterson-Brown

# BREAST SURGERY

**FOURTH EDITION**

## Edited by

## J. Michael Dixon
BSc MB ChB MD FRCS FRCS(Ed) FRCP

Professor of Surgery
School of Molecular and Clinical Medicine
University of Edinburgh
Consultant Surgeon and Clinical Director, Breakthrough Research Unit
Edinburgh Breast Unit
Western General Hospital
Edinburgh, UK

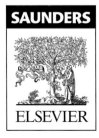

SAUNDERS

ELSEVIER

Edinburgh   London   New York   Oxford   Philadelphia   St Louis   Sydney   Toronto   2009

# SAUNDERS
## ELSEVIER

Fourth edition © 2009 Elsevier Limited. All rights reserved.

First edition 1997
Second edition 2001
Third edition 2005
Fourth edition 2009
 Reprinted 2010, 2011

ISBN 9780702030123

**British Library Cataloguing in Publication Data**
A catalogue record for this book is available from the British Library

**Library of Congress Cataloging in Publication Data**
A catalog record for this book is available from the Library of Congress

**Notice**

Knowledge and best practice in this field are constantly changing. As new research and experience broaden our knowledge, changes in practice, treatment and drug therapy may become necessary or appropriate. Readers are advised to check the most current information provided (i) on procedures featured or (ii) by the manufacturer of each product to be administered, to verify the recommended dose or formula, the method and duration of administration, and contraindications. It is the responsibility of the practitioner, relying on their own experience and knowledge of the patient, to make diagnoses, to determine dosages and the best treatment for each individual patient, and to take all appropriate safety precautions. To the fullest extent of the law, neither the Publisher nor the Editors assumes any liability for any injury and/or damage to persons or property arising out of or related to any use of the material contained in this book.

*The Publisher*

**ELSEVIER** your source for books,
journals and multimedia
in the health sciences
**www.elsevierhealth.com**

Working together to grow
libraries in developing countries

www.elsevier.com | www.bookaid.org | www.sabre.org

**ELSEVIER**   **BOOK AID** International   Sabre Foundation

The Publisher's policy is to use paper manufactured from sustainable forests

Printed in China

*Commissioning Editor:* Laurence Hunter
*Development Editor:* Elisabeth Lawrence
*Project Manager:* Andrew Palfreyman
*Text Design:* Charlotte Murray
*Cover Design:* Kirsteen Wright
*Illustration Manager:* Gillian Richards
*Illustrators:* Martin Woodward and Richard Prime

# Contents

# Contents

# Contributors

Douglas J.A. Adamson, MB, ChB, MD,
PhD, FRCP, FRCR
Consultant Clinical Oncologist
Department of Oncology
Ninewells Hospital
Dundee, UK

Monica Arnedos, MD
The Breast Unit
Royal Marsden Hospital
London, UK

Andrew D. Baildam, BSc, MB, ChB,
MD, FRCS
Consultant Oncoplastic Breast Surgeon
Withington Hospital;
Honorary Senior Lecturer in Surgical Oncology
University of Manchester
Manchester, UK

Nicola L.P. Barnes, MB, ChB, MRCS
Surgical Research Fellow
Academic Department of Surgery
University of Manchester
Manchester, UK

Tom Bates, MB, BS, FRCS
Consultant Surgeon
Breast Unit
William Harvey Hospital
Ashford, UK

Nigel J. Bundred, MD, FRCS
Professor of Surgical Oncology
Education and Research Centre
University of Manchester;
Consultant Surgeon
South Manchester University Hospital
Manchester, UK

Massimiliano Cariati, MBBS, PhD
Department of Academic Oncology
Guy's Hospital
Guy's and St Thomas' NHS Foundation
Trust
London, UK

Krishna B. Clough, MD
Chief of Surgery
Paris Breast Center
Paris, France

Tim Davidson, ChM, MRCP, FRCS
Consultant Surgeon
Breast Unit
University Department of Surgery
Royal Free Hospital
London, UK

John Dewar, BM, BCh, FRCP, FRCR
Department of Radiotherapy and Oncology
Ninewells Hospital
Dundee, UK

J. Michael Dixon, BSc, MB, ChB, MD, FRCS,
FRCS(Ed), FRCP
Professor of Surgery
School of Molecular and Clinical Medicine
University of Edinburgh
Consultant Surgeon and Clinical Director,
Breakthrough Research Unit
Edinburgh Breast Unit
Western General Hospital
Edinburgh, UK

William C. Dooley, MD, FACS
G. Rainey Williams Professor of Surgical
Oncology and Chair
University of Oklahoma Breast Institute;
Director, Division of Surgical Oncology
University of Oklahoma Health Sciences Center
Oklahoma City, OK, USA

Ian O. Ellis, BM, BS, BMedSc, MRCPath, FRCPath
Professor of Cancer Pathology
University of Nottingham School of Medicine;
Honorary Consultant Pathologist
City Hospital
Nottingham, UK

D. Gareth R. Evans, MB, ChB, FRCS
Professor of Medical Genetics
Academic Unit of Medical Genetics
St Mary's Hospital
Manchester, UK

Lesley Fallowfield, BSc, DPhil
Professor in Psycho-oncology
Cancer Research UK
Psychosocial Oncology Group
Brighton and Sussex Medical School
University of Sussex
Brighton, UK

# Contributors

**Valerie A. Jenkins, BSc, DPhil**
Senior Research Fellow
Cancer Research UK
Psychosocial Oncology Group
Brighton and Sussex Medical School
University of Sussex
Brighton, UK

**Gabriel J. Kaufman, MD**
Department of breast cancer and reconstructive
surgery
Paris Breast Center
Paris, France

**Pamela Levack, MB, ChB, MRCP**
Consultant in Palliative Care
Ninewell's Hospital
Dundee, UK

**R. Douglas Macmillan, MD, FRCS**
Consultant Surgeon and Associate Clinical
Director
Nottingham Breast Institute
Nottingham City Hospital
Nottingham, UK

**Monica Morrow, MD, FACS**
Chief of the Breast Surgery Service
Co-Chief of the Breast Program
Memorial Sloan-Kettering Cancer Center
New York , NY, USA

**Claude Nos, MD**
Department of breast cancer and reconstructive
surgery
Paris Breast Center
Paris, France

**Tawakalitu Oseni, MD**
Surgical Oncology Fellow
Fox Chase Cancer Center
Philadelphia, PA, USA

**Arnie D. Purushotham, MBBS, FRCS, MD**
Professor of Breast Cancer
Department of Academic Oncology
Guy's Hospital
Guy's and St Thomas' NHS Foundation Trust
London, UK

**Richard M. Rainsbury, BSc, MS, FRCS**
Consultant Oncoplastic Breast Surgeon
Royal Hampshire County Hospital
Winchester, UK

**Emad A. Rakha, MD, PhD**
Nottingham Breast Institute
City Hospital
Nottingham, UK

**Rajendra S. Rampaul, MB, ChB, MD, FRCS**
Specialist Registrar in Surgery
Nottingham Breast Institute
City Hospital
Nottingham, UK

**John F.R. Robertson, MB, ChB, FRCS**
Professor of Surgery
University of Nottingham;
Consultant Surgeon
City Hospital
Nottingham, UK

**Gillian Ross, MB, ChB, FRCP**
Senior Lecturer and Honorary Consultant Clinical
Oncologist
Royal Marsden Hospital
London, UK

**Ian E. Smith, MD, FRCP, FRCPE**
Professor of Cancer Medicine and
Consultant Clinical Oncologist
The Breast Unit
Royal Marsden Hospital and Institute of
Cancer Research
London, UK

**Alastair M. Thompson, BSc, MB ChB, MD,
FRCSEd (Gen)**
Professor of Surgical Oncology
Department of Surgery and Molecular Oncology
University of Dundee
Ninewells Hospital and Medical School
Dundee, UK

**Steven Thrush, MBBS, FRCS(Gen Surg)**
Consultant Surgeon
Breast Unit
Worcester Royal Hospital
Worcester, UK

**Eva M. Weiler-Mithoff, MD, FRCS(Ed),
FRCS(Glasg), FRCS(Plast)**
Consultant Plastic and Reconstructive Surgeon
Canniesburn Plastic Surgery Unit
Glasgow Royal Infirmary
Glasgow, UK

**A. Robin M. Wilson, MB, ChB, FRCR, FRCP**
Consultant Radiologist
King's College Hospital
London, UK

**Virginia Wolstenholme, MB**
Consultant Clinical Oncologist
Barts and the London NHS Trust
London, UK

# Series preface

Since the publication of the first edition in 1997, the *Companion to Specialist Surgical Practice* series has aspired to meet the needs of surgeons in higher training and practising consultants who wish contemporary, evidence-based information on the subspecialist areas relevant to their general surgical practice. We have accepted that the series will not necessarily be as comprehensive as some of the larger reference surgical textbooks which, by their very size, may not always be completely up to date at the time of publication. This Fourth Edition aims to bring relevant state-of-the-art specialist information that we and the individual volume editors consider important for the practising subspecialist general surgeon. Where possible, all contributors have attempted to identify evidence-based references to support key recommendations within each chapter.

We remain grateful to the volume editors and all the contributors of this Fourth Edition. Their enthusiasm, commitment and hard work has ensured that a short turnover has been maintained between each of the editions, thereby ensuring as accurate and up-to-date

content as possible. We remain grateful for the support and encouragement of Laurence Hunter and Elisabeth Lawrence at Elsevier Ltd. We trust that our aim of providing up-to-date and affordable surgical texts has been met and that all readers, whether in training or in consultant practice, will find this fourth edition an invaluable resource.

**O. James Garden** MB, ChB, MD, FRCS(Glas), FRCS(Ed), FRCP(Ed), FRACS(Hon), FRCSC(Hon)

Regius Professor of Clinical Surgery, Clinical and Surgical Sciences (Surgery), University of Edinburgh, and Honorary Consultant Surgeon, Royal Infirmary of Edinburgh

**Simon Paterson-Brown** MB, BS, MPhil, MS, FRCS(Ed), FRCS

Honorary Senior Lecturer, Clinical and Surgical Sciences (Surgery), University of Edinburgh, and Consultant General and Upper Gastrointestinal Surgeon, Royal Infirmary of Edinburgh

# Editor's preface

The late, great John Bostwick compared writing a textbook to running a marathon. He pointed out that a surgeon is like a marathon runner who must constantly reassess their record and continue to set new goals. My goal for the Third Edition was to provide trainees in surgery with a text setting out the body of knowledge that is necessary for the specialist breast surgeon together with a perspective of how breast surgery could evolve.

Since the Third Edition, science has continued to move forward and the art of breast surgery has continued to progress. This volume reassesses current practices in breast surgery and the goal has been to extend the scope of the book, to add new topics, including how to perform a good mastectomy, and to cover some areas more comprehensively, such as benign disease, locally advanced and metastatic breast cancer.

The new volume builds on the changes that were introduced in the Third Edition. The chapters on imaging, pathology and ductoscopy have been revised and updated. An area that continues to advance is the use of oncoplastic techniques to produce better outcomes for patients undergoing breast-conserving surgery. The chapter on breast-conserving surgery has been rewritten and extended, and the previous chapter on partial breast reconstruction has been split into two. This now includes a completely new text on the wide range of oncoplastic techniques that can be used to excise a cancer from different quadrants of the breast. For many countries mastectomy is the most commonly performed operation for patients with breast cancer and yet little is included in textbooks on how to excise all the breast tissue while at the same time producing a satisfactory mastectomy scar. Thus the decision to add a new chapter on this subject. There continues to be major changes in the management of the axilla and this chapter has been rewritten by new authors.

There have been numerous advances in our understanding of the genetics of breast cancer, with increasing emphasis on screening and improved management of patients carrying genes known to be associated with an increased breast cancer risk. These new advances are reflected in the revised chapter on this topic. The chapter on breast reconstruction now includes details of the extended latissimus dorsi flap, a procedure which is being used increasingly for autologous whole-breast reconstruction. There have been extensive revisions to the chapters on common breast cancer conditions and ductal carcinoma in situ. Previously there was a single large chapter on the systemic therapy of breast cancer and a second chapter on palliative care. There have been such advances in these areas that three completely new chapters have been included. One deals with adjuvant systemic therapy in patients with operable breast cancer, a second covers locally advanced disease and a third metastatic breast cancer incorporating palliative care. Partial breast radiotherapy after breast-conserving surgery has gained increasing popularity in the USA. There remains controversy as to which patients benefit from postoperative chest wall radiotherapy after mastectomy and new data in both these areas are included in the revised chapter on radiotherapy. The chapter on psychosocial issues has been updated.

Although this book concentrates on breast cancer management, a large percentage of a breast surgeon's time is involved in looking after patients with benign breast disease. For this reason the chapter on benign disease, which appeared for the first time in the Third Edition, has been rewritten and extended to include a wider range of conditions. Litigation in breast disease continues to accelerate at an alarming rate and the chapter covering this topic, which has been one of the few chapters present in all four editions, has received a thorough revision.

Ideas and concepts for this book have evolved over many years. The desire to share insights and lessons learnt from clinical experience whilst building on the cumulative experience of others has been the main motivation for this book. Putting together such a book has involved many people. Seeing the edition emerge from its many outlines brings its own reward. Ultimately, however, its success will be judged by you the reader and you will decide whether I have achieved the goals set out above and whether the efforts of the many authors involved have been worthwhile.

Your feedback is welcome. If there are topics we should have covered which have been omitted, or this text fails to meet your expectations, please let me know. If you enjoy this book, please tell your friends and colleagues.

# Acknowledgements

Firstly I would like to say a big thank you to all those who have contributed to this fourth edition. As in previous editions I have hassled and bullied various authors, who despite this have produced consistently high-quality work. I would specifically like to thank my PA, Mrs Jan Mauritzen, who has not only coordinated with the authors and Liz Lawrence, the Editorial Project Manager at Elsevier, but has made the many changes to the text that I have requested. I would like to acknowledge the many individuals who have trained and taught me over so many years. My enthusiasm in breast disease was ignited by Professor David Page, a pathologist from Nashville.

Professor Page was spending a sabbatical in Edinburgh during the year I spent in pathology and his enthusiasm for his topic was the major reason I pursued a career in breast disease. The surgeons who have influenced me the most include the late John Bostwick III and my contemporary and friend, Krishna Clough. I pay tribute to their foresight and surgical skills. What has underpinned my career in breast surgery over so many years is the enormous positive feedback I have received from the many patients who I have been fortunate enough to care for. Their ability to cope with their disease and the treatments they receive remains my inspiration.

J. Michael Dixon
Edinburgh

# Evidence-based practice in surgery

Critical appraisal for developing evidence-based practice can be obtained from a number of sources, the most reliable being randomised controlled clinical trials, systematic literature reviews, meta-analyses and observational studies. For practical purposes three grades of evidence can be used, analogous to the levels of 'proof' required in a court of law:

1. **Beyond all reasonable doubt.** Such evidence is likely to have arisen from high-quality randomised controlled trials, systematic reviews or high-quality synthesised evidence such as decision analysis, cost-effectiveness analysis or large observational datasets. The studies need to be directly applicable to the population of concern and have clear results. The grade is analogous to burden of proof within a criminal court and may be thought of as corresponding to the usual standard of 'proof' within the medical literature (i.e. $P < 0.05$).

2. **On the balance of probabilities.** In many cases a high-quality review of literature may fail to reach firm conclusions due to conflicting or inconclusive results, trials of poor methodological quality or the lack of evidence in the population to which the guidelines apply. In such cases it may still be possible to make a statement as to the best treatment on the 'balance of probabilities'. This is analogous to the decision in a civil court where all the available evidence will be weighed up and the verdict will depend upon the balance of probabilities.

3. **Not proven.** Insufficient evidence upon which to base a decision, or contradictory evidence.

Depending on the information available, three grades of recommendation can be used:

a. Strong recommendation, which should be followed unless there are compelling reasons to act otherwise.

b. A recommendation based on evidence of effectiveness, but where there may be other factors to take into account in decision-making, for example the user of the guidelines may be expected to take into account patient preferences, local facilities, local audit results or available resources.

c. A recommendation made where there is no adequate evidence as to the most effective practice, although there may be reasons for making a recommendation in order to minimise cost or reduce the chance of error through a locally agreed protocol.

## Strong recommendation

Evidence where a conclusion can be reached **'beyond all reasonable doubt'** and therefore where a **strong recommendation** can be given.

This will normally be based on evidence levels:

- Ia. Meta-analysis of randomised controlled trials
- Ib. Evidence from at least one randomised controlled trial
- IIa. Evidence from at least one controlled study without randomisation
- IIb. Evidence from at least one other type of quasi-experimental study.

## Expert opinion

Evidence where a conclusion might be reached **'on the balance of probabilities'** and where there may be other factors involved which influence the recommendation given. This will normally be based on less conclusive evidence than that represented by scalpel icons:

- III. Evidence from non-experimental descriptive studies, such as comparative studies and case–control studies
- IV. Evidence from expert committee reports or opinions or clinical experience of respected authorities, or both.

Evidence in each chapter of this volume which is associated with either a strong recommendation or expert opinion is annotated in the text by either a **scalpel** or **pen-nib** icon as shown above. References associated with **scalpel** evidence will be highlighted in the reference lists, along with a short summary of the paper's conclusions where applicable.

# 1

# The role of imaging in breast diagnosis including screening and excision of impalpable lesions

A. Robin M. Wilson
R. Douglas Macmillan

## Introduction

Breast cancer is a major health problem. Worldwide it has an increasing incidence, with over 1 million newly diagnosed cases each year, and is the commonest cancer to affect women and the commonest cause of cancer death in women. Breast cancer mortality in the UK is among the highest in the world, with approximately 28 deaths per 100 000 women per annum. This equates to around 35 000 new breast cancers diagnosed and 14 500 deaths attributable to breast cancer each year. Approximately 1 in 9 women in the UK will develop breast cancer at some time during their life.[1]

Strategies for diagnosing and managing breast cancer are based on our current understanding of breast disease epidemiology. Around 5% of breast cancer is hereditary, mainly associated with the *BRCA1* and *BRCA2* gene defects. This type of breast cancer tends to occur in younger women. The remaining 95% of breast cancer is sporadic and its incidence increases with age. Breast cancer is very rare under the age of 35 years and over 80% of breast cancer occurs in women over the age of 50. The causes of sporadic breast cancer are largely believed to be environmental factors. Recognised risk factors include early menarche, late menopause, nulliparity, and long-term use of the contraceptive pill and hormone replacement therapy (HRT). Less than 1% of breast cancer occurs in men.

As there is a poor understanding of the causes of breast cancer, primary prevention is currently not a realistic or achievable option. It is known that earlier diagnosis of breast cancer is more likely to result in a favourable outcome. Tumour size at diagnosis, grade and lymph node stage are the best predictors of outcome. Regardless of tumour type or grade, the smaller a breast cancer is at the time of diagnosis, the more likely it is that it has not spread beyond the breast. As a result the current strategy for reducing breast cancer mortality is to seek diagnosis as early as possible.

 Early detection and improvements in treatment have led to a 30% reduction in breast cancer mortality in the UK in all age groups over the past 20 years.[2]

Early diagnosis is achieved by encouraging women to present as early as possible to breast clinics when they develop breast symptoms and through regular breast cancer screening. Breast imaging is fundamental to both.

## Imaging in symptomatic breast practice

Based on mortality statistics from the 1980s and 1990s, although the UK did not have the highest incidence of breast cancer it did have the highest death rate.

Recognising that breast cancer diagnosis and treatment required significant improvement, in 1995 the UK Department of Health published guidelines for improving outcomes in breast cancer. These guidelines were updated in 2002 by the National Institute for Clinical Excellence (NICE).[3] The guidelines emphasise the following three key issues in breast cancer care:

- accurate and timely diagnosis;
- appropriate treatment decided by accurate staging of disease;
- appropriate follow-up of patients undergoing treatment.

Imaging is required at all three stages of this process, and mammography and ultrasound have a pivotal role to play. Around 200 specialist breast units in the NHS deal with the diagnosis of symptomatic breast problems. About 60% of breast cancer is detected by symptomatic breast referral clinics. These clinics follow national protocols that define the triple test, i.e. the combination of clinical assessment, imaging (mammography and ultrasound) and needle cytology or core biopsy, as the required standard. 'One-stop' clinics are recommended at which all the necessary tests required to make a diagnosis, including needle biopsy, are performed at one clinic visit. In order to achieve the earliest possible diagnosis of symptomatic breast cancer, women are encouraged through a variety of health promotion methods to present to these clinics as soon as they develop any change in their breasts.

# Breast imaging techniques

## Mammography

X-ray mammography has been the basis of breast imaging for more than 30 years. The sensitivity of mammography for breast cancer is age dependent. The denser the breast, the less effective this method is for detecting early signs of breast cancer. Breast density tends to be higher in younger women and increased density obscures early signs of breast cancer. The sensitivity of mammography for breast cancer in women over 60 years of age approaches 95%, while mammography can be expected to detect less than 50% of breast cancers in women under 40 years of age.[4]

Mammography uses ionising radiation to obtain an image and therefore should only be used where there is

likely to be a clinical benefit. Consensus is that the benefits of mammography in women over the age of 40 years are likely to far outweigh any oncogenic effects of repeated exposure. Screening of women over the age of 40 by mammography is accepted practice. However, in symptomatic practice there is rarely an indication for performing mammography in women under the age of 35 unless there is a strong clinical suspicion of malignancy. In many centres, all women over the age of 35 presenting to breast clinics undergo mammography as a routine. Practice is changing and ultrasound is being increasingly used for the assessment of women with focal breast symptoms in this age range. Mammography is routine in all women in the screening age group attending symptomatic clinics who have not had a screening mammogram in the past year.

Most mammography in the UK has been carried out using conventional analogue X-ray films. Film/screen mammography has been refined over the years but has now reached the limits of this technology. Film/screen mammography is a difficult technique to maintain at the quality levels required for optimal diagnosis because of the narrow latitude of operation of these systems and because it requires labour-intensive quality-control measures to maintain the necessary diagnostic standards. The future of mammography lies in digital acquisition of the image, so digital mammography is now being introduced in the UK.[5–8] There are major benefits from acquiring mammograms in direct digital format.[8] The resolution required for digital mammography has only recently become available. Compared with conventional mammography, the benefits of full-field digital mammography include better imaging of the dense breast, the application of computer-aided detection and a number of logistical advantages providing potential for more efficient mammography services.[9,10] The much wider dynamic range of digital mammography means that visualisation of the entire breast density range on a single image is easily achievable. In the clinical setting, comparative studies have shown that digital mammography performs in general as well as film/screen mammography but is better in younger women and in women with dense breasts.[5,6]

Mammography is the basis of stereotactic breast biopsy. Stereotactic biopsy can be carried out using a dedicated prone biopsy table or by using an add-on device to a conventional upright mammography unit. This technique is used for biopsy of impalpable lesions that are not clearly visible on ultrasound (e.g. microcalcifications).

## Ultrasound

High-frequency (≥10 MHz) ultrasound is a very effective diagnostic tool for the investigation of focal breast symptoms.[11] Ultrasound does not involve ionising radiation and is a very safe imaging technique. It has a high sensitivity for breast pathology and also a very high negative predictive value.[12]

 High-resolution ultrasound easily distinguishes between most solid and cystic lesions and can differentiate benign from malignant lesions with a high degree of accuracy. However, in most circumstances, solid lesions seen on ultrasound require needle sampling for accurate diagnosis.

Ultrasound is the technique of choice for the further investigation of focal symptomatic breast problems at all ages. Under 35 years of age, when the risk of breast cancer is very low, it is usually the only imaging technique required. Over 35, when the risk of breast cancer begins to increase, it is often used in conjunction with mammography. Ultrasound is less sensitive than mammography for the early signs of breast cancer and is therefore not used for population screening. However, ultrasound does increase the detection of small breast cancer in women who have a dense background pattern on mammography.[4] In the screening setting, there is currently insufficient evidence of any mortality benefit and insufficient resources to allow for routine ultrasound screening of women with dense mammograms.[13] Ultrasound is the technique of first choice for biopsy of both palpable and impalpable breast lesions visible on scanning.

Ultrasound is now used routinely to assess the axilla in women with breast cancer in most units. Axillary nodes that show abnormal morphology can be sampled accurately by fine-needle aspiration (FNA) or needle core biopsy.

 Up to 50% of patients with axillary metastatic disease can be diagnosed using this method, avoiding the need for sentinel node biopsy in women with pathologically proven nodal involvement.[14]

Doppler ultrasound adds little to breast diagnosis and is not widely used. Three-dimensional ultrasound of the breast is said to increase the accuracy of biopsy and the detection of multifocal disease but

again is not widely available. Elastography is a new application of ultrasound technology that allows the accurate assessment of the stiffness of breast tissue. It is being evaluated at present and may prove to be a useful tool in excluding significant abnormalities, for instance in assessment of asymptomatic abnormalities detected by ultrasound screening.

## Magnetic resonance mammography

Magnetic resonance imaging (MRI) is now widely available. However, magnetic resonance mammography (MRM) of the breast requires dedicated breast coils and these are much less widely available. In order to image the breast the patient is scanned prone and injection of intravenous contrast is required. MRM is the most sensitive technique for detection of breast cancer, approaching 100% for invasive cancer and up to 92% for ductal carcinoma in situ (DCIS), but it has high false-positive rates.[15,16] Rapid acquisition of images facilitates assessment of signal enhancement curves that can be helpful in distinguishing benign and malignant disease. However, significant overlap in the enhancement patterns usually means that needle sampling is required. Magnetic resonance-guided breast biopsy is available in a few centres but most breast lesions seen on MRM that are larger than 5 mm can be seen on ultrasound if they are clinically significant.

 MRM is likely to prove the best method for screening younger women (under 40 years) at increased risk of breast cancer but, because of cost, it is unlikely to be used for general population screening.[17–20]

MRM is the best technique for imaging women with breast implants. It is also of benefit in identifying recurrent disease where conventional imaging and biopsy have failed to exclude recurrence. Provided it is carried out more than 18 months after surgery, MRI will accurately distinguish between scarring and tumour recurrence. MRI is being used increasingly to examine women for multifocal disease prior to conservation surgery, although there is a lack of evidence of its efficacy and value so it is not routine in this clinical setting. Breast MRI is of value in assessing response of large or locally advanced breast cancers to neoadjuvant chemotherapy.

MRI of the axilla can demonstrate axillary metastatic disease but its sensitivity is not sufficient for it to replace surgical staging of the axilla. For advanced breast cancer, MRI is the technique of choice for assessing spinal metastatic disease.

## Computed tomography

Computed tomography (CT) has no role in primary imaging of the breast. CT is used to diagnose and stage systemic spread of breast cancer and to assess response of metastatic disease to treatment, particularly lung, pleural and liver metastases. Some patients with breast cancer do have their cancers diagnosed incidentally during a routine CT scan.

## Isotope imaging

Breast scintigraphy is not widely used because of its lack of sensitivity compared with other techniques. It is used in a few centres to stage the breast prior to surgery and to assess response to treatment. Scintigraphy is widely used to diagnose and assess the presence of skeletal metastatic disease.

Positron emission scintigraphy, particularly when combined with CT, is a new technology that may have a role in future in staging breast cancer and monitoring response to treatment. At present, it is regarded as a research tool and its specific uses and indications are still being defined.

# Breast cancer screening

## Aim

The aim of breast screening is to reduce mortality through early detection. Randomised controlled trials and case–control studies carried out between the 1960s and 1980s demonstrated that population screening by mammography can be expected to reduce overall breast cancer mortality by around 25% and by 35–40% in those who participate.

The validity of these trials was questioned in 2000–2002 but subsequent reviews by the Swedish combined trials group and a World Health Organisation International Agency for Research on Cancer committee of experts have reaffirmed the mortality benefit of mammographic screening and determined that criticisms of the mammographic screening trials were unjustified.[21–26]

The mortality benefit of screening is greatest in women aged 55–70 years.[23,24] The mortality benefit of screening women aged between 40 and 55 is approximately 20%. Screening women under the age of 40 has not been shown to provide any mortality benefit.[23,24]

## Population screening

Breast screening has been introduced in many countries over the past 20 years. In most countries, screening is recommended in all women aged 40 and over but in countries that provide population-based screening, women of 50 and over are specifically targeted. Breast cancer screening was introduced in the UK in 1987 and provides screening by invitation, free at the point of delivery, to all women between the ages of 50 and 70.[1] Women over 70 can attend but are not invited. Over 70% of the invited population need to attend for a significant overall mortality benefit to be achieved. Women under the age of 50 are not offered screening in the UK unless they are at increased risk. From 2009 the screening invitation age range will be extended to include women aged 47–73 years.

## Method and frequency

The screening method is two-view mammography; clinical examination of the breast and breast self-examination have not been shown to contribute to mortality reduction through early detection and so are not included.[8,27,28]

Women are invited every 3 years. There has been some concern that this screening interval is too long. Mammography can be expected to detect breast cancer approximately 2 years before it becomes clinically apparent. The frequency of mammographic screening is determined by the lead-time of breast cancer. Based on the average growth time of breast cancer according to age, this means that mammographic screening should ideally be carried out yearly in women aged 40–50, every 2 years in women aged 50–60 and every 3 years thereafter. However, the breast screening frequency trial completed in 1995 did not show any predicted benefit for women aged 50–64 screened every year compared with those screened every 3 years.[29] Screening once every 3 years can be expected to detect approximately two-thirds of breast cancer that will arise during the 3-year screening interval.

One-third of breast cancers will present in the interval between screens, so-called interval cancers. Half of these present in the third year after screening.

## Factors affecting the effectiveness of screening

HRT increases breast density and in a proportion of women this treatment reduces the sensitivity of mammography for breast cancer.[8,28–36] Up to 25% of women taking combined estrogen/progestogen preparations continuously show increased density on mammography. This effect is significantly less with other HRT preparations. The use of HRT has been shown to significantly reduce the sensitivity and specificity of mammographic screening. HRT also increases the risk of developing breast cancer.[30]

## Quality assurance

Breast screening programmes should have in-built quality assurance; the NHS Breast Screening Programme is subject to comprehensive quality assessment and all 100 screening units across the country have to comply with nationally defined standard guidelines. There are national targets for screening set by a central Department of Health Advisory Committee (Table 1.1).

## The screening process

Women invited for screening attend either a static or mobile screening unit where two-view mammography is performed. The images are then double read within a few days. The vast majority of women

Table 1.1 • NHS Breast Screening Programme: screening targets, September 2003

| Objective | Criteria | Minimum standard | Target |
|---|---|---|---|
| To maximise the number of eligible women who attend for screening | Percentage of eligible women who attend for screening | • ≥70% of invited women to attend for screening | • 80% |
| To maximise the number of cancers detected | (a) Rate of invasive cancers detected in eligible women | • Prevalent screen ≥2.7 per 1000<br>• Incident screen ≥3.1 per 1000 | • Prevalent screen >3.6 per 1000<br>• Incident screen ≥4.2 per 1000 |
| | (b) Rate of cancers detected that are in situ carcinoma | • Prevalent screen ≥0.4 per 1000<br>• Incident screen ≥0.5 per 1000 | |
| | (c) Standardised detection ratio | • ≥0.85 | • ≥1.0 |
| To maximise the number of small invasive cancers | Rate of invasive cancers less than 15 mm in diameter detected in eligible women invited and screened | • Prevalent screen ≥1.5 per 1000<br>• Incident screen ≥1.7 per 1000 | • Prevalent screen >2.0 per 1000<br>• Incident screen ≥2.5 per 1000 |
| To achieve optimum image quality | (a) High-contrast spatial resolution | • ≥12 lp/mm | |
| | (b) Minimal detectable contrast:<br>5–6 mm detail<br>0.5 mm detail<br>0.25 mm detail | • ≤1.2%<br>• ≤5%<br>• ≤8% | • ≤0.8%<br>• ≤3%<br>• ≤5% |
| | (c) Aim film density | • 1.5–1.9 | |
| To limit radiation dose | Mean glandular dose per film for a standard breast at clinical settings | • ≤2.5 mGy | |
| To minimise the number of women undergoing repeat examinations | Number of repeat examinations | • <3% of total examinations | • <2% of total examinations |

(Continued)

Table 1.1 • NHS Breast Screening Programme: screening targets, September 2003—Cont'd

| Objective | Criteria | Minimum standard | Target |
|---|---|---|---|
| To minimise the number of women screened who are referred for further tests* | (a) Percentage of women who are referred for assessment | • Prevalent screen <10%<br>• Incident screen <7% | • Prevalent screen <7%<br>• Incident screen <5% |
| | (b) Percentage of women screened who are placed on early recall | • <0.5% | • ≤0.25% |
| To ensure that the majority of cancers, both palpable and impalpable, receive a non-operative tissue diagnosis of cancer | Percentage of women who have a non-operative diagnosis of cancer by cytology or needle histology after a maximum of two visits | • ≥80% | • >90% |
| To minimise the number of unnecessary operative procedures | Rate of benign biopsies | • Prevalent screen <3.6 per 1000<br>• Incident screen <2.0 per 1000 | • Prevalent screen <1.8 per 1000<br>• Incident screen <1.0 per 1000 |
| To minimise the number of cancers in the women screened presenting between screening episodes | Rate of cancers presenting in screened women:<br>(a) in the 2 years following a normal screening episode<br>(b) in the third year following a normal screening episode | *Expected standard*<br>• 1.2 per 1000 women screened in the first 2 years<br>• 1.4 per 1000 women screened in the third year | |
| To ensure that women are recalled for screening at appropriate intervals | Percentage of eligible women whose first offered appointment is within 36 months of their previous screen | • >90% | • 100% |
| To minimise anxiety for women awaiting the results of screening | Percentage of women who are sent their result within 2 weeks | • >90% | • 100% |
| To minimise the interval from the screening mammogram to assessment | Percentage of women who attend an assessment centre within 3 weeks of attendance for the screening mammogram | • >90% | • 100% |
| To minimise diagnostic delay for women who are diagnosed non-operatively | Proportion of women for whom the time interval between non-operative biopsy and result is 1 week or less | • >90% | • 100% |
| To minimise the delay for women who require surgical assessment | Proportion of women for whom the time interval between the decision to refer to a surgeon and surgical assessment is 1 week or less | • ≥90% | • 100% |
| To minimise any delay for women who require treatment for screen-detected breast cancer | Percentage of women who are admitted for treatment within 2 months of their first assessment visit | • >90% | • 100% |

(95%) are informed by letter within 2 weeks of attendance that their mammograms show no evidence of breast cancer. Those women in the appropriate age range will be invited for screening 3 years later. They are advised to contact their general practitioner as soon as possible if they become aware of any change in their breasts in the meantime.

The screening process includes a fully integrated multidisciplinary assessment process for all screen-detected mammographic abnormalities; screening programmes should ideally retain responsibility through to definitive diagnosis. Approximately 5% of women screened are recalled for further assessment of a problem identified at screening. Some women are recalled for further assessment of a clinical sign or symptom identified at the time of screening but the vast majority of women are recalled because of a mammographic abnormality.

 The most important cancers detected at screening are high-grade DCIS, as most cases of this type will progress to grade 2 or 3 invasive breast cancer within the following 3 years, and grade 2 and 3 invasive breast cancers under 10 mm in diameter, as at this size these tumours are much less likely to have metastasised.[37,38]

The common types of mammographic abnormality and their positive predictive value for cancer are shown in Table 1.2. Well-defined masses are almost always benign and do not require recall, whereas ill-defined masses and spiculated lesions always require further assessment (**Figs 1.1** and **1.2**). Clustered microcalcifications account for a high proportion of recalls that result in needle biopsy. More than 20% of screen-detected breast cancer is DCIS, mostly high or intermediate grade, and most of this type of cancer is detected by the presence of clustered microcalcifications (**Fig. 1.3**). Invasive cancer is usually represented on mammography by either an ill-defined or spiculated mass. It is essential to detect these lesions at small size as they more commonly represent grade 2 or 3 invasive cancer.

Three-quarters of women recalled simply require further imaging (mammography and/or ultrasound) and clinical assessment before being reassured and discharged. The remaining 25% will undergo a needle biopsy procedure in order to diagnose around 6 cancers per 1000 women screened. Interval follow-up of uncertain mammographic findings is discouraged,

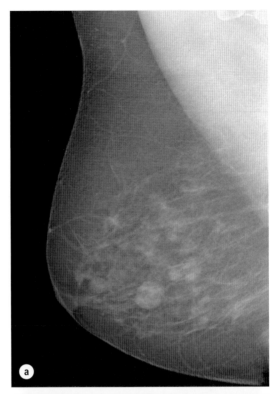

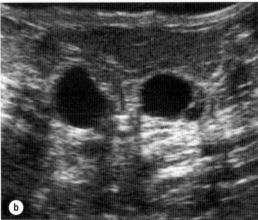

**Figure 1.1** • **(a)** Digital mammogram showing well-defined masses, the typical appearance of simple breast cysts. **(b)** Ultrasound image showing typical features of simple cysts, i.e. well-circumscribed anechoic masses with distal acoustic enhancement.

Table 1.2 • Positive predictive value (PPV) for malignancy of mammographic signs

| Sign | PPV (%) |
| --- | --- |
| Well-defined mass | <1 |
| Ill-defined mass | 35–50 |
| Spiculated mass | 50–90 |
| Architectural distortion | 20–40 |
| Asymmetric density | <2 |
| Clustered microcalcifications | 15 |

the emphasis being on obtaining a definitive diagnosis by the use of image-guided breast biopsy, with an achievable standard of over 90% of breast cancers diagnosed prior to first surgery. Despite advances in breast needle biopsy techniques a small proportion of women still require open surgical biopsy for diagnosis (up to 0.25% of women screened).

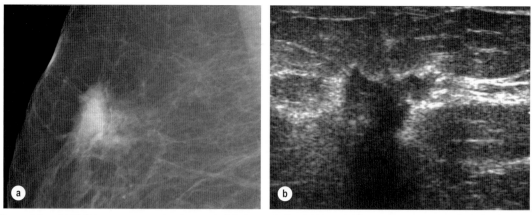

**Figure 1.2** • **(a)** Digital mammogram showing a spiculated mass in the right breast. The appearances are typical of an invasive carcinoma. The mass contains microcalcifications and there is evidence of skin tether. **(b)** Ultrasound image showing the typical features of an invasive carcinoma with an irregular mass with intraduct tumour extension and causing acoustic shadowing.

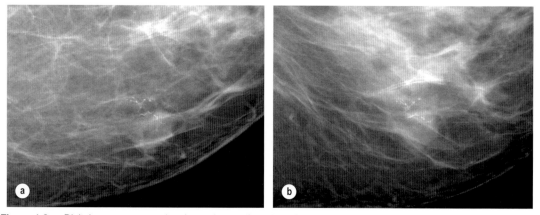

**Figure 1.3** • Digital mammograms showing a cluster of casting microcalcifications in the lower inner quadrant of the left breast. The appearances are typical of high-grade ductal carcinoma in situ.

The performance of the NHS Breast Screening Programme in 2003 is shown in Table 1.3. The screening programme is predicted to produce a 25% reduction in mortality (1750 cancers per year) directly attributable to early detection through screening by the year 2010.

## Adverse effects

Receiving an invitation for screening and attending for mammography are not associated with any significant anxiety. However, recall for further assessment does cause measurable anxiety, although this has largely subsided after 3 months.

The numbers of women who undergo open surgical biopsy for what proves to be benign disease should be kept to a minimum. Considerable training and investment in equipment has resulted in a four-

fold decline in benign surgical biopsies generated through the screening programme. False-positive recall and benign surgical biopsy are both more likely in younger women.

Overdiagnosis refers to the detection via screening of breast cancers that require treatment but which would never have threatened the life of the woman. There is considerable debate about what proportion if any of screen-detected breast cancers fall into this category. It is likely that most low-grade DCIS and some special low-grade invasive cancers do represent overdiagnosis, and detection of these results in unnecessary treatment and unnecessary morbidity associated with knowledge of the diagnosis of cancer. The consensus view is that overdiagnosis applies to no more than 10% of screen-detected breast cancer and that at this level this does not negate the overall mortality benefit of breast screening. Women attending

Table 1.3 • NHS Breast Screening Programme: results 2003

|  | 2005/2006 | 2006/2007 |
| --- | --- | --- |
| Total number of women invited | 2,381,122 | 2,437,531 |
| Acceptance rate | 74.9% | 73.8% |
| Number of women screened (invited) | 1,782,381 | 1,797,219 |
| Number of women screened (self-referral) | 107,666 | 101,855 |
| Total number of women screened | 1,891,408 | 1,901,233 |
| Number of women recalled for assessment | 87,469 | 83,728 |
| Percentage of women recalled for assessment | 4.7% | 4.5% |
| Number of benign surgical biopsies | 1,751 | 1,676 |
| Number of cancers detected | 14,841 | 14,753 |
| Cancers per 1000 women screened | 7.8 | 7.7 |
| Number of in situ cancers detected | 3,019 | 3,168 |
| Number of cancers less than 15 mm | 6,184 | 6,151 |
| Standardised detection ratio (invited only) | 1.41 | 1.41 |

From NHS Breast Screening Programme Annual Review 2008. Available at http:\\www.cancerscreening.nhs.uk.

for screening must be informed fully about both the likely positive and negative effects of screening.

## Screening women at increased risk

Women at increased risk of developing breast cancer due to a proven inherited predisposing genetic mutation, family history (with no proven genetic mutation), previous radiotherapy (e.g. mantle radiotherapy for Hodgkin's lymphoma) or benign risk lesions (atypical hyperplasia, lobular carcinoma in situ) may be selected for screening at young age. Whether it is possible to identify other substantially increased risk groups by summating various other epidemiological factors (e.g. age at menarche, body mass index, age at first pregnancy, alcohol intake) continues to be debated. The cut-off point at which clinical management of a woman is altered is often referred to as moderate risk. Those likely or proven to be carriers of a predisposing genetic mutation are termed high risk.

NICE guidelines have been produced (latest version 2006) to classify risk groups and guide care.[39] They state that women at or near population risk should be managed in primary care (defined as <3% risk for women aged 40–49). Women at moderate risk are those with a 10-year risk of 3–8% between 40 and 49 years or a lifetime risk >17%, and those at high risk are defined as those with a 10-year risk of >8% between 40 and 49 years or a lifetime risk >30%.

Such cut-offs are useful as guidelines for specialist referral but most risk factors require clinical interpretation before a risk management policy is discussed.

Unfortunately, the underlying problem with screening young women at increased risk of breast cancer is that no screening test has yet been shown to reduce mortality in such women. Screening in this group is therefore a management option for which an exact benefit cannot be quoted to an individual woman. Screening should not be offered to those who fall below the moderate-risk cut-off.

## Methods of screening young women at increased risk: mammography

A national evaluation study of mammographic screening for young women with a family history of breast cancer is being conducted (FH01 study). The study compares screening in women aged 40–44 who are at least moderate risk with the control arm of the age trial (population-based trial of screening women in their forties as yet unreported).

Mammography has a greater positive predictive value in young women at high risk compared with age matched controls but lacks sensitivity. This may be a particular problem in women with BRCA1 mutations.[20,40–43]

BRCA1-related breast cancer is usually high grade and often has a 'pushing' margin. It rarely presents with associated DCIS. The mammographic features

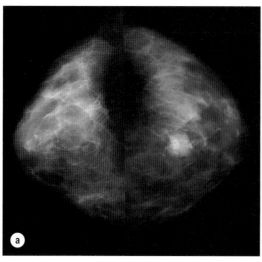
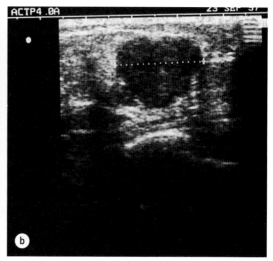

**Figure 1.4** • **(a)** Conventional mammogram showing a circumscribed mass in the central part of the left breast. **(b)** Ultrasound image of the same mass. Core biopsy showed an invasive carcinoma.

are therefore usually of a mass lesion with no associated microcalcification and no architectural distortion (**Fig. 1.4a**). Such cancers often present symptomatically as interval cases. *BRCA2*-related cancers are more similar to sporadic cases and may be more likely to be detected by mammography. Ultrasound screening significantly improves sensitivity when there is a dense mammographic background pattern but has lower positive predictive value and has not been shown to be a useful screening modality. Ultrasound features of *BRCA1* cancers are often benign or indeterminate (**Fig. 1.4b**). If mammographic screening is selected, it should be repeated annually in women under age 50.

### Methods of screening young women at high risk: MRI

There is evidence that MRI is the most sensitive method of imaging young women but has significant resource implications.[40,44] The specificity of MRI has been a concern, although with second-look recall (after which many potentially abnormal findings may resolve), targeted ultrasound and the slowly increasing availability of MRI-guided biopsy this may be less of a problem than initially thought. The MARIBS study evaluating MRI in addition to mammography and several other studies have shown that MRI may be the most sensitive screening test for young high-risk women, but it is arguable whether the prognosis of cancers detected is sufficiently influenced.[45] On the basis of its better performance over mammography in terms of sensitivity,

NICE recommended annual MRI surveillance for women aged 30–39 years with a 10-year risk of >8% and women aged 40–49 years with a 10-year risk >20%.[39] MRI is also recommended in high-risk women with a dense mammographic background pattern.

### Age to start screening in young women at increased risk

The age for starting screening should be based on risk rather than the age of affected relatives. For women at moderate risk, screening should start at age 40. This can seem paradoxical if the reason moderate risk has been established is because there is one first-degree relative affected in their thirties. However, if no other affected relatives can be identified, then the individual only just qualifies as moderate risk and the emphasis of management should be on reassurance rather than screening. For women at high risk, screening may be started at age 30–35. Such high-risk women should ideally be managed in a specialist setting where experience with MRI screening is available. Women must be advised about the limitations of screening at young age. This is particularly relevant to known mutation carriers for whom there is no evidence that screening can improve survival (cf. risk-reducing surgery).

## Image-guided breast biopsy

Needle biopsy is highly accurate in determining the nature of most breast lesions.[46–49] Patients with benign conditions avoid unnecessary surgery; carrying out open surgical biopsy for diagnosis should be regarded as a failure of the diagnostic process. For patients who prove to have breast cancer, needle biopsy provides accurate understanding of the type and extent of disease so ensuring that patients, and the doctors treating them, are able to make informed treatment choices. Needle biopsy not only provides accurate information on the nature of malignant disease, such as histological type and grade, but also facilitates pretreatment assessment of tumour biology.

## Which biopsy technique?

The current methods available for breast tissue diagnosis are FNA for cytology, needle core biopsy for histology, vacuum-assisted mammotomy (VAM) and open surgical biopsy.

### FNA versus needle core biopsy

There has been much debate about the comparative benefits of FNA and core biopsy,[46–49] but 14G 22-mm automated core biopsy provides significantly greater sensitivity, specificity and positive predictive value. Results with core biopsy are particularly superior to FNA in stereotactic biopsy of microcalcifications and architectural distortions.

The overall better performance achievable with core biopsy compared with FNA is illustrated in the performance of the NHS Breast Screening Programme in the UK. In 1994, using FNA as the primary diagnostic technique, fewer than 10% of 90 units were able to achieve the target of 70% preoperative diagnosis rate for cancer. By 2003, most units had converted to automated core biopsy and all units achieved the minimum standard and the majority exceeded the expected standard of 90% preoperative diagnosis rate.[1]

### Vacuum-assisted mammotomy

The predominant reasons for not achieving an accurate diagnosis by needle biopsy are sampling error and failure to retrieve sufficient representative material. These problems have been largely addressed by the development of larger directional core techniques that yield significantly greater volumes of tissue.[50–52]

VAM is a very successful method for improving the diagnostic accuracy of borderline breast lesions and lesions at sites in the breast difficult to biopsy using other techniques. VAM has been shown to understage both in situ and invasive cancer approximately half as often as conventional core biopsy

(typically 10% vs. 20%).[53,54] The VAM technique has a higher sensitivity because it allows sampling of lesions at sites that are difficult to biopsy using either FNA or core biopsy and because the amount of tissue harvested is at least five times greater per core specimen.

The indications for VAM include:

- very small mass lesions;
- architectural distortions;
- failed 'conventional' core biopsy;
- small clusters of microcalcifications;
- papillary and mucocele-like lesions;
- diffuse non-specific abnormality;
- excision of benign lesions;
- sentinel node sampling.

Core biopsy and VAM are now the recommended techniques for sampling calcifications and mammographic architectural distortions.[55] For calcifications it is imperative that there is proof of representative sampling with specimen radiography. If calcification is not demonstrated on the specimen radiograph and the histology is benign, then management cannot be based on this result as there is a high risk of sampling error; the procedure must either be repeated or open surgical biopsy carried out.

## Guidance techniques for breast needle biopsy

Ultrasound guidance is the technique of choice for biopsy of both palpable and impalpable breast lesions; it is less costly, easy to perform and more accurate than freehand or other image-guided techniques.[46]

Ultrasound provides real-time visualisation of the biopsy procedure and visual confirmation of adequate sampling. Between 80% and 90% of breast abnormalities will be clearly visible on ultrasound and amenable to biopsy using this technique. For impalpable abnormalities not visible on ultrasound, stereotactic X-ray-guided biopsy is required. A few lesions are only visible on MRI and require magnetic resonance-guided biopsy.[56] A number of different approaches have been developed for this procedure using both closed and open magnets. FNA, core biopsy and VAM may all be used for magnetic resonance-guided sampling.

The negative predictive value of combined normal mammography and ultrasound is extremely high; where there is a clinically palpable abnormality and mammography and ultrasound are entirely normal, the likelihood of malignancy is low (<1%). However, in these circumstances it remains prudent in the presence of a localised clinical abnormality to carry out freehand needle biopsy to exclude the occasional diffuse malignant process, such as classical lobular carcinoma or low-grade DCIS, that may be occult on both mammography and ultrasound.

For stereotactic procedures it is prudent to mark the biopsy site for future reference. Gel pellets or cellulose can be placed during the procedure to mark the biopsy site. These markers have the advantage of being visible on ultrasound so that repeat biopsy or localisation for surgery can be subsequently performed under ultrasound rather than X-ray guidance. These markers dissolve and are reabsorbed in a few weeks, leaving a small metal marker in case delayed X-ray identification of the biopsy site is required.

## Number of samples

A simple rule for satisfactory sampling using needle techniques is to obtain sufficient material to achieve a diagnosis.[55,57] For ultrasound-guided core biopsy, a diagnosis may be possible on a single core. Showing on ultrasound that the needle has passed through the centre of the abnormality and by examining the sample with the naked eye, it is usually, but not always, possible to confirm whether a satisfactory sample has been obtained. As some lesions are heterogeneous, sensitivity does increase with more extensive sampling of a lesion. The number of core specimens obtained should reflect the nature of the abnormality being sampled. For ultrasound-guided biopsy where there is a suspicion of carcinoma, it is recommended that multiple core specimens are obtained.

As stereotactic biopsy is used for abnormalities that are difficult to define on ultrasound and are therefore more difficult to sample, a minimum of five core specimens should be obtained. Ensuring that calcification is present in at least three separate cores and/or five separate flecks of calcification are retrieved from the area of suspicion is essential to ensure an accurate diagnosis.

When there is still diagnostic uncertainty, 8G VAM can be used to obtain larger tissue volumes (approximately 300 mg per core). An 8G mammotomy probe is preferred for therapeutic removal of breast lesions such as fibroadenomas.

## Biopsy results

It is important that the result of needle breast biopsy is always correlated with the clinical and imaging findings before clinical management is discussed with the patient. This is best achieved by reviewing each case at prospective multidisciplinary meetings.[46]

# Surgery for clinically occult breast lesions

## Wire-guided excision

The number of impalpable, clinically occult breast lesions detected by screening is increasing. Accurate localisation techniques are required to facilitate their surgical excision. The hooked wire is the most commonly employed technique and has proved very reliable but does have inherent associated problems. There are various designs of localisation wire in common use. All have some form of anchoring device such as a hook with a splayed or barbed tip. The wire is deployed under stereotactic or ultrasound guidance within a rigid over-sheath cannula, which is then removed once positioning is satisfactory (**Fig. 1.5**). The patient is then transferred to the operating theatre with the wire in situ. Most wires are very flexible and when the cannula is removed the wire may assume a quite circuitous course, especially after stereotactic insertion when the breast is released from compression. This may lead to difficulty in resheathing of the wire with the cannula in theatre. In order to achieve resheathing the wire needs to be pulled gently and as straight as possible. In a very fatty breast in which there is no solid lesion or the wire has not transfixed the lesion, care must be taken to avoid displacing the wire. Wire kinking can also occur if the over-sheath is forced over the wire. The purpose of the over-sheath is to enable palpability of the wire tip by ballottement. This can be difficult in fibrous breasts or for lesions deep in the breast. After resheathing, a cosmetically considered incision is placed near to the tip of the wire and an excision performed. Accurate wire

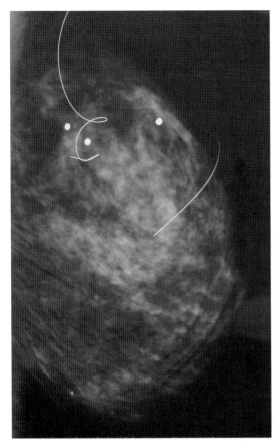

**Figure 1.5** • Conventional mammogram showing a Nottingham wire marking a small impalpable mass.

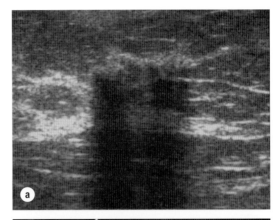

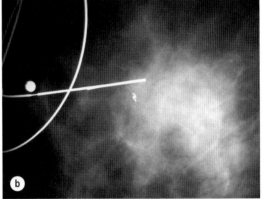

**Figure 1.6** • **(a)** Ultrasound showing a cluster of gel pellets placed at the site of a previous stereotactic biopsy. The clear visibility of the pellets facilitates ultrasound localisation for surgery of abnormalities that would normally require X-ray localisation. **(b)** Mammogram after ultrasound localisation in the same case showing accurate placement of the marker wire.

placement is essential and ideally the shortest possible length of wire should be within the breast. In recent practice this has been greatly facilitated by the use of radio-opaque markers placed at the time of initial stereotactic biopsy such that wire localisation can be performed under ultrasound guidance (**Fig. 1.6**). In addition, for superficial lesions a skin marker may be more appropriate.

Although lesions may be clinically occult prior to surgery, most mass lesions will be palpable intraoperatively. Procedures that can be surgically more challenging are wide local excisions for DCIS with no mass lesion. In such cases, where the distribution of disease is often more eccentric, careful excision planning is necessary. Inserting more than one wire and even bracketing the lesion with three or four wires can be useful.

If the procedure is being performed to establish a diagnosis, a small representative portion of the lesion is excised through a small incision, so leaving a satisfactory cosmetic result if the lesion proves to be benign (the European surgical quality assurance guidelines require such diagnostic surgical excision specimens to weigh less than 30 g). For diagnostic excisions of very small lesions, a therapeutic wide excision may (after discussion with the patient) be considered appropriate, as the resulting cosmetic effect of removing an extra rim of tissue may be insignificant. Protocols vary for therapeutic excisions, but in general the lesion should be excised with a 10-mm macroscopic margin of normal tissue. Intraoperative specimen radiography is essential, both to check that the lesion has been removed and, if cancer has been diagnosed, to ensure that adequate wide local excision has been achieved.

Some surgeons experienced in this imaging technique have also used intraoperative ultrasound. Not only can excision be guided but the margins of a wide local excision specimen can also be assessed intraoperatively using ultrasound.

## Radioisotope occult lesion localisation

Radioisotope occult lesion localisation (ROLL) has been advocated as an alternative to the hooked-wire technique.[58] ROLL was first described by the Milan group using $^{99m}$Tc-labelled human macroaggregate albumin, check scintigraphy and a hand-held gamma probe to guide surgical excision. The Nottingham method has modified the Milan technique and uses radio-opaque contrast injected with the radiolabel and immediate check mammography (**Fig. 1.7**). Subsequently some centres have combined ROLL with sentinel node biopsy. ROLL uses essentially the same equipment as sentinel node biopsy. It has been described using macroaggregate (which does not migrate from the injection site) or low-molecular-weight colloid (which does migrate and is normally used for sentinel node biopsy). In both situations it is radiolabelled with $^{99m}$Tc and injected directly into the lesion. The threshold of the signal processor on the gamma detector is then adjusted so that an audible signal is only heard when the probe is directly over the lesion. The probe then directs excision intraoperatively.

In a randomised trial of ROLL versus wire localisation, 2% of ROLL patients had a failed technique due to intraductal injection of radiolabelled colloid and dye that gave a ductogram appearance on check mammography in both cases.[59,60] As the radio-opaque dye is absorbed rapidly, both cases were successfully converted to wire localisation.

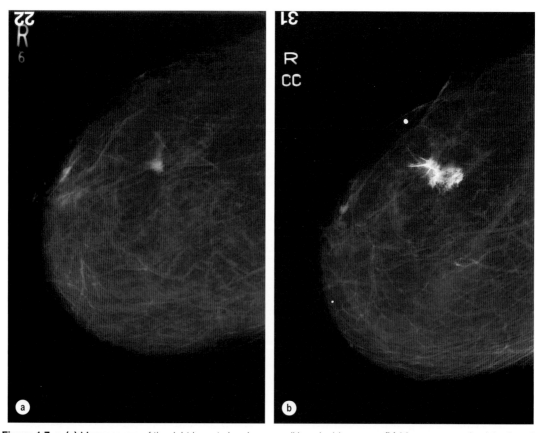

**Figure 1.7 • (a)** Mammogram of the right breast showing a small impalpable cancer. **(b)** Mammogram after injection of radionuclide mixed with X-ray contrast confirming satisfactory localisation (ROLL).

The main differences between ROLL and wire guidance were that both surgeons and radiologists found ROLL easier to perform overall and patients found ROLL less painful. There was no significant difference in accuracy of marking, operating time, mean specimen weight, intraoperative re-excision or second therapeutic operation. Other studies have suggested that obtaining clear margins may be significantly easier with ROLL. In essence there is little to choose between ROLL and wire localisation, although ROLL may be the more suitable technique in the localisation of non-mass lesions (e.g. DCIS).

There are various methods described for combining ROLL with sentinel node biopsy.[61–63] Low-molecular-weight colloid can be injected at a different site, at the same site with a different radiolabel, or into the tumour. With intratumoral injection of $^{99m}$Tc nanocolloid, only one injection is required and high success rates have been reported. Combined with radio-opaque contrast, this modification of the Nottingham method has proved successful.

# Oncoplastic considerations for screen-detected lesions

Oncoplastic surgery aims to provide optimum effectiveness of surgical treatment for breast cancer with minimum effect on quality of life. As the 10-year survival of screen-detected disease is estimated at 87%, women do live a long time with the effects of breast cancer surgery on body image, quality of life and self-esteem. The degree to which these outcomes are affected is strongly related to the cosmetic outcome of surgery.

When assessing a woman for surgery for screen-detected cancer, thought should be given to the following: scar placement (within skin tension lines or periareolar); reconstruction of breast defects; whether the woman may have quality-of-life benefits from breast reduction; and whether taking a larger margin may be desirable and still achievable with excellent cosmesis. The latter consideration may be particularly relevant for DCIS, for which over 30% or women require further surgery after attempts at breast-conserving surgery because of involved excision margins.

## Key points

- Breast imaging is an essential part of modern multidisciplinary breast diagnosis.
- Mammography is the technique of choice for population breast screening.
- Screening is targeted at women aged 50–70 years and can be expected to reduce mortality through early detection by 30%.
- The aim should be to achieve as near as possible 100% non-operative diagnosis of breast problems.
- Both palpable and impalpable breast lesions are best sampled under image guidance.
- Automated core biopsy is the sampling technique of first choice.
- Ultrasound is the guidance technique of first choice.
- Digital stereotactic core biopsy should be reserved for sampling lesions not visible on ultrasound.
- A 14G core biopsy can provide a definitive diagnosis in more than 90% of cases and should be the preferred method.
- Mammotomy can provide the diagnosis in most of the remainder.
- Stereo-guided vacuum-assisted mammotomy (VAM) is particularly effective for small clusters of indeterminate microcalcifications and calcifications in sites difficult to access with core biopsy.
- VAM is an effective and well-tolerated sampling device for breast diagnosis and can also be used to completely excise benign lesions.
- All breast needle biopsy results should be discussed at prospective multidisciplinary meetings where the pathology results are correlated with the clinical and imaging findings.
- Accurate image-guided localisation and skills in wide local excision are required for the surgical treatment of impalpable breast lesions.

# References

1. NHS Cancer Screening Programmes. Available at http:\\www.cancerscreening.nhs.uk/breastscreen/index.html.

2. Blanks RG, Moss SM, McGahan CE et al. Effects of NHS breast screening programme on mortality from breast cancer in England and Wales, 1990–8: comparison of observed with predicted mortality. Br Med J 2000; 321:1724–31.

3. National Institute for Clinical Excellence. Guidance on cancer services. Improving outcomes in breast cancer: manual update. London: National Institute for Clinical Excellence, 2002. Available at http:\\www.nice.org.uk.

4. Kolb TM, Lichy J, Newhouse JH. Comparison of the performance of screening mammography, physical examination, and breast US and evaluation of factors that influence them: an analysis of 27,825 patient evaluations. Radiology 2002; 225:165–75.

5. Skaane P, Young K, Skjennald A. Comparison of film-screen mammography and full-field mammography with soft-copy reading in a population-based screening program: the Oslo II study. Radiology 2002; 225:267.

6. Pisano ED, Gatsonis C, Hendrick E et al. Diagnostic performance of digital versus film mammography for breast cancer screening. N Engl J Med 2005; 353:1773–83.

7. James JJ. The current status of digital mammography. Clin Radiol 2004; 59:1–10.

8. Committee on Technologies for the Early Detection of Breast Cancer. Mammography and beyond: developing technologies for the early detection of breast cancer. Washington, DC: National Academy Press, 2001.

9. Legood R, Gray A. A cost comparison of full-field digital mammography with film-screen mammography in breast cancer screening. NHSBSP Equipment Report 0403. Sheffield: NHS Breast Screening Programme Publications, 2004.

10. Gur D, Sumkin JH, Rockette HE et al. Changes in breast cancer detection and mammography recall rates after the introduction of a computer-aided detection system. J Natl Cancer Inst 2004; 96:185–90.

11. Wilson ARM, Teh W. Mini symposium: Imaging of the breast. Ultrasound of the breast. Imaging 1998; 9:169–85.

12. Lister D, Evans AJ, Burrell HC et al. The accuracy of breast ultrasound in the evaluation of clinically benign discrete breast lumps. Clin Radiol 1998; 53:490–2.

13. Teh W, Wilson ARM. The role of ultrasound in breast cancer screening: a consensus statement for the European Group for Breast Cancer Screening. Eur J Cancer 1998; 34:449–50.

14. Damera A, Evans AJ, Cornford EJ et al. Diagnosis of axillary nodal metastases by ultrasound guided core biopsy in primary operable breast cancer. Br J Cancer 2003; 89:1310–13.

15. Kuhl C. The current status of breast MR imaging. Part 2. Clinical applications. Radiology 2007; 244:672–91.

16. Kuhl CK, Schrading S, Bieling HB et al. MRI for diagnosis of pure ductal carcinoma in situ: a prospective observational study. Lancet 2007; 370:485–92.

17. Kuhl CK, Schmutzler RK, Leutner CC et al. Breast MR imaging screening in 192 women proved or suspected to be carriers of a breast cancer susceptibility gene: preliminary results. Radiology 2000; 215:267–79.

18. Warner E, Plewes DB, Shumak RS et al. Comparison of breast magnetic resonance imaging, mammography, and ultrasound for surveillance of women at high risk for hereditary breast cancer. J Clin Oncol 2001; 19:3524–31.

19. Stoutjesdijk MJ, Boetes C, Jager GJ et al. Magnetic resonance imaging and mammography in women with a hereditary risk of breast cancer. J Natl Cancer Inst 2001; 93:1095–102.

20. Brekelmans CTM, Seynaeve C., Bartels CCM et al. Effectiveness of breast cancer surveillance in BRCA1/2 gene mutation carriers and women with high familial risk. J Clin Oncol 2001; 19:924–30.

21. Olsen O, Gotzsche PC. Cochrane review on screening for breast cancer with mammography. Lancet 2001; 358:1340–2.

22. Olsen O, Gotzsche PC Systematic review of screening for breast cancer mammography. Available at http://image.thelancet.com/lancet/extra/fullreport.pdf.

23. WHO handbook on cancer prevention, 7th edn. Lyons: IARC Press, 2002.

   A comprehensive review of all the available data on the effectiveness of breast cancer screening in reducing breast cancer mortality.

24. Nystrom L, Andersson I, Bjurstam N et al. Long-term effects of mammographic screening: update overview of the Swedish randomised trials. Lancet 2002; 359:909–19.

   Long-term follow-up of the combined Swedish trials showing significant mortality benefit after more than 20 years.

25. Tabar L, Vitak B, Tony HH et al. Beyond randomised controlled trials: organised mammographic screening substantially reduces breast carcinoma mortality. Cancer 2001; 91:1724–31.

26. Duffy S, Tabar L, Chen HH et al. The impact of organised mammographic screening on breast carcinoma mortality in seven Swedish counties. Cancer 2002; 95:458–69.

27. Hackshaw AK, Paul EA. Breast self-examination and death from breast cancer: a meta-analysis. Br J Cancer 2003; 88:1047–53.

28. Smith RA, Saslow D, Sawyer KA et al. American Cancer Society guidelines for breast cancer screening: update 2003. CA Cancer J Clin 2003; 53:141–69.

29. Breast Screening Frequency Trial Group. The frequency of breast cancer screening: results from the UKCCCR randomized trial. Eur J Cancer 2002; 38:1458–64.

30. Million Women Study Collaborators. Breast cancer and hormone replacement therapy in the Million Women Study. Lancet 2003; 362:419–27.

   Report of significantly increased risk of breast cancer in women taking HRT in the UK.

31. Perrson I, Thurfjell E, Holmberg I. Effect of estrogen and estrogen–progestin replacement regimes on mammographic breast parenchymal density. J Clin Oncol 1997; 15:3201–7.

32. Sendag F, Cosan Terek M, Ozsener S et al. Mammographic density changes during different postmenopausal hormone replacement therapies. Fertil Steril 2001; 76:445–50.

33. Evans A. Hormone replacement therapy and mammographic screening. Clin Radiol 2002; 57:563–4.

34. Litherland JC, Stallard S, Hole D et al. The effect of hormone replacement therapy on the sensitivity of screening mammograms. Clin Radiol 1999; 54:285–8.

35. Kavanagh AM, Mitchell H, Giles GG. Hormone replacement therapy and accuracy of mammographic screening. Lancet 2000; 355:270–4.

36. Litherland JC, Evans AJ, Wilson ARM. The effect of hormone replacement therapy on recall rate in the National Health Breast Screening Programme. Clin Radiol 1997; 52:276–9.

37. Evans AJ, Pinder SE, Ellis IO et al. Screen detected ductal carcinoma in situ (DCIS): over-diagnosis or obligate precursor of invasive disease? J Med Screen 2001; 8:149–51.

38. Evans AJ, Burrell HE, Pinder SE et al. Detecting which invasive cancers at mammographic screening saves lives? J Med Screen 2001; 8:86–90.

39. National Institute for Clinical Excellence. Guidance on cancer services. Familial breast cancer. London: National Institute for Clinical Excellence, 2006. Available at http:\\www.nice.org.uk

40. Robson M. Breast cancer surveillance in women with hereditary risk due to BRCA1 or BRCA2 mutations. Clin Breast Cancer 2004; 5:260–8.

41. Tilanus-Linthorst M, Verhoog L, Obdeijn I-M et al. A BRCA1/2 mutation, high breast density and prominent pushing margins of a tumour independently contribute to a frequent false-negative mammography. Int J Cancer 2002; 102:91–5.

42. Warner E, Plewes DB, Hill KA et al. Surveillance of BRCA1 and BRCA2 mutation carriers with magnetic resonance imaging, ultrasound, mammography, and clinical breast examination. JAMA 2004; 292:1317–25.

43. Hamilton LJ, Evans AJ, Wilson ARM et al. Breast imaging findings in women with BRCA1- and BRCA2-associated breast cancer. Clin Radiol 2004; 59:895–902.

44. Kriege M, Brekelmans CTM, Boetes C et al. Efficacy of MRI and mammography for breast cancer screening in women with a familial or genetic predisposition. N Engl J Med 2004; 351:427–37.

45. Leach MO, Boggis CR, Dixon AK et al. Screening with magnetic resonance imaging and mammography of a UK population at high familial risk of breast cancer: a prospective multicentre cohort study (MARIBS). Lancet 2005; 365:1769–78.

46. Teh W, Wilson ARM. Definitive non-surgical breast diagnosis: the role of the radiologist. Clin Radiol 1998; 53:81–4.

47. Britton PD. Fine needle aspiration or core biopsy. Breast 1999; 8:1–4.

48. Britton PD, McCann J. Needle biopsy in the NHS Breast Screening Programme 1996/7: how much and how accurate? Breast 1999; 8:5–11.

49. Vargas HI, Agbunag RV, Khaikhali I. State of the art of minimally invasive breast biopsy: principles and practice. Breast Cancer 2000; 7:370–9.

50. Heywang-Kobrunner SH, Schaumloffel U, Viehweg P et al. Minimally invasive stereotaxic vacuum core breast biopsy. Eur Radiol 1998; 8:377–85.

51. Brem RF, Schoonjans JM, Sanow L et al. Reliability of histologic diagnosis of breast cancer with stereotactic vacuum-assisted biopsy. Am Surg 2001; 67:388–92.

52. Parker SH, Klaus AJ, McWey PJ et al. Sonographically guided directional vacuum-assisted breast biopsy using a handheld device. Am J Roentgenol 2001; 177:405–8.

53. Kettritz U, Rotter K, Murauer M et al. Stereotactic vacuum biopsy in 2874 patients: a multicenter study. Cancer 2004; 100:245–51.

54. Brenner RJ, Bassett LW, Fajardo LL et al. Stereotactic core needle breast biopsy: a multi-institutional prospective trial. Radiology 2001; 218:866–72.

55. Bagnall MJC, Evans AJ, Wilson ARM et al. When have mammographic calcifications been adequately sampled at needle core biopsy? Clin Radiol 2000; 55:548–53.

56. Kuhl CK, Morakkabati N, Leutner CC et al. MR imaging-guided large-core (14-gauge) needle biopsy of small lesions visible at breast MR imaging alone. Radiology 2001; 220:31–9.

57. Fishman JE, Milikowski C, Ramsinghani R et al. US-guided core-needle biopsy of the breast: how many specimens are necessary? Radiology 2003; 226:779–82.

58. Luini A, Zurrida S, Paganelli G et al. Comparison of radioguided excision with wire localisation of occult breast lesions. Br J Surg 1999; 86:522–5.

59. Rampaul RS, Bagnall M, Burrell H et al. Radio-isotope for occult lesion localisation: results from a prospective randomised trial of ROLL versus wire guidance in occult lesions of the breast. Br J Surg 2004; 91:1575–7.

60. Rampaul RS, Burrell H, Macmillan RD et al. Intraductal injection of the breast: a potential pitfall of radioisotope occult lesion localisation. Br J Radiol 2002; 76:425–6.

61. Patel A, Pain SJ, Britton P et al. Radioguided occult lesion localisation (ROLL) and sentinel node biopsy for impalpable invasive breast cancer. Eur J Surg Oncol 2004; 30:918–23.

62. Tanis PJ, Deurloo EE, Valdes Olmos RA et al. Single intralesional tracer dose for radio-guided excision of clinically occult breast cancer and sentinel node. Ann Surg Oncol 2001; 8:850–5.

63. Gray RJ, Giuliano R, Dauway EL et al. Radio-guidance for nonpalpable primary lesions and sentinel lymph node(s). Am J Surg 2001; 182:404–6.

# 2

# Pathology and biology of breast cancer

Rajendra S. Rampaul
Emad A. Rakha
John F.R. Robertson
Ian O. Ellis

## Introduction

Management of women with breast carcinoma has undergone significant changes over the past 20 years. The pathology and biology of breast cancer influences diagnosis, selection of primary and adjuvant treatment, formulation of follow-up protocols, prognosis, and provision of counselling and reassurance. Screening and public education have accounted for a major shift in the number and type of the breast carcinomas detected today. Cancers are now of smaller size and more often lymph node negative. There is an increasing need to discriminate accurately the risk of recurrence and select appropriate adjuvant systemic therapies. Modern clinical practice employs a significant input from histopathological data to assist in the decision-making process for selecting treatments. This can be achieved by identifying accurate prognostic and predictive factors. A prognostic factor is defined as any patient or tumour characteristic that is predictive of the patient's outcome. Outcome is usually measured in terms of cancer-specific survival or disease-free survival. A predictive factor is defined as any patient or tumour characteristic that is predictive of the patient's response (outcome) to a specified treatment. The factors currently employed in breast cancer prognostication and prediction each possess independent prognostic information and predictive power and may be combined into an index, making it more 'user friendly', informative and reproducible. A prognostic index is defined as quantitative set of values based on results of a prognostic model. There are several reasons for the use of such prognostic indices in breast cancer, which include the ability:

1. to separate patients into groups with significantly differing survival probabilities;
2. to separate patients into groups which include a 'cured' group and a group with poor survival;
3. to place a sufficient percentage of cases into each group;
4. to be applicable for all operable breast cancers – small, screen detected as well as symptomatic and young age;
5. to be prospectively validated;
6. to be capable of use in all units and to be inexpensive.

In this chapter common pathological features of breast cancer are reviewed and their role in guiding patients' management considered.

## Traditional factors

### Lymph node stage

Involvement of local and regional lymph nodes by metastatic carcinoma is one of the most important prognostic factors in breast cancer. The revised TNM staging system for breast cancer has confirmed that the absolute number of axillary lymph nodes involved by metastatic cancer ('positive lymph nodes') is one of the most important prognostic factors in breast cancer.[1] Lymph node stage has been used consistently as a guide for therapy. However, lymph node stage is considered as a time-dependent factor: the longer the tumour has been growing, the more likely it is that lymph nodes are involved by spread. It has also been reported that when taken alone lymph node stage is incapable of defining either a (cured) group or one with close to 100% mortality from breast cancer.

Clinical assessment of nodal status (as in TNM classification) is unreliable.[2,3] Palpable nodes may be enlarged because they show benign reactive changes whilst nodes bearing tumour deposits can be impalpable. Although axillary sonography is a moderately sensitive and fairly specific technique in the diagnosis of axillary metastatic involvement,[4] histological examination of the lymph nodes from the axilla should be carried out in all patients with primary operable invasive breast cancer. It is well known that patients who have histologically confirmed lymph node involvement have a significantly poorer prognosis than those without nodal metastases. The 10-year survival is reduced from 75% for patients with no nodal involvement to 25–30% for those with involvement of multiple nodes. Prognosis worsens the greater the number of nodes involved, and the level of nodal involvement can provide useful information; metastasis to the higher level nodes (level II or III) in the axilla and particularly those at the apex (level III) carries a worse prognosis (**Fig. 2.1**).

Additionally, studies suggest that overall survival is decreased as the number of nodes that are involved increases.[5–7]

Optimal management of the axilla is discussed in Chapter 7. At Nottingham, the protocol is a blue dye-assisted four-node axillary sample.

Four-node axillary sampling has been shown to provide accurate prognostic information and has an extremely low rate of lymphoedema.[2] Of 1275 patients, only 0.04% suffered symptomatic complaints of arm swelling and lymphoedema.

A refinement of lymph node sampling is provided by the technique of sentinel lymph node (SLN) biopsy. There have been several studies to examine the validity of this technique. The Axillary Lymphatic Mapping Against Nodal Axillary Clearance (ALMANAC) trial provides level I evidence for UK-based practice.[3]

From a pathological perspective, there are unresolved questions about how to optimally assess the sentinel node. Studies have shown that the mean number of sentinel nodes is close to 3. As the number of nodes removed during SLN biopsy is fewer, pathologists are now challenged to process these few nodes optimally. Several methods have been studied: routine paraffin histology, intraoperative frozen section, immunohistochemistry and more intensive methods such as serial sectioning and molecular methods, including polymerase chain reaction (PCR) and reverse transcription–PCR (RT–PCR).

Presently there is no consensus for the optimal handling of the SLN in the laboratory. Most centres have developed their own 'in-house' protocols, which are invariably tied to the institution's research ambitions. This ad hoc approach can influence interpretation of results, as the amount of material assessed between centres is not uniform, even ignoring methodological differences. In a number of large studies, using different histopathological techniques, the SLN false-negative rate (defined as how often the SLN is negative for malignancy when cancer is present in the rest of the axilla) varies between 0% and 11%.

In Nottingham the MRC ALMANAC protocol is employed to assess all sentinel node biopsies. These nodes are cut into slices about 3 mm thick, taken perpendicular to the long axis of the node to maximise the assessment of the marginal sinus, with one

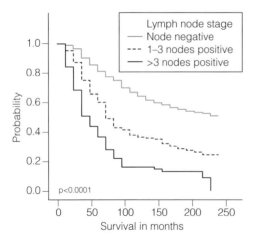

**Figure 2.1** • Overall survival for patients in the NTPBCS according to lymph node stage ($P < 0.0001$).

node per cassette. The majority of nodes can be completely embedded in one cassette. Larger nodes have alternate slices embedded and may require more than one cassette. Large, obviously involved nodes have one section taken. This approach is consistent with National Health Service Breast Screening recommendations.

Intraoperative frozen sections or imprint cytology of axillary lymph nodes have been advocated by some authors. Conventional frozen sections have a high false-negative rate of between 10% and 30%. More intensive intraoperative assessment with serial sections and immunohistochemistry has been described,[8] but is time-consuming and labour intensive. Frozen section is best applied to selected cases; for example, if the node is macroscopically abnormal and this is confirmed histologically to be metastatic carcinoma, further axillary surgery can be performed immediately. Some studies have found low false-negative rates of 2–3% with intraoperative imprint cytology,[9] but not all have been able to achieve this level of accuracy. Lymph node status can be assessed preoperatively using ultrasound combined with fine-needle aspiration or core biopsy and this reduces the need for perisoperative frozen section and imprint cytology to assess axillary nodes intraoperatively.

RT–PCR is more sensitive than immunohistochemistry at detecting metastatic tumour in axillary nodes. Two types of methods have been used to detect tumour cells with molecular techniques. First a genetic defect such as chromosomal rearrangement or mutation can be used. The problem with this is that no single genetic defect is seen in all breast carcinomas. The second method is to use a molecular marker that is present in tumour cells but not in the adjacent tissue. To identify a marker that has this specificity and is expressed in the majority of tumours is difficult. It may be necessary to use a panel of markers. A major problem with PCR is the potentially high false-positive rate due to the sensitivity of the method and potential for contamination. In addition, it is not possible with PCR to determine whether the DNA comes from cells which are viable. An advantage of haematoxylin/eosin sections and immunohistochemistry is that the morphology of the cells can be examined and malignancy confirmed. A major unresolved question is whether carcinoma detected only by PCR or RT–PCR has the same prognostic significance as haematoxylin/eosin positivity.

The detection rate of micrometastases in axillary lymph nodes has been reported to range from 9% to 46%.[10] Studies have used serial sectioning with or without immunohistochemical stains to detect micrometastatic foci and these methods have increased detection rates. However, repeatedly studies on SLN micrometastases have not had sufficient follow-up to see any survival effects and so the prognostic significance of such occult metastasis at this time is unknown.

The European Working Group for Breast Screening Pathology[11] has formulated working guidelines for the assessment and pathological work-up of SLNs in breast cancer. From a literature review, the committee concluded that it was not possible to determine the significance of micrometastasis or isolated tumour cells. They noted that approximately 18% of cases are associated with other nodal (non-sentinel node) metastases. False-negative rates are most often determined via immunohistochemistry (IHC). However, at present it is recommended that an intensive work-up is not justified on a population level. The committee did suggest multilevel assessment and, where resources permit, intraoperative assessment.

## Tumour size

Tumour size is one of the most powerful predictors of prognosis in breast cancer.[12,13] The frequency of nodal metastases in patients with tumours <10 mm is 10–20%,[13] and node-negative patients with tumours <10 mm have a 10-year disease-free survival rate of about 90%.[14] Tumour size is a time-dependent prognostic factor that depends on the period between tumour development and detection, and on the balance between tumour cell proliferation and death (tumour growth rate). It is well known that the association between increasing tumour size and increasing number of positive lymph nodes and worse outcome is highly statistically significant.[13] Therefore, the main aim of population screening with mammography is to detect smaller tumours which are likely to have a better outcome than those that present symptomatically (of a larger size). Patients with smaller tumours have a better long-term survival than those with larger tumours (**Fig. 2.2**). Estimation of tumour size has assumed particular importance since the introduction of population screening. In most studies the frequency of axillary lymph node metastasis in small

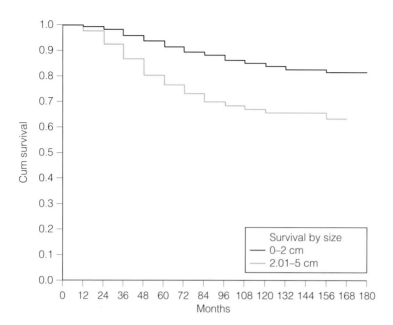

**Figure 2.2** • Overall survival according to size.

Survival by size
— 0–2 cm
— 2.01–5 cm

(so-called minimally invasive carcinoma (MIC)) invasive carcinomas is 15–20%,[15–17] compared with over 40% in tumours measuring 15 mm or more.[18] During the prevalent round of breast screening even more favourable results are obtained, with the frequency of axillary lymph node metastasis ranging from 0% to 15%.[19–22] The Nottingham Tenovus Primary Breast Cancer Study (NTPBCS) has generated data that suggests the cut-off point of 10 mm is not the best discriminator for MIC. Life-table analysis of survival curves found no difference between tumours measuring up to 9 mm and those measuring 10–14 mm. This indicates that <15 mm may be a more realistic watershed in defining small, invasive carcinomas of good prognosis. It is clear that pathological tumour size is a valuable prognostic factor and it has become an important quality assurance measure for breast screening.[21,23–26] It is also used in part to judge the ability of radiologists to detect small impalpable invasive carcinomas.

## Differentiation

Modern pathologists have recognised that invasive carcinomas can be divided according to their degree of differentiation. There are two ways to achieve this: (i) by allocating a histological type according to the architectural pattern of the tumour; (ii) by assigning a grade of differentiation based on semi-quantitative evaluation of structural characteristics.

Certain histological types of invasive carcinoma carry a favourable prognosis. Tubular, mucinous, invasive cribriform, medullary and tubulolobular types, together with rare tumour types such as adenoid cystic carcinoma, adenomyoepithelioma and low-grade and squamous carcinoma, have all been reported to have a more favourable outcome than invasive carcinoma of no special type (ductal NST). Undoubtedly, assessment of histological type provides prognostic information in breast cancer. However, this effect is relatively small in a multivariate analysis[27] when compared with the prognostic value of histological grade; histological type may prove to be more useful in increasing our understanding of the biology of breast cancers.[28]

Invasive lobular carcinoma (ILC) is of particular importance. It comprises approximately 5–15% of breast cancers and appears to have a distinct biology. It is less common than invasive carcinoma of no special type, also called invasive ductal carcinoma (IDC).

Recently, Rakha et al. examined a large group of 5680 breast tumours (415 patients (8%) with pure ILC and 2901 (55.7%) with IDC (no special type)) and demonstrated that, compared to IDC, patients with ILC tended to be older and have tumours that are more frequently of lower grade (typically, grade 2; 84%), hormone receptor positive (86% compared to 61% in IDC), of larger size and with absence of vascular invasion. More patients with ILC compared with IDC were placed in the good Nottingham Prognostic Index group (40% compared to 21% in IDC). ILC showed indolent but progressive behavioural characteristics with nearly linear survival curves which crossed those of IDC after approximately 10 years of follow-up, thus eventually exhibiting a worse long-term outcome. Interestingly, ILC showed a better response to adjuvant hormonal therapy with improvement in survival in patients who received hormonal therapy compared with matched patients with IDC.[29]

## Tumour grade

Bloom and Richardson made a useful contribution by adding numerical scoring to the method of tumour grading devised by Patey and Scarfe.[30] The former system did not provide clear guidance on cut-off points. The Nottingham method was therefore devised to provide greater objectivity of the grading system.

In brief, assessment of grade considers three tumour characteristics: tubule formation, nuclear pleomorphism and mitotic counts. A numerical scoring system of 1–3 is used for each factor individually.

The three scores are added together to produce scores of 3–9, on which an overall tumour grade is assigned:

- Grade 1 – well differentiated = score 3–5 points.
- Grade 2 – moderately differentiated = score 6–7 points.
- Grade 3 – poorly differentiated = score 8–9 points.

It should be noted that grade is valuable irrespective of morphological type.

There is a highly significant correlation with long-term prognosis (**Fig. 2.3**); patients with grade 1 tumours have an 85% chance of surviving 10 years after diagnosis, whereas in patients with grade 3 tumours this is reduced to 45%. It has now been shown conclusively that the Nottingham method, with its more objective criteria, has excellent reproducibility when used by experienced pathologists.

Interestingly, grade is not included in the recent revision of the TNM staging system of breast cancer as its value is questioned in certain settings such as lobular type.

These issues were addressed by Rakha et al. in a large study of grade and overall survival in a large and well-characterized consecutive series of operable breast cancer (*n* = 2219 cases), with a long-term follow-up (median 111 months) using the Nottingham histological grading system. Histological grade was strongly associated with both breast cancer-specific survival (BCSS) and disease-free survival (DFS) in the whole series, as well as in different subgroups based on tumour size (pT1a, pT1b, pT1c and pT2) and lymph node stage (pN0 and pN1 and pN2). The authors were able to demonstrate differences in survival between different individual grades (1, 2 and 3). In multivariate analyses histological grade was an independent predictor of both BCSS and DFS.[31]

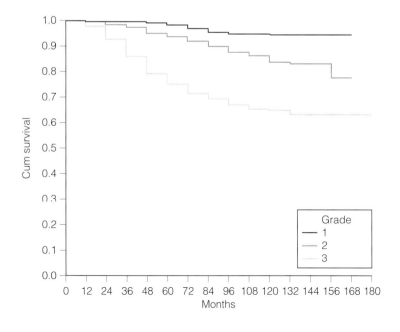

**Figure 2.3** • Overall survival according to grade.

Additionally, the usefulness of routinely assessing grade in invasive lobular cancer was also examined by this group in 4987 patients,[32] of whom 517 were pure ILC cases. The majority of ILC was of classical type or mixed lobular variants (89%). Most ILC cases were moderately differentiated (grade 2) tumours (76%), while a small proportion of tumours were either grade 1 or 3 (12% each). There were positive associations between histological grade and other clinicopathological variables of poor prognosis, such as larger tumour size, positive lymph node status, vascular invasion, estrogen receptor and androgen receptor negativity, and p53 positivity. Multivariate analyses showed that histological grade was an independent predictor of BCSS and disease-free interval.

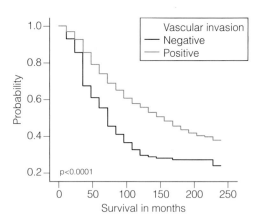

**Figur 2.4** • LVI and breast cancer-specific survival.

## Vascular invasion

The presence of tumour emboli in vascular and lymphatic spaces has emerged as an important prognostic factor. Several studies have now shown that the presence of vascular invasion correlates closely with local and regional lymph node involvement.[33,34] It has been suggested that it can provide prognostic information as powerful as lymph node stage. Reproducibility is the limiting factor in its widespread adoption and routine clinical assessment. In a Nottingham study assessing vascular invasion, the issue of reproducibility was specifically addressed. Of the 1704 cases examined, a subset of 400 cases was examined by two or more pathologists. Analysis of inter-observer variation showed a 77% overall agreement on histological features and an 85.8% overall agreement in the classification of vascular invasion. Other studies have reported a similarly high concurrence between pathologists.[35,36] The assessment of vascular invasion must be regarded as subjective, but despite this there is good evidence that a high rate of concurrence can be obtained as long as strict criteria are used. Lymphatic and vascular invasion is considered to be a valuable surrogate for lymph node stage in cases where nodes have not been removed for examination. Even in patients whose axillary nodes are tumour free on histological examination there is a correlation between the presence of lymphovascular invasion (LVI) and early recurrence.

 Recently, Lee et al.[37] assessed the prognostic value of LVI in a group of 2760 patients with node-negative breast cancer with long-term follow-up (median 13 years). This study demonstrated a strong association between poor histological grade and younger age with LVI-positive cancers. LVI was prognostically significant and was independent of grade, size and type for overall survival (see **Fig. 2.4**).

# Molecular/predictive factors

Despite the overall association of molecular markers with prognosis and outcome, they are limited in their ability to capture the nuances of the complex cascade of events that drive the clinical behaviour of breast cancer. Morphological factors are unable to predict response to systemic treatments and tumours of apparently homogeneous morphological characters still vary in response to therapy and have distinct outcomes. The use of strategies ranging from hormone therapy to chemotherapy and recently to novel receptor-directed therapies and vaccines relies on the expression of predictive factors by the cancer, either individually (e.g. estrogen receptors, progesterone receptors, human epidermal growth factor receptor 2 (HER-2) and epidermal growth factor receptor (EGFR)) or globally (e.g. high-throughput gene expression assays). These molecular markers are used not only to guide treatments, but are also being used to monitor response and detect relapse. It is envisaged that molecular predictive markers may form the basis of tailoring an individual's adjuvant therapy based on the genetic fingerprint of the cancer.

## Estrogen receptors (ERs)/ progesterone receptors (PRs)

Knowledge of the expression of hormone receptors and their subcellular regulatory pathways is one of the classic examples of the use of translational medicine in breast cancer to further diagnosis and treatment of this disease. The degree of ER expression is used to predict an individual's response to hormone therapy. Both ERs and PRs are steroid receptors which are located in the cell nucleus. Estrogen and progesterone are considered to diffuse into cells, or be transported, to the nucleus. Genes, regulated by steroid receptors, are involved in controlling cell growth and it is currently believed that these effects are the most relevant to ERs and that ER expression influences the behaviour and treatment of breast cancer.[38] Elucidation of the downstream effect on genes which are known to be influenced by hormones has led to the inclusion of these ER-regulated genes in high-density oligonucleotide array panels.[39] This may better define those pathways that are endocrine responsive. This should lead to improved therapies with reduced side-effects and a greater potential for cure.[40]

In unselected patients approximately 30% will respond to endocrine therapy. A tumour with both ER and PR expression carries a 78% chance of responding to hormone therapy, while those cancers that are ER/PR negative respond rarely, if ever.[41–43] Due to its close relationship with histological grade, ERs are not of independent prognostic significance.[43]

## Methods of measuring ERs and PRs

There are a multitude of methods available; however, in clinical practice most are based on two distinct strategies. The first is ligand-binding methods, i.e. radiolabelled steroid ligand is used to detect the receptor. The second relies on the recognition of the receptor protein by specific antibodies. Several studies have examined the correlation between assay and outcome/response and at present there is no clear advantage to any one method; however, some studies have suggested that IHC analyses may have a slight advantage.[42] IHC is currently the most commonly used method because it can be performed on paraffin-embedded material.

## Interpretation of assays

The optimal way to score IHC for ERs and PRs remains controversial. One method is to use an 'H' score (histo score) which takes into account the frequency of positive cells as well as intensity of staining and multiplies the two. The Allred score categorises the percentage of cells (0–5) and the intensity (0–3) and adds these two scores to give a numerical score from 0 to 8. Others simply estimate the percentage of positively stained tumour nuclei. It is important to appreciate that all methods are subjective and, at best, semiquantitative. ER/PR status in the histopathological report has a clearly defined role as a predictive factor for the response of systemic endocrine therapy. ERs and PRs should be assessed on all breast tumour specimens. As these assays have become simpler, and less costly, they are gradually becoming available for all patients. Progress still needs to be made in standardisation of assay technique, objectivity and reproducibility.

## Type 1 growth factor receptors

Activation of growth factor receptors was first found to be important in human cancers by identifying the homology between the viral oncogene v-*erbB* and EGFR. Sequence similarity between the *ERBB1* gene which encodes EGFR resulted in the isolation of a second growth factor receptor, the human orthologue *neu*, HER-2 (erbB-2). Screening of genomic DNA and messenger RNAs with probes allowed isolation of two additional relatives of the human *ERB1* gene. They were subsequently named erbB-3 (HER-3) and erbB-4 (HER-4).

To date there are four known receptors which belong to this growth factor receptor family: HER-1–4 and ligands for some of these have been identified. The family works in a co-receptor dimerisation type activation pathway.

The first two members of this family have been studied extensively in breast cancer. There are limited data on the role of HER-3 and HER-4 as well as their ligands. This family of signalling molecules is currently of immense clinical interest as the first two members are targets against which novel bioreceptor agents have been developed, including Iressa, Tarveca, Herceptin and lopatinib.

### EGFR

EGFR expression has been well studied in breast cancer. Consequent on major differences in study designs the EGFR assay used and confounding factors such as adjuvant therapy, there is no consensus on its prognostic value. With the development of tyrosine kinase inhibitor- and EGFR-directed biotherapies, there is now a growing impetus to not only standardise assays for detecting EGFR but also to delineate accurately its prognostic and predictive potential.

### Methods of testing

Several techniques directed at DNA, RNA, protein (including functionally activated protein) or serum can be employed to identify EGFR expression in breast cancer.

Of all such methods, IHC is the most practical. The advantages of IHC in EGFR as in HER-2 testing include reproducibility, ease of interpretation and the low cost compared to other techniques. It can also be employed on archival tissue. Protein levels can be quantified by Western analysis or enzyme immunoassay; however, architecture of tissue is lost in these procedures and there may be contamination by normal tissue cells or ductal carcinoma in situ. Serum EGFR levels have been examined in breast carcinoma; however, few data are available.[44,45] Due to the paucity of relevant data, it is difficult to draw conclusions on the current value of measuring EGFR in the serum of patients.

### Prognostic and predictive value

The prognostic value of EGFR in breast cancer has been examined in several large studies. There remains no consensus on its prognostic value. The lack of a clear picture has been attributed to several factors: lack of a standard assay (monoclonal vs. polyclonal), lack of a cut-off for positivity and great variation in study designs (size, follow-up and influence of adjuvant therapy). Klijn et al. reviewed data from over 5000 patients where EGFR had been assessed.[46] Findings from this review demonstrated a great heterogeneity of study design, levels of cut-offs for positive and negative and, not surprisingly, differences in its prognostic value in these various studies.

Recently, Tsutsui et al.[47] reported on a large series of 1029 patients (with adjuvant therapy) and found EGFR to be of independent prognostic value irrespective of nodal status. In contrast, studies by Rampaul et al.[48] and Ferrero et al.[49] (without adjuvant therapy) showed EGFR to be of no prognostic value (these latter series also incorporated grade and had longer follow-up).

The predictive value of this marker for hormone resistance or responsiveness is better defined. EGFR tumours are considered more resistant to endocrine therapy, and there exists an inverse relationship with EGFR-negative cancers (they are more likely ER positive) being more often sensitive to endocrine manipulation. Although some studies have been able to demonstrate that EGFR status is a predictor of tamoxifen failure and even response rates,[50] there are conflicting data from well-designed level II studies[51] that have shown no value of EGFR in predicting the efficacy of tamoxifen in high-risk postmenopausal women.

Perhaps the most exciting use of EGFR status, and indeed the driving impetus for clinicians and scientists to measure it accurately, is its putative role in defining those who should respond to novel EGFR-directed therapies.

## HER-2

HER-2 remains an important target in the development of a variety of new cancer therapies, which include monoclonal antibody (mAb)-based therapy, small-molecule drugs directed at the internal tyrosine kinase portion of the HER-2 oncoprotein, and vaccines. The most widely known HER-2-directed therapy is trastuzumab (Herceptin; Genentech, South San Francisco, CA, USA). Trastuzumab is a humanised recombinant mAb that specifically targets the HER-2 extracellular domain. There are a variety of techniques available to determine HER-2 status in breast cancer, some of which are employed for research purposes only. In diagnostic pathology laboratories HER-2 status is assessed routinely either by IHC, which assesses expression of the HER-2 oncoprotein, and fluorescence in situ hybridisation (FISH), which measures the number of *HER2* gene copies per chromosome 17 or gene amplification. Modifications of ISH using colorimetric detection are being developed, including chromogenic in situ hybridisation (CISH) and silver-enhanced in situ hybridisation (SISH).

### Methods of HER-2 testing

Current guidelines for HER-2 testing[52] specify the methods which are suitable to detect either the HER-2 protein (by IHC) or gene amplification (using FISH or other in situ methods). Guidelines stress the need for stringent, reproducible and consistent criteria for testing.

#### *Immunohistochemistry (IHC) for HER-2 testing*

Among the methods in use for determining HER-2 status, IHC is the most widely used. In studies employing various commercially available antibodies, a wide variety of sensitivity and specificity in fixed paraffin-embedded tissues is seen.[53, 54] Antigen retrieval techniques are not currently standardised and they introduce the potential for false-positive staining. Nonetheless, IHC possesses many advantages to support its widespread adoption: (i) it allows for the preservation of tissue architecture and so can be used to identify local areas of overexpression within a heterogeneous sample, and can distinguish between HER-2 positivity in in-situ and invasive cancer; (ii) it is applicable to routine patient samples, facilitating use as a diagnostic test, and this allows prospective and retrospective research studies of HER-2 status to be undertaken.

Two Food and Drug Administration (FDA)-approved IHC tests for determining HER-2 status are available: HercepTest (DAKO, Carpeteria, CA, USA), based upon a polyclonal antibody; and CB11 (Pathway, Ventana Medical Systems, Tucson, AZ, USA), based upon a monoclonal antibody. The National Comprehensive Cancer Network guidelines[55] classify an IHC score of 0 or 1+ as representing HER-2-negative status, 3+ as positive while 2+ is equivocal. Positive staining is defined as strong, continuous membranous expression of HER-2 in at least 10% of tumour cells. However, a joint report from the American Society of Clinical Oncology (ASCO) and the College of American Pathologists (CAP)[52] specified a threshold of >30% strong circumferential membrane staining for a positive result. If both uniformity and a homogeneous, dark circumferential pattern are seen, the resultant cases are likely to be amplified by FISH as well as positive for HER-2 protein expression. The equivocal range for IHC (score 2+), which may include up to 15% of samples, is defined as complete membrane staining that is either non-uniform or weak in intensity but with obvious circumferential distribution in at least 10% of cells. Equivocal or inconclusive results should be tested by FISH. Consistent with previous guidelines, a negative HER-2 test is defined as either an IHC result of 0 or 1+ for cellular membrane protein expression (no staining or weak, incomplete membrane staining in any proportion of tumour cells).

### In situ hybridisation for HER-2 testing

FISH and CISH measure directly the number of *HER2* genes per chromosome 17, and when there is a chromosome centromeric enumeration probe (CEP) included, the copy number of chromosome 17 gene amplification is defined as an increase in HER-2/CEP17 ratio above 2.0. ISH results are semiquantitative, counting the number of signals in non-overlapping interphase nuclei of the lesion using either single-colour (HER-2 probe only, e.g. Ventana Inform) or dual-colour hybridisation (using HER-2 and chromosome 17 centromere probes

simultaneously, e.g. Abbott, Chicago, USA, DAKO, Copenhagen, Denmark, etc.), the latter making it easier to distinguish true HER-2 amplification from chromosomal aneuploidy. ISH allows simultaneous morphological assessment, where evaluation of gene amplification can be restricted to invasive carcinoma cells. Many studies have compared FISH and IHC in the evaluation of HER-2 and have demonstrated concordance between the two techniques of up to 91%. Two studies have shown that FISH predicts HER-2 positivity more accurately than IHC when applied to molecularly characterised breast cancers.[56,57]

Three FISH tests are FDA-approved for selecting patients for treatment with trastuzumab. The Path Vysion (Vysis Inc., Downers Grove, IL, USA) and PharmDx (Dako) tests require a ratio (HER-2 to CEP17) of 2.0 or greater for the sample to be considered amplified and both include an *HER2* gene probe and a chromosome 17 probe. The INFORM test (Ventana Medical Systems) requires that at least 5.0 gene copies of *HER2* be present if a sample is to be considered amplified as this kit uses a single *HER2* gene probe without a chromosome 17 probe.

Recommended guidelines for HER-2 assessment in the UK have recently been updated and the reader is referred to these guidelines for further details.[58]

In brief, a two-phase testing algorithm based on IHC assay as the primary screen with FISH being reserved for equivocal cases is currently recommended. This is based on evidence showing very good concordance between IHC and FISH results on breast carcinomas from 37 laboratories when tested in experienced reference centres.[59]

### Chromogenic in situ hybridisation (CISH/SISH)

Chromogenic in situ hybridisation (CISH) and the silver-based variant (SISH) are colorimetric methods to detect gene amplification which can be viewed using a standard light microscope. Concordance between FISH and SISH for the validation of *HER2* gene status is about 96% (kappa = 0.754, 95% CI).

### Prognostic significance and association with other prognostic factors

The seminal work by Slamon et al. in 1987 showed that *HER2* gene amplification independently predicted overall survival (OS) and disease-free survival (DFS) in a multivariate analysis in node-positive patients.[60] Since then most large studies have confirmed this relationship in multivariate analysis.

It is now well established that there is a significant correlation between HER-2 overexpression/amplification and poor prognosis for patients with nodal metastasis. At present, there is no consensus on the prognostic value of HER-2 in node-negative breast cancer patients, a group most often diagnosed through screening and representing a subgroup which could potentially benefit from appropriate adjuvant therapy.

Rilke et al. reported on the prognostic significance of HER-2 expression and its relationship with other prognostic factors.[61] Using specimens from 1210 consecutive patients treated between 1968 and 1971 at a single institution (National Cancer Institute of Milan), with no systemic adjuvant therapy and 20-year follow-up, overexpression of HER-2 was found in 23% and showed a negative impact on survival of node-positive but not node-negative patients. Analysis of HER-2 in relation to the presence of lymphoplasmacytic infiltrate (LPI; favourable prognosis) and nodal status demonstrated that in node-negative, LPI-negative patients, HER-2 overexpression showed the same level of correlation with poor prognosis as in those patients with nodal metastasis. However, in the patients with node-negative disease and LPI positivity, HER-2 overexpression correlated with good prognosis. Some studies have reported a prognostic value for HER-2 in node-negative patients in selected subgroups,[62,63] whereas others have shown no correlation.[64,65]

Mirza et al. have published a systematic review of prognostic factors in node negative disease.[66] Data for HER-2 showed a lack of standardisation of assays and no association with survival.[66] However, HER-2 status was shown to be of independent prognostic significance in two large studies with long-term follow-up.[68,69] These findings need to be validated prospectively by an independent dataset.

There is at present no agreement on the association between HER-2 and other prognostic factors. Several studies have shown a lack of association between HER-2 status and tumour size,[60,70,71] although some do report a correlation.[61,72–76]

### Prediction of response to therapy
#### Hormonal therapy
Transfection of normal breast cancer cells with the *HER2* gene has been shown to result in acquisition of estrogen-independent growth, that is insensitive to tamoxifen.[77,78]

A number of clinical studies, using various end-points such as time to relapse, more rapid spread to other sites and disease-free survival or overall survival, have reported an association between HER-2 positivity and resistance to hormonal therapy.[79–83] Some reports have described specific resistance to tamoxifen in HER-2-overexpressing tumours.[81,82] The 20-year update of the Naples GUN trial[81] found that HER-2 overexpression not only predicted resistance to tamoxifen, but that HER-2-positive patients had a worse outcome on tamoxifen therapy compared with those who were untreated.

Several studies have also shown a reduction in response rates to hormonal therapy. Metastatic breast cancer which overexpressed HER-2, measured by high plasma levels of extracellular domain, demonstrated a substantial reduction in response rate to hormonal therapy.[84] Other studies have failed to find an association or even a trend between HER-2 status and response to hormonal therapy.[85,86] Elledge et al. examined the response to tamoxifen in 205 tumours with ER-positive disease. In HER-2-positive compared to HER-2-negative patients, they found no significant evidence for a poorer response, time to treatment failure or survival.[87] In a more recent study, the relationship between HER-2 overexpression and response to tamoxifen was examined in the adjuvant setting in 741 (650 ER positive, 91 ER negative/PR positive) of the total of 1572 patients in the CALGB 8541 trial who had HER-2 measured.[88] Tamoxifen significantly improved response, DFS and OS irrespective of HER-2 status. However, tamoxifen was not randomised within this trial and all patients received one of three regimens of doxorubicin. Thus these data on tamoxifen resistance have limitations to their interpretation.

With regards to HER-2 and prognosis, not only is there clinical value in its positive expression but also in its absence – in so-called 'triple negative' cancers, i.e. cancers which are HER-2, ER and PR negative. It also denotes a biologically different subgroup. The recognition of basal phenotype in these triple negative cancers is of growing importance, with several lines of evidence supporting the view that triple negative tumours and basal phenotype are not interchangeable but rather distinct entities. An in-depth discussion of these issues is beyond the scope of this work and the reader is directed to the excellent detailed reviews by Rakha et al.[89]

## Histopathology of patients with *BRCA1* and *BRCA2* mutations

The cancers which develop in patients with a genetic predisposition to breast cancer as a result of mutations in the breast cancer susceptibility genes *BRCA1* and *BRCA2* are of great clinical interest. Identification of histological features that could indicate a genetic predisposition would be useful in providing an insight into the function of these genes and may aid in identifying those in whom screening for genetic mutations would be useful. There is a general agreement that *BRCA1*-related cancers are more frequently 'medullary-like' carcinomas and are high grade compared to those in patients without this genetic alteration. Cancers associated with *BRCA1* mutations have a significantly higher mitotic rate, a larger proportion of tumour with a continuous pushing margin and more lymphocytic infiltration than sporadic breast cancers.[90,91] These are also likely to be less positive for ER and PR and are more often aneuploid, have a high S-phase fraction, show greater accumulation of p52 protein and have greater expression of basal cytokeratins (CK5/6, CK14 and CK17) than do sporadic breast cancers.[92–97] However, none of these features alone or in combination can be used to identify a cancer as being from a *BRCA1* gene mutation carrier. Pathological features reported in *BRCA2*-related breast cancer have been less consistent. Marcus et al.[92] noted a significantly higher proportion of tubulo-lobular cancers in *BRCA2* mutation carriers than in other patients. However, it has been reported in another study that tubular carcinomas are less common in *BRCA2* mutation carriers.[94] Ames et al.[97] investigated the histological phenotypes of breast carcinoma in women under 40 years of age with and without *BRCA1* and *BRCA2* germline mutations. It was found that the pleomorphic variant of invasive lobular carcinoma was more common in patients with *BRCA2* mutations. Others have reported that *BRCA2*-related cancers tend to be of high histological grade,[94,98] whereas others

have not noted any significant difference in grade between *BRCA2*-related cancers and controls.[99]

## High-throughput molecular techniques as prognostic and predictive tools in breast cancer

### Genomics

#### Mechanisms of genetic aberrations

The sequencing of the entire human genome has permitted the introduction of high-throughput technologies which allows survey of thousands of genes and their products in a single assay. Together with powerful analytical tools this has opened new avenues for classifying breast cancer into biologically and clinically distinct groups based on DNA copy number alterations and gene expression patterns.

Cancer development is driven by the accumulation of DNA changes within the genome. DNA repair defects lead to a genome-wide genetic instability and this can drive further cancer progression. **Genomics** (*the study of the human genome*), **transcriptomics** (*the study of the transcriptome* (mRNAs)) and **proteomics** (*the analysis of the protein complement of the genome*) are the three branches of molecular biology that are being explored in an effort to improve understanding, diagnosis, prognostication and provide new therapeutic targets for the treatment of breast cancer.

The genetic fingerprint provides information on normal cellular processes and morphological/phenotypic expression. When this message is altered, it forms the nidus for the development and progression of cancer. These alterations can be caused by DNA mutations, chromosomal aberrations, epigenetic modification and protein interactions. DNA mutations can lead to a change in gene function. These mutations are often due to base substitutions which may directly cause a stop codon. As a result the gene is only partly transcribed and any functional protein production terminated. Chromosomal instability can be due to DNA modification, mutation or viral genome integration. Changes in chromosome numbers are also seen and cancers can be aneuploid (60–90 chromosomes) or near diploid (46 chromosomes). In solid tumours virtually all chromosomal rearrangements are unbalanced, the net result being loss or gain in certain parts of the chromosome. By screening the genome, current losses and gains can be identified. This information can be used to investigate regions of overlap to reveal the genes that are involved in malignant transformation and cancer progression. In some situations, the DNA copy number and code remain intact but the accessibility of this DNA for transcription is affected by epigenetic modifications. This process can occur through DNA methylation. It directly silences genes and interferes with the binding of transcription factors by changing the chromatin structure around the gene. Global hypomethylation is a characteristic feature of the genome of a cancer cell. However, some sequences can be hypermethylated such as CpG islands, which tend to lie around the transcription start sites of approximately half of all human genes. DNA hypomethylation has been shown to correlate with chromosome instability. Chromatin architecture remodelling is essential for gene transcription, thus the prognostic significance of quantitative chromatin changes.[100,101]

## Assessment of genomic status in breast cancer

Several high-throughput molecular techniques have been developed to assess the status of the genome in a given cell population, in terms of copy number, DNA sequencing and structure. Large-scale DNA or gene copy number alterations can be assessed using loss of heterozygosity (LOH) and comparative genomic hybridisation (CGH) studies, as well as other techniques. LOH can be used to identify chromosomal regions where allelic losses are more frequent. In one study,[102] a panel of 150 polymorphic microsatellite markers from throughout the whole genome was used to identify such regions. These data were correlated with clinico-pathological features and showed that four specific loci that correlated with lymph node metastasis (11q23–24, 13q12, 17p13.3 and 22q13). Microsatellites can also be used to check the ability of cells to repair DNA replication errors. Microsatellite instability can be employed to identify both genetic and epigenetic modification. It has been shown that both genetic and epigenetic alterations of *hMSH2* and *hMLH1* contribute to genomic instability and tumour progression in sporadic breast cancer.

Chromosome-based CGH can be used to identify the loss of one or both copies of a given gene as well as regions of amplification. In addition, the technique provides information on the number of copies of any part of each chromosome throughout the whole genome. There have been several studies using CGH in breast carcinoma,[103,104] and those with clinical follow-up have led to the identification of genetic changes related to prognosis. However, the resolution of chromosome-based CGH is limited to approximately 10 million base pairs (Mbp). This limitation makes it difficult to link copy number changes to the genes involved. Another limitation to this technique is the need to perform karyotyping for target identification in every experiment.

Therefore, array CGH has been developed to overcome the problems of chromosome-based CGH. Array CGH does not require a normal metaphase spread but rather an array of DNA fragments (100 bp to 100 kb) and their precise chromosomal locus. This approach can provide resolutions up to 1 Mb. Albertson et al. utilised this technique to map the recurrent breast cancer amplicon at chromosome 20q12.3. They were able to demonstrate that what was previously described as a single amplicon is in fact two distinct amplicons (ZNF217 and CYP24). A novel amplicon at 17q21.3 which is implicated in the amplification and overexpression of the *HOXB7* gene in breast cancer has also been recently characterised using array CGH.[105]

## Assessment of gene expression in breast cancer

In gene expression profiling, each gene is usually represented by a single element (created with a complementary DNA (cDNA) or oligonucleotide for the gene studied) and with high-density oligonucleotide cDNA microarrays technology, many thousands of gene-specific mRNAs can be measured in parallel in a single tissue sample. The principal of gene expression cDNA array is comparable to array CGH other than that it uses cDNA generated from mRNA. Similar to the two main types of expression microarrays (cDNA microarrays and oligonucleotide microarrays), serial analysis of gene expression can provide profiling of the transcriptome by taking a raw count of sequence tags, each representing a transcript in an RNA population, with each one representing one gene.

Broadly speaking, molecular profiling of breast cancers by gene expression microarrays can be performed in one of two ways: unsupervised or supervised analysis. Unsupervised analysis is used mainly for partitioning tumour samples into groups or classes on the basis of gene expression profiles regardless of other features. The main objective of this approach is to determine whether discrete subsets of cancers can be defined on the basis of gene expression profiles and whether new classes can be identified (class discovery) that may have clinical significance and to develop a new molecular taxonomy. Supervised analysis, on the other hand, is used to allocate tumours to specific groups based on clinical or pathological features (e.g. clinical outcome or response to therapy). There are two main types of supervised analysis: class comparison and class prediction. The former aims to identify the transcriptomic differences between two classes of tumours, whereas the development of a 'gene signature' is the ultimate goal of the latter.

In breast cancer, the class discovery studies were pioneered by the Stanford group,[106] which proved the principle that breast cancer could be classified into molecularly distinct groups based upon gene expression profiles and their similarity to normal cell counterparts. Multiple independent studies have confirmed and expanded the original results. According to these studies, breast cancer was classified into two main classes (ER-positive and ER-negative tumours) and each one can be classified into multiple molecularly distinct subclasses. For example, the ER-negative tumours encompass three subgroups, one overexpressing HER-2, one with tumours expressing genes characteristic of basal/myoepithelial cells (basal-like cancer), and one with a gene expression profile similar to normal breast tissue. cDNAs have also been used to distinguish cancers with *BRCA1/BRCA2* mutations[107,108] and to determine ER status,[109] lymph node status[110,111] and prognostic subgroups in node-negative breast cancer.[112] These recent studies demonstrate the ability of cDNA to have a direct translational use in clinical practice.

## Proteomics

The genetic code does not inform on which proteins are expressed by a cancer, or whether they are functional, if expressed. Post-translational modifications such as glycosylations or phosphorylation of proteins affect their expression and function at the protein level, which cannot be detected by assessing the status of the genome or transcriptome in a given cell population. Therefore, proteomics aims to assess changes at the protein level in which the proteome is displayed. Proteomics is quickly evolving to provide supportive and critical information

to data generated through genomic approaches in high-throughput formats. This can be achieved by using different techniques such as two-dimensional polyacrylamide gel electrophoresis, isotope-coded affinity tagging, surface-enhanced laser desorption ionisation and matrix-associated laser desorption ionisation – time of flight.

These global expression profiling approaches yield candidate proteins and related genes that require verification through application of other techniques. Tissue microarrays (TMAs) provide a method for high-throughput protein expression analysis of large cohorts of archival samples that can be readily linked to clinico-pathological and long-term follow-up databases. TMAs have expedited the validation of the prognostic and predictive significance of several candidate biomarkers. The technique allows for a composite slide of up to 1000 cores of tissue to be constructed into one paraffin block. The advantages are obvious in screening for novel protein expression. There are concerns on the validity of the cores as being representative samples and indeed this aspect has not been well studied, with only one study examining a large sample size with correlation to corresponding larger histology sections.[103] This technology and its application has been extensively reviewed recently.[89,113]

## Clinical use of the high-throughput molecular techniques

It is envisaged that gene expression profiles may be able to guide decisions on the choice of hormonal, chemotherapeutic or targeted agents for each individual in the future. Presently, one of the best examples of the use of genomics and proteomics in clinical practice is the use of HER-2 expression/amplification to select patients for trastuzumab. Such profiles are useful to identify prognostically significant genes, which studies have demonstrated can perform better than traditional markers.[104,114] In metastatic disease, expression patterns can be used to establish the primary lesion in patients with more than one primary. Transcription profiling has also been shown to differentiate accurately breast cancers with germ-line mutations in *BRCA1/BRCA2* from those without such mutations. Such findings, if validated in other studies, open the way for molecular phenotyping in high-risk families. In addition, gene expression profiling has been used to develop expression predictors (class prediction studies) that can be used for many types of clinical management decisions, including risk assessment, diagnostic testing, prognostic stratification and treatment selection. There are two types of class prediction studies in breast cancer: prognostic and predictive class prediction. Prognostic class prediction includes (i) poor-prognosis gene signatures that can discriminate between a good and a poor outcome by comparison between highly aggressive and less aggressive primary tumours, and (ii) recurrence score gene signatures by defining tumours based on the risk of disease relapse. The predictive class prediction includes predictors of response to therapy.[115,116]

An example of prognostic class prediction study is that reported by Van't Veer et al. Expression profiles of 117 primary breast cancers were compared with known prognostic factors and matched with 5 years of follow-up data; 25 000 genes were used to generate expression profiles, which separated the tumours into two groups. Group 1 developed distant metastasis in 34% and in group 2,70% developed distant metastasis. From the 25 000-gene set, 70 genes had great accuracy in predicting recurrent disease. Multivariate analysis with grade, size, LVI, age and ER showed the poor-prognosis micro-array profile to be an independent predictor of recurrent disease. This approach was further tested in 295 patients and again the use of gene profiling was able to accurately identify a poor-prognosis group.[101,109] MammaPrint® assay, which is based on the Amsterdam 70-gene gene signature, is currently used as a molecular diagnostic test for breast cancer prognostication and prediction. Another predictor calculates a recurrence score on the basis of the expression of 21 known genes, with the use of RT–PCR in formalin-fixed, paraffin-embedded tissue. 'The Oncotype DX assay' has been developed by researchers at Genomic Health. Oncotype DX is currently used as a diagnostic test to quantify the likelihood of disease recurrence in women with early-stage breast cancer and assesses the likely benefit from tamoxifen and certain types of chemotherapy. Oncotype DX employs a mathematical algorithm called the recurrence score (range 1–100) to calculate continuous risk for relapse and death for patients receiving adjuvant tamoxifen, and has recently been shown in a large population-based case–control study to be an effective predictive test for ER-positive, node-negative breast cancer patients

treated or untreated with tamoxifen and no chemotherapy.[117] In addition, a number of microarray studies have been published which identified other prognostic signatures with clinical significance. For example, Chang et al.[118] have used a 'wound-response gene expression signature' to stratify breast cancer patients based on the hypothesis that features of the molecular programme of normal wound healing might play an important role in cancer metastasis. They found that this gene signature can improve the risk stratification of early breast cancer over that provided by standard clinicopathological features. A gene expression signature of hypoxia response, derived from studies of cultured mammary epithelial cells' 'hypoxia gene signature', was a strong predictor of clinical outcomes in breast cancer.[119]

Although proteomics has a long history that predates profiling at the RNA level, difficulties in protein identification and the lack of reproducibility of several assay platforms have limited the utility of such profiling systems. In breast cancer research, however, proteomics has begun to take on a role in the monitoring of response, prediction of resistance and relapse in patients treated with novel bio-directed therapies.[120]

# Clinical use of prognostic factors in patient management

Prognosis in breast cancer depends on the presence of spread of disease and on the inherent aggressiveness of the tumour. The latter depends on a number of intrinsic biological characteristics, some of which have already been evaluated, such as morphological features, growth rate and hormone responsiveness. Accurate prognostication is now required on an individual patient basis and this can only be achieved by using a prognostic index that includes both time-dependent and biological factors. The best way to obtain such an index is to take potential factors that have been shown to have some value in univariate analysis and submit them to multivariate analysis. This has been the approach in deriving the Nottingham Prognostic Index (NPI), which is based on three factors using the following formula:

NPI = pathological tumour size(cm) × 0.2
    + lymph node stage(Scored 1,2 or 3)
    with 1 being node negative, 2 being 1–3
    involved nodes and 3 more than 3 nodes

involved + histological grade(Scored 1,2 or 3) based on the 3 grades

Arbitrary cut-off points of 3.4 and 5.4 are used to divide patients into six prognostic groups: excellent (EPG), good (GPG), moderate (MPG) I and II, poor (PPG) and very poor (VPG) (Tables 2.1–2.3, **Figs 2.5** and **2.6**).

The NPI provides extremely powerful prognostic information and has demonstrated utility and reproducibility in studies from other centres. In this respect Henson et al., in a retrospective analysis of prognostic data in over 22 000 women from the SEER Programme of the National Cancer Institute in the USA, confirmed that a combination of lymph node stage and histological grade improved prediction of prognosis. In a similar way Chevallier et al.[121] have identified 'young' age, tumour size and histological grade as factors which added to lymph node stage in the prediction

of recurrence; these factors were used to divide lymph node-negative patients into three prognostic groups.

Table 2.1 • NPI showing percentage in each prognostic group

| | Percentage in prognostic group | |
|---|---|---|
| | 1980–86 | 1990–99 |
| EPG | 12 | 14 |
| GPG | 19 | 21 |
| MPG I | 29 | 28 |
| MPG II | 24 | 22 |
| PPG | 11 | 11 |
| VPPG | 5 | 4 |

Prognostic groups: EPG, excellent prognosis; GPG, good prognosis; MPG, moderate prognosis; PPG, poor prognosis; VPG, very poor prognosis.

Table 2.2 • Differences in 10-year survival for each prognostic group

| | 10-year survival (%) | ±95% CL | P (log rank) |
|---|---|---|---|
| EPG | 96 | 2 | |
| GPG | 93 | 4 | 0.14 |
| MPG I | 82 | 4 | <0.0001 |
| MPG II | 75 | 4 | 0.0007 |
| PPG | 53 | 8 | <0.0001 |
| VPG | 39 | 12 | 0.003 |
| All | 80 | 2 | |

Prognostic groups: EPG, excellent prognosis; GPG, good prognosis; MPG, moderate prognosis; PPG, poor prognosis; VPG, very poor prognosis.
CL, confidence limit.

Table 2.3 • Relative risk reduction by NPI

| | 1980–86 | ±95% CL | 1990–99 | ±95% CL | RRR (death) | % ARR (death) |
|---|---|---|---|---|---|---|
| EPG | 88 | 6 | 96 | 2 | 0.67 | 8 |
| GPG | 72 | 8 | 93 | 4 | 0.75 | 21 |
| MPG I | 61 | 6 | 82 | 4 | 0.54 | 21 |
| MPG II | 42 | 6 | 75 | 4 | 0.57 | 35 |
| PPG | 14 | 8 | 53 | 8 | 0.45 | 39 |
| VPG | 12 | 10 | 39 | 12 | 0.31 | 27 |
| All | 55 | | 80 | | 0.56 | 25 |

Prognostic groups: EPG, excellent prognosis; GPG, good prognosis; MPG, moderate prognosis; PPG, poor prognosis; VPG, very poor prognosis.
ARR, absolute risk reduction; CL, confidence limit; RRR, relative risk reduction.

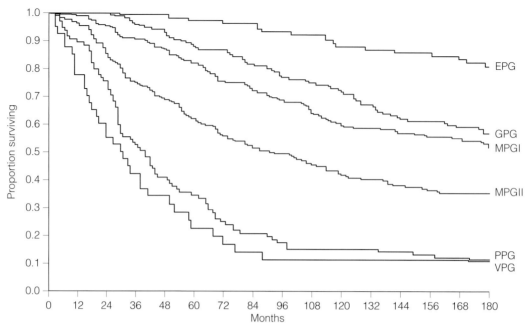

**Figure 2.5** • Survival by NPI (1980–86).

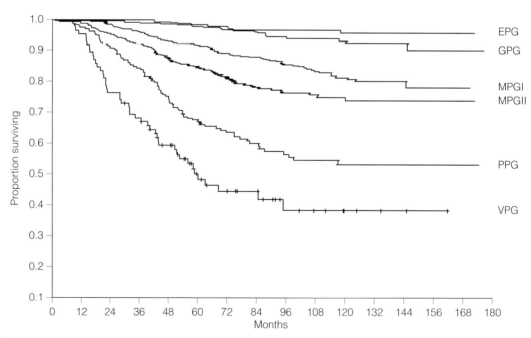

**Figure 2.6** • Survival by NPI (1990–99).

Breast cancer histopathology minimum dataset.

Surname.......................Forenames...........................Date of birth............

Sex...... Hospital............ Hospital No............ NHS No............

Date of receipt....................... Date of reporting ........... Report No.....................

Side: [ ] Right  [ ] Left              Pathologist.................. Surgeon .......................

Specimen type: [ ] Diagnostic localisation biopsy      [ ] Diagnostic open biopsy

[ ] Therapeutic excision                [ ] Mastectomy

Specimen weight .................................g

Axillary procedure: [ ] Lymph node sample [ ] Axillary clearance [ ] Sentinel node biopsy

-------------------------------------------------------------------------------------------------------

**Non-invasive malignant lesion** [ ] Not present

[ ] Ductal,high grade              [ ] Ductal,intermediate grade        [ ] Ductal,low grade

Growth pattern(s):  [ ] Solid       [ ] Cribriform  [ ] Micropapillary  [ ] Papillary

[ ] Apocrine    [ ] Flat/ clinging   [ ] Other

Size (pure DCIS only).........................mm

[ ] Paget's disease of the nipple

[ ] Lobular neoplasia

Microinvasion: [ ] Not present  [ ] Present  [ ] Possible

-------------------------------------------------------------------------------------------------------

**Invasive carcinoma**    [ ] Not present

Grade: [ ] I       [ ]II  [ ]III  [ ] Not assessable

[ ] Ductal / no specific type (NST)      [ ] Tubular carcinoma              [ ] Lobular carcinoma

[ ] Mucinous carcinoma          [ ] Medullary type carcinoma

[ ] Mixed (please tick component types present)            [ ] Not assessable

[ ] Other primary carcinoma (please specify).................................................................

[ ] Other malignant tumour (please specify)...................................................................

Maximum diameter of invasive tumour .........................mm

Whole size of tumour (to include DCIS extending >1mm beyond invasive area)...........mm

Vascular invasion (blood or lymphatic)  [ ] Present            [ ] Possible            [ ] Not seen

-------------------------------------------------------------------------------------------------------

**For DCIS and invasive carcinoma**

Excision margins:   [ ] Reaches margin  [ ] Uncertain   [ ] Does not reach margin

Nearest (surgically relevant) margin .........................mm

Axillary nodes received: [ ] Yes [ ] No  Number positive........... Total number...........

Other nodes received:   [ ] Yes [ ] No  Number positive........... Total number...........

Site of the nodes......................................................

Estrogen receptor status:      [ ] Positive            [ ] Negative            [ ] Not known

**Figure 2.7** • Breast cancer histopathology minimum dataset.

One of the strengths of the NPI is the fact that it has been verified prospectively. Further confirmation of its value has been provided by its validation in two large multicentre studies involving nearly 11 000 patients in total.[121–123] Such studies demonstrate the inherent power of the pathological factors used in the NPI, which has become the most widely used index for the management of patients with breast cancer, certainly in the UK.

Other pathology-based prognostic indices used in breast cancer include AdjuvantOnline (AO)[124] and the St Gallen criteria.[125] AO is a programme that is available through the web and is used to assess risk for the development of breast cancer metastases using traditional prognostic factors that include age, lymph node status, tumour size, tumour grade and hormone receptor status. It has the distinct advantage over the NPI in that it integrates treatment and for this reason AO is the programme most commonly used by oncologists. It is constantly evolving and being updated. The current St Gallen-derived algorithm for selection of adjuvant systemic therapy for early breast cancer patients includes tumour size and grade, nodal status, menopausal status, peritumoural vessel invasion, endocrine status and HER-2 status.

# Contents of the final surgical pathology report: the minimum dataset

The Royal College of Pathologists minimum dataset for breast cancer was originally developed in recognition that certain histopathological features of both in situ and invasive carcinoma are directly related to clinical outcome and may therefore be important in deciding the most appropriate treatment, including extent of surgery and use of and choice of adjuvant therapy. In addition histopathological features can be used to monitor breast screening programmes, the success of which is reflected by more favourable prognostic features of the cancers detected and also changing patterns of disease, particularly identified by cancer registries.

The minimum set of data should be used by pathologists reporting all breast cancers, both screen detected and those presenting symptomatically.

The Royal College of Pathologists minimum dataset has been approved by the NHS BSP and the European Commission Working Group, the British Association of Surgical Oncologists, the British Breast Group and the United Kingdom Association of Cancer Registries (**Fig. 2.7**).

## Key points

- Histopathological features such as size, grade and lymph node stage are key to prognosticating and guiding adjuvant therapy in breast cancer patients.
- The type 1 growth factor family (e.g. EGFR and HER-2) are becoming key molecular features in the design of novel biologically targeted therapies.
- The combination of standard pathological features and each cancer's genetic fingerprint will enable us in the future to individually tailor each patient's therapy.

# References

1. Singletary SE, Allred C, Ashley P et al. Revision of the American Joint Committee on Cancer staging system for breast cancer. J Clin Oncol 2002; 20:3628–36.

2. Rampaul RS, Mullinger K, Macmillan RD et al. Incidence of clinically significant lymphoedema as a complication following surgery for primary operable breast cancer. Eur J Cancer 2003; 39(15):2165–7.

3. Mansel RE, Fallowfield L, Kissin M et al. Randomized multicenter trial of sentinel node biopsy versus standard axillary treatment in operable breast cancer: the ALMANAC Trial. J Natl Cancer Inst 2006; 98(9):599–609.

4. Alvarez S, Anorbe E, Alcorta P et al. Role of sonography in the diagnosis of axillary lymph node metastases in breast cancer: a systematic review. Am J Roentgenol 2006; 186:1342–8.

5. Rampaul RS, Evans AJ, Ellis IO et al. Long term regional recurrence and survival after axillary nodal sampling for breast cancer. Eur J Cancer 2003; 1(4):23 (Abstr.).

6. Shukla HS, Melhuish J, Mansel RE et al. Does local therapy affect survival rates in breast cancer? Ann Surg Oncol 1999; 6(5):455–60.

7. Macmillan RD, Rampaul RS, Lewis S et al. Preoperative ultrasound-guided node biopsy and sentinel node augmented node sample is best practice. Eur J Cancer 2004; 40(2):176–8.

8. Veronesi U, Galimberti V, Zurrida S et al. Sentinel lymph node biopsy as an indicator for axillary dissection in early breast cancer. Eur J Cancer 2001; 37(4):454–8.

9. Veronesi U, Paganelli G, Viale G et al. Sentinel lymph node biopsy and axillary dissection in breast cancer: results in a large series. J Natl Cancer Inst 1999; 91(4):368–73.

10. Schwartz GF, Guiliano AE, Veronesi U. Consensus Conference Committee. Proceeding of the consensus conference of the role of sentinel lymph node biopsy in carcinoma of the breast April 19–22, 2001, Philadelphia, PA, USA. Breast J 2002; 8(3):124–38.

11. Cserni G, Amendoeira I, Apostolikas N et al. Discrepancies in current practice of pathological evaluation of sentinel lymph nodes in breast cancer. Results of a questionnaire based survey by the European Working Group for Breast Screening Pathology. J Clin Pathol 2004; 57(7):695–701.

12. Fisher ER, Fisher B, Sass R et al. 1984. Pathologic findings from the National Surgical Adjuvant Breast Project (Protocol No. 4). XI. Bilateral breast cancer. Cancer 1984; 54:3002–11.

13. Carter CL, Allen C, Henson DE. Relation of tumor size, lymph node status, and survival in 24,740 breast cancer cases. Cancer 1989; 63:181–7.

14. Rosen PP, Groshen S, Kinne DW et al. Factors influencing prognosis in node-negative breast carcinoma: analysis of 767 T1N0M0/T2N0M0 patients with long-term follow-up. J Clin Oncol 1993; 11:2090–100.

15. Foulkes WD, Grainge MJ, Rakha EA et al. Tumor size is an unreliable predictor of prognosis in basal-like breast cancers and does not correlate closely with lymph node status. Breast Cancer Res Treat 2008 (Epub ahead of print).

16. O'Dwyer PJ. Editorial. Axillary dissection in primary breast cancer; the benefits of node clearance warrant reappraisal. Br Med J 1992; 302:360–1.

17. Blamey RW. Clinical aspects of malignant disease. In: Elston CW, Ellis IO (eds) Systemic pathology. The breast, 3rd edn. London: Churchill Livingstone; 1998; pp. 501–13.

18. Henson DE, Ries L, Freedman LS et al. Relationship among outcome stage of disease and histologic grade for 22,616 cases of breast cancer. Breast Cancer Res Treat 1991; 22:207–19.

19. Kutianawala MA, Sayed M, Stotter A et al. Staging the axilla in breast cancer: an audit of lymph-node retrieval in one UK regional centre. Eur J Surg Oncol 1998; 24:280–2.

20. Steele RJC, Forrest APM, Gibson T. The efficacy of lower axillary sampling in obtaining lymph node status in breast cancer: a controlled randomized trial. Br J Surg 1985; 72:368–9.

21. Dixon JM, Dillon P, Anderson TJ et al. Axillary sampling in breast cancer: an assessment of its efficacy. Breast 1998; 7:206–8.

22. Cabanas RM. An approach for the treatment of penile carcinoma. Cancer 1977; 39:456–66.

23. Royal College of Radiologists. Quality Assurance Guidelines for Radiologists. NHS BSP Publications no. 15, 1990.

24. Royal College of Radiologists. Quality Assurance Guidelines for Radiologists. NHSBSP Publications no. 15, January 1997.

25. European Commission. European Guidelines for Quality Assurance in Mammography Screening, 2nd edn. Luxembourg: Office for Official Publications of the European Communities, 1996.

26. Mansel RE, Goyal A, Newcombe RG. ALMANAC Trialist Group. Internal mammary node drainage and its role in sentinel lymph node biopsy: the initial ALMANAC experience. Clin Breast Cancer 2004; 5(4):279–84.

27. Rosen PP, Groshen S, Saigo S et al. Pathological prognostic factors in stage I (T1N0M0) and stage II (T1N1M0) breast carcinoma: a study of 644 patients with median follow-up of 18 years. J Clin Oncol 1989; 7:1239–51.

28. Parker C, Rampaul RS, Pinder SE et al. E-Cadherin as a prognostic indicator in primary breast cancer. Br J Cancer 2001; 14(85):1958–63.

29. Rakha EA, El-Sayed ME, Powe DG et al. Invasive lobular carcinoma of the breast: response to hormonal therapy and outcomes. Eur J Cancer 2008; 44(1):73–83.

30. Elston CW, Ellis IO. Pathological prognostic factors in breast cancer. I. The value of histological grade in breast cancer: experience from a large study with long-term follow-up. Histopathology 2002; 41(3A):154–61.

31. Rakha EA, El-Sayed ME, Lee AH et al. Prognostic significance of Nottingham histologic grade in invasive breast carcinoma. J Clin Oncol 2008; 26(19):3153–8.

32. Rakha EA, El-Sayed ME, Menon S et al. Histologic grading is an independent prognostic factor in invasive lobular carcinoma of the breast. Breast Cancer Res Treat 2008; 111(1):121–7.

33. Pinder SE, Ellis IO, Galea M et al. Pathological prognostic factors in breast cancer. III. Vascular invasion: relationship with recurrence and survival in a large study with long-term follow-up. Histopathology 1994; 24(1):41–7.

34. Truong PT, Yong CM, Abnousi F et al. Lymphovascular invasion is associated with reduced locoregional control and survival in women with node-negative

breast cancer treated with mastectomy and systemic therapy. J Am Coll Surg 2005; 200(6):912–21.

35. Haybittle JL, Blamey RW, Elston CW et al. A prognostic index in primary breast cancer. Br J Cancer 1982; 45:361–6.

36. Ellis IO, Bell J, Todd J et al. Evaluation of immuno-reactivity with monoclonal antibody NCRC-II in breast carcinoma. Br J Cancer 1987; 56:295–9.

37. Lee AH, Pinder SE, Macmillan RD et al. Prognostic value of lymphovascular invasion in women with lymph node negative invasive breast carcinoma. Eur J Cancer 2006; 42(3):357–62.

38. Gee J, Eloranta J, Ibbitt J et al. Overexpression of TFAP2C in invasive breast cancer correlates with a poorer response to anti-hormone therapy and reduced patient survival. J Pathol 2008 (Epub ahead of print).

39. Sarwar N, Kim JS, Jiang J et al. Phosphorylation of ERalpha at serine 118 in primary breast cancer and in tamoxifen-resistant tumours is indicative of a complex role for ERalpha phosphorylation in breast cancer progression. Endocr Relat Cancer 2006; 13(3):851–61.

40. Gee JM, Shaw VE, Hiscox SE et al. Deciphering antihormone-induced compensatory mechanisms in breast cancer and their therapeutic implications. Endocr Relat Cancer 2006; 13(Suppl 1):S77–88.

41. Dowle CS, Owainati A, Robins A et al. The prognostic significance of the DNA content of human breast cancer. Br J Surg 1987; 74:133–6.

42. Putti TC, El-Rehim DM, Rakha EA et al. Estrogen receptor-negative breast carcinomas: a review of morphology and immunophenotypical analysis. Mod Pathol 2005; 18(1):26–35.

43. Dowsett M, Allred C, Knox J et al. Relationship between quantitative estrogen and progesterone receptor expression and human epidermal growth factor receptor 2 (HER-2) status with recurrence in the Arimidex, Tamoxifen, Alone or in Combination trial. J Clin Oncol 2008; 26(7):1059–65.

44. Kumar RR, Meenakshi A et al. Enzyme immunoassay of human epidermal growth factor. Human Antibodies 2001; 10:143–7.

45. Eberhard DA, Huntzicker E et al. Epidermal growth factor receptor immunohistochemistry: assay selection and amplification to breast cancers (abstr.). ASCO, 2002, no. 1791.

46. Klijn JGM, Berns PMJ, Schmitz PI et al. The clinical significance of epidermal growth factor receptor in human breast cancer: a review of 5232 patients. Endocr Rev 1992; 13:3–17.

47. Tsutsui S, Ohno S, Murakami S et al. Prognostic value of epidermal growth factor and its relationship to the ER status of 1029 patients with breast cancer. Breast Cancer Res Treat 2002; 71:67–75.

48. Rampaul RS, Pinder SE, Robertson JF et al. EGFR expression in operable breast cancer: is it

of prognostic significance? Clin Cancer Res 2004; 10(7):2578.

49. Ferrero JM, Ramaioli A, Largillier R et al. Epidermal growth factor receptor expression in 780 breast cancer patients: a reappraisal of the prognostic value based on an eight-year median follow-up. Ann Oncol 2001; 12(6):835–41.

50. Nicholson RI, McCelland RA, Gee JMW et al. Epidermal growth factor receptor expression in breast cancer. Association with response to endocrine therapy. Breast Cancer Res Treat 1994; 29:117–25.

51. Knoop A, Bentzen SM, Nielsen MM et al. Value of epidermal growth factor receptor, HER-2, p53 and steroid receptors in predicting the efficacy of Tamoxifen in high risk postmenopausal breast cancer patients. J Clin Oncol 2001; 19:3376–84.

52. Wolff AC, Hammond ME, Schwartz JN et al. American Society of Clinical Oncology/College of American Pathologists guideline recommendations for human epidermal growth factor receptor 2 testing in breast cancer. J Clin Oncol 2007; 25:118–45.

53. Ratcliffe N, Wells W, Wheeler K et al. The combination of in situ hybridization and immunohistochemical analysis: an evaluation of Her2/neu expression in paraffin-embedded breast carcinomas and adjacent normal-appearing breast epithelium. Mod Pathol 1997; 10:1247–52.

54. Busmanis I, Feleppa F, Jones A et al. Analysis of cerbB2 expression using a panel of 6 commercially available antibodies. Pathology 1994; 26:261–7.

55. Carlson RW, Moench SJ, Hammond ME et al. (2006) HER2 testing in breast cancer: NCCN Task Force report and recommendations. J Natl Compar Cancer Network 2006; 4(Suppl 3):S1–22; quiz S23–4.

56. Bartlett JM, Going JJ, Mallon EA et al. Evaluating HER2 amplification and overexpression in breast cancer. J Pathol 2001; 195:422–8.

57. Press MF, Slamon DJ, Flom KJ et al. Evaluation of HER-2/neu gene amplification and overexpression: comparison of frequently used assay methods in a molecularly characterized cohort of breast cancer specimens. J Clin Oncol 2002; 20:3095–105.

58. Walker RA, Bartlett JM, Dowsett M et al. HER2 testing in the UK: further update to recommendations. J Clin Pathol 2008; 61(7):818–24.

59. Dowsett M, Bartlett J, Ellis IO et al. Correlation between immunohistochemistry (HercepTest) and fluorescence in situ hybridization (FISH) for HER-2 in 426 breast carcinomas from 37 centres. J Pathol 2003; 199:418–23.

60. Slamon DJ, Clark GM, Wong SG et al. Human breast cancer: correlation of relapse and survival with amplification of the HER-2/neu oncogene. Science 1987; 235(4785):177–82.

61. Rilke F, Colnaghi MI, Cascinelli N et al. Prognostic significance of HER-2/neu expression in breast

cancer and its relationship to other prognostic factors. Int J Cancer 1991; 49(1):44–9.

62. Viani GA, Afonso SL, Stefano EJ et al. Adjuvant trastuzumab in the treatment of her-2-positive early breast cancer: a meta-analysis of published randomized trials. BMC Cancer 2007; 7:153.

63. Carter P, Presta L, Gorman CM et al. Humanization of an anti-p185HER2 antibody for human cancer therapy. Proc Natl Acad Sci USA 1992; 89:4285–9.

64. Disis ML, Knutson KL, Schiffman K et al. Pre-existent immunity to the HER-2/neu oncogenic protein in patients with HER-2/neu overexpressing breast and ovarian cancer. Breast Cancer Res Treat 2000; 62:245–52.

65. Ward RL, Hawkins NJ, Coomber D et al. Antibody immunity to the HER-2/neu oncogenic protein in patients with colorectal cancer. Hum Immunol 1999; 60:510–15.

66. Mirza AN, Mirza NQ, Vlastos G et al. Prognostic factors in node-negative breast cancer: a review of studies with sample size more than 200 and follow-up more than 5 years. Ann Surg 2002; 235(1):10–26.

67. Bernards R, Destree A, McKenzie S et al. Effective tumor immunotherapy directed against an oncogene-encoded product using a vaccinia virus vector. Proc Natl Acad Sci USA 1987; 84:6854–8.

68. Disis ML, Gralow JR, Bernhard H et al. Peptide-based, but not whole protein, vaccines elicit immunity to HER-2/neu, oncogenic self-protein. J Immunol 1996; 156:3151–8.

69. Nagata Y, Furugen R, Hiasa A et al. Peptides derived from a wild-type murine proto-oncogene c-erbB-2/HER2/neu can induce CTL and tumor suppression in syngeneic hosts. J Immunol 1997; 159:1336–43.

70. Kraus MH, Popescu NC, Amsbaugh SC et al. Overexpression of the EGF receptor-related proto-oncogene erbB-2 in human mammary tumor cell lines by different molecular mechanisms. Embo J 1987; 6:605–10.

71. Ring CJ, Blouin P, Martin LA et al. Use of transcriptional regulatory elements of the MUC1 and ERBB2 genes to drive tumour-selective expression of a prodrug activating enzyme. Gene Ther 1997; 4:1045–52.

72. Yu DH, Hung MC. Expression of activated rat neu oncogene is sufficient to induce experimental metastasis in 3T3 cells. Oncogene 1991; 6:1991–6.

73. Bria E, Cuppone F, Fornier M et al. Cardiotoxicity and incidence of brain metastases after adjuvant trastuzumab for early breast cancer: the dark side of the moon? A meta-analysis of the randomized trials. Breast Cancer Res Treat 2008; 109(2):231–9.

74. Chang H, Riese DJ 2nd, Gilbert W et al. Ligands for ErbB-family receptors encoded by a neuregulin-like gene. Nature 1997; 387:509–12.

75. Juhl H, Downing SG, Wellstein A et al. HER-2/neu is rate-limiting for ovarian cancer growth. Conditional depletion of HER-2/neu by ribozyme targeting. J Biol Chem 1997; 272:29482–6.

76. Deshane J, Siegal GP, Wang M et al. Transductional efficacy and safety of an intraperitoneally delivered adenovirus encoding an anti-erbB-2 intracellular single-chain antibody for ovarian cancer gene therapy. Gynecol Oncol 1997; 64:378–85.

77. Schmidt M, Hynes NE, Groner B et al. A bivalent single-chain antibody-toxin specific for ErbB-2 and the EGF receptor. Int J Cancer 1996; 65:538–46.

78. Park JW, Hong K, Carter P et al. Development of anti-p185HER2 immunoliposomes for cancer therapy. Proc Natl Acad Sci USA 1995; 92:1327–31.

79. Chen SY, Yang AG, Chen JD et al. Potent antitumour activity of a new class of tumour-specific killer cells. Nature 1997; 385:78–80.

80. Newby JC, Johnston SRD, Smith I et al. Expression of epidermal growth factor and C-erb-2 during the development of tamoxifen resistance in human breast cancer. Clin Cancer Res 1997; 3:1643–51.

81. Nicholson RI, McCelland RA, Finlay P et al. Relationship between EGF-R, C-erb-2 protein expression and Ki67 immunostaining in breast cancer and hormone sensitivity. Eur J Cancer 1993; 29A:1018–23.

82. Giai M, Roagna R, Ponzone R et al. Prognostic and predictive relevance of C-erb-2 and ras expression in node positive and negative breast cancer. Anticancer Res 1994; 14:1441–50.

83. Archer SG, Eliopoulos SA, Spandidos D et al. Expression of ras p21, p53 and C-erb-2 in advanced breast cancer and response to first line hormonal therapy. Br J Cancer 1995; 72:1259–66.

84. Pegram MD, Konecny GE, O'Callaghan C et al. Rational combinations of trastuzumab with chemotherapeutic drugs used in the treatment of breast cancer. J Natl Cancer Inst 2004; 96(10):739–49.

85. Muss H, Berry D, Thor A et al. Lack of interaction of tamoxifen (T) use and ErbB-2/ HER-2/neu (H) expression in CALGB 8541: a randomized adjuvant trial of three different doses of cyclophosphamide, doxorubicin and fluorouracil (CAF) in node-positive primary breast cancer (BC). Proc Am Soc Clin Oncol 1999; 18:68a.

86. Paik S, Bryant J, Park C et al. ErbB-2 and response to doxorubicin in patients with axillary lymph node positive, hormone receptor-negative breast cancer. J Natl Cancer Inst 1998; 90:1361–70.

87. Elledge RM, Green S, Ciocca D et al. HER-2 expression and response to tamoxifen in estrogen receptor-positive breast cancer: a Southwest Oncology Group Study. Clin Cancer Res 1998; 4(1):7–12.

88. Ravin PM, Green S, Albain V et al. Initial report of the SWOG biological correlative study of CerbB-2 expression as a predictor of outcome in a trial comparing adjuvant CAF with tamoxifen (T) alone. Proc Am Soc Clin Oncol 1998; 17:97a.

89. Rakha EA, Reis-Filho JS, Ellis IO. Basal-like breast cancer: a critical review. J Clin Oncol 2008; 26(15):2568–81.

90. Johannsson OT, Idvall I, Anderson C et al. Tumour biological features of BRCA1-induced breast and ovarian cancer. Eur J Cancer 1997; 33:362–71.

91. Chappuis PO, Nethercot V, Foulkes WD. Clinico-pathological characteristics of BRCA1- and BRCA2-related breast cancer. Semin Surg Oncol 2000; 18:287–95.

92. Marcus JN, Watson P, Page DL. Hereditary breast cancer. Pathobiology, prognosis and BRCA 1 and BRCA 2 linkage. Cancer 1996; 77:967.

93. Marcus JN, Page DL, Watson P et al. BRCA 1 and BRCA 2 hereditary breast cancer phenotypes. Cancer 1997; 80:543.

94. Breast Cancer Linkage Consortium. Pathology of familial breast cancer: differences between breast cancer in carriers of BRCA 1 or BRCA 2 mutational and sporadic cases. Lancet 1997; 349:1505.

95. Robson M, Gilewski T, Haas B et al. BRCA-associated breast cancer in young women. J Clin Oncol 1998; 16:1642.

96. Karp SE, Tonin PN, Begin LR et al. Influence of BRCA 1 mutations on nuclear grade and oestrogen receptor status of breast carcinoma in Ashkenazi Jewish women. Cancer 1997; 80:435.

97. Ames JE, Egan AJM, Southey MC et al. The histologic phenotypes of breast carcinoma occurring before age 40 in women with and without BRCA 1 or BRCA 2 germline mutations. Cancer 1998; 83:2335.

98. Agnarsson BA, Jonasson JG, Bjornsdottir IB et al. Inherited BRCA 2 mutation associated with high grade breast cancer. Breast Cancer Res Treat 1998; 47:121.

99. Marcus JN, Watson P, Page DL et al. BRCA 2 hereditary breast cancer phenotype. Breast Cancer Res Treat 1997; 44:275.

100. Baak JP, Colpaert CG, van Diest PJ et al. Multivariate prognostic evaluation of the mitotic activity index and fibrotic focus in node-negative invasive breast cancers. Eur J Cancer 2005; 41(14):2093–101.

101. Baak JPA, Vooiji GP, Brugal G. Nuclear image cytometry: quantitation of chromatin pattern, steroid receptor content and Ki-67. In: Baale JPA (ed.) Manual of quantitative pathology in cancer diagnosis and prognosis. Heidelberg: Springer-Verlag, 1991; pp. 232–43.

102. Palcic B, Garner DM, MacAulay CE. Image cytometry and chemoprevention in cervical cancer. J Cell Biochem 1995; 23(Suppl):43–54.

103. Nagahata T, Hirano A, Utada Y et al. Correlation of allelic losses and clinicopathologic factors in 504 primary breast cancers. Breast Cancer 2002; 9:208–15.

104. Hermsen MAJA, Baak JPA, Weiss J et al. Genetic analysis of 513 lymph node negative breast carcinomas by CGH and relation to clinical, pathologic, morphometric and DNA cytometric prognostic factors. J Pathol 1998; 186:356–62.

105. Janssen EAM, Baak JPA, Guervos MA et al. Lymph node negative breast cancer, specific chromosomal aberrations are strongly associated with high mitotic activity and predict outcome more accurately than grade, tumour diameter and oestrogen receptor. J Pathol (in press).

106. Hyman E, Kauraniemi P, Hautaniemi S et al. Impact of DNA amplification on gene expression patterns in breast cancer. Cancer Res 2002; 62:6240–5.

107. Hu Z, Fan C, Oh DS et al. The molecular portraits of breast tumors are conserved across microarray platforms. BMC Genomics 2006; 7:96.

108. Hedenfalk I, Duggan D, Chen Y et al. Gene expression profiles in hereditary breast cancer. N Engl J Med 2001; 344:539–48.

109. Van't Veer LJ, Dai H, van de Vijer MJ et al. Expression profiling predicts outcomes in breast cancer. Breast Cancer Res 2002; 5:57–8.

110. Gruvberger S, Ringner M, Chen Y et al. Oestrogen receptor status in breast cancer is associated with remarkably distinct gene expression profiles. Cancer Res 2001; 61:5979–84.

111. West M, Blanchette C, Dressman H et al. Predicting the clinical status of human breast cancer by using gene expression profiles. Proc Natl Acad Sci USA 2001; 98:11462–7.

112. Ahr A, Kam T, Solbach S et al. Identification of high risk breast cancer by gene expression profiling. Lancet 2002; 359:131–2.

113. Van de Vijver MJ, He YD, van't Veer LJ et al. A gene expression signature as a predictor of survival in breast cancer. N Engl J Med 2002; 347:1999–2009.

114. Rampaul RS, Pinder SE, Blamey RW et al. Evaluation of a high throughput approach to assess HER-2 using tissue microarray and ACIS technology. Breast Cancer Res Treat 2001; 54:4.

115. Bertucci F, Viens P, Hingamp P et al. Breast cancer revisited using DNA array-based gene expression profiling. Int J Cancer 2003; 103(5):565–71.

116. Perou CM, Sorlie T, Eisen MB et al. Molecular portraits of human breast tumours. Nature 2000; 406:747–52.

117. Habel LA, Shak S, Jacobs MK et al. A population-based study of tumor gene expression and risk of breast cancer death among lymph node-negative patients. Breast Cancer Res 2006; 8:R25.

118. Chang HY, Nuyten DS, Sneddon JB et al. Robustness, scalability, and integration of a wound-response gene expression signature in predicting breast cancer survival. Proc Natl Acad Sci USA 2005; 102:3738–43.

119. Chi JT, Wang Z, Nuyten DS et al. Gene expression programmes in response to hypoxia: cell type specificity and prognostic significance in human cancers. PLoS Med 2006; 3:e47.

120. McCelland CM, Gullick WJ. Identification of surrogate markers for determining drug activity using proteomics. Biochem Soc Trans 2003; 31(6):1488–90.

121. Chevallier B, Mossen V, Dauce JP et al. A prognostic score in histological node negative breast cancer. Br J Cancer 1990; 61:436–40.

122. Brown JM, Benson EA, Jones M. Confirmation of a long term prognostic index in breast cancer. Breast 1993; 2:144–7.

123. Balslev I, Axesson CK, Zedelev K et al. The Nottingham Prognostic Index applied to 9,149 patients from the studies of the Danish Breast Cancer Cooperative Group (DBCG). Breast Cancer Res Treat 1994; 32:281–90.

124. Ravdin PM, Siminoff LA, Davis GJ et al. Computer programme to assist in making decisions about adjuvant therapy for women with early breast cancer. J Clin Oncol 2001; 19:980–91.

125. Goldhirsch A, Glick JH, Gelber RD et al. Meeting highlights: international expert consensus on the primary therapy of early breast cancer 2005. Ann Oncol 2005; 16:1569–83.

# 3

# Ductoscopy and the intraductal approach to breast cancer

William C. Dooley

## New developments

The last 2 years has seen rapid evolution of submillimetre endoscopy and its application to breast ducts. Optics have improved, allowing manufacturers the ability to devote a smaller cross-sectional diameter to light and image capture and leave available larger working channels for visually directed biopsy. These new smaller scopes and new vacuum-assisted biopsy techniques have begun to allow investigators to serially sample up and down the ductal tree and truly begin to map pathological changes.[1,2] The value of this is confirmed by Hunerbein and colleagues at Berlin, who have now been able to find extensive intra-ductal carcinoma beyond what could be seen by traditional external imaging techniques.[3]

The further development of autofluorescence techniques by Jacobs and colleagues from Munich opens the potential of being able to distinguish visually benign from more suspicious lesions on the basis of simple biological differences in the ductal lining tissue.[4] The confusion over the overlap in appearance of benign and malignant intraductal lesions has led some authors to question the value of ductoscopy as a current clinical tool.[5-7] The application of autofluorescence as in bronchoscopy will enhance our abilites to use this technique and separate confusing intraluminal growths into those visually recognisable as being more or less suspicious. Combining ductoscopic findings with results of other imaging techniques seems already to offer substantial benefits in determining the presence

and extent of small cancers.[6-8] As the techniques of ductoscopy continue to evolve, some are using scopes introduced not just through the nipple but also through direct cyst puncture.[9] Further refinements of both instrumentation and techniques will further expand both the clinical and research utility of ductoscopy in the near future.[10,11]

## Historical development of ductoscopy

The intraductal approach to breast cancer diagnosis was recognised early by cytologists such as George Papanicolau.[12] Unfortunately few breast cancers could be diagnosed from the few micro litres of cell-poor fluid which could be elicited from most women's breasts.[13] In the 1960s, Wrensch and colleagues began a series of studies on women in the San Francisco region to determine if the presence of nipple fluid or its cytological characteristics could predict future breast cancer risk.[14] Published data of more than 30-year follow-up on more than 7000 women has shown that the relative risk of women who had nipple fluid expressible was 1.88 times that of women with no fluid for the development of cancer in the following decade. Furthermore if there was cytological atypia in that fluid the relative risk jumped to 4.9 for the development of breast cancer within a decade. Interestingly, in other series of cytological or histological breast epithelial atypia the risk for subsequent cancer fell rapidly in the second and third decades after its initial detection. Fine-needle aspiration studies from Fabian et al. showed similar risk levels associated with cellular atypia.[15] Dupont et al. defined both the current histological criteria for atypical ductal hyperplasia (ADH) and its natural history with a series of papers in the 1980s.[16,17] Each of these series confirm the increased risk for cancer associated with epithelial atypia in breast ducts independent of sampling method and confirm the time-dependent nature of that elevated risk.

Japanese surgeons such as Okazaki began investigating the use of ductoscopy in the early 1990s.[18–20] Endoscope technologies had greatly improved optics and reduced the diameter of scope needed for both illumination and image capture. Early studies on Japanese patients with bloody nipple discharge using a solid rigid scope <2 mm in diameter showed value in identifying the cause for the discharge, but the scopes were fragile and expensive and rarely advanced more than 3 cm into the breast. Persistence with this technology and improved optics and designs resulted in submillimetre multifibre scopes and with the addition of a working channel this improved success in the mid-1990s in the Orient.[21–25] The technique of ductal endoscopy for the evaluation and management of symptomatic nipple discharge has now spread to Korea and Hong Kong. The Oriental approach still has several drawbacks. First, the scopes used were usually rigid with the camera mounted as a heavy object at the end of a delicate optical fibre. The torque caused by such a long lever arm makes manipulating the scope around tight turns in the breast difficult. Second, the working channel is used primarily to instil air into the ductal system. This does not relax the smooth muscle of the ductal walls and affords little distension for investigation of more distal branches. It also causes sharp bright boundaries between fluid and air interfaces, leading to optical distortion and degraded images secondary to light reflection. In spite of these difficulties, Oriental investigators have moved to cyst endoscopy and other uses beyond nipple discharge alone.[26–28]

Early attempts in the USA with submillimetre scopes were unsuccessful in patients with central tumours.[29] Cells recovered from distending the major ducts with saline showed promise in improving cytology yield over those from simple nipple aspiration or expression. Combining this experience with the prior data from Wrensch and colleagues, an attempt was made to develop a way to cannulate fluid-producing ducts and to maximise the recovery of shed intraluminal ductal cells. Recent data from the NSABP P-01 study suggested that high-risk patients with ductal atypia had the greatest reduction in future breast cancer incidence with tamoxifen chemoprevention. Increasing the cell yield of nipple aspiration is necessary to have a viable test to screen for ADH.[30] The initial ductal lavage study enrolled women with prior contralateral breast cancer or who were defined as high risk by the Gail model and had normal mammograms and no abnormality on physical examination.[31] The majority (85%) had fluid expressed from at least one duct per breast. Atypia was present in 24% of the patients who successfully had a fluid-producing duct cannulated and lavaged with saline. At least 7% of this atypia was severe and bordering on malignancy. Subsequent series of severe atypia detected by lavage suggest that 50–70% of the atypia is from a mammographically occult malignancy. Ongoing studies will determine the natural history of lavage-detected atypia, the correlation of atypia clearance on chemoprevention agents and future risk reduction of breast cancer, and the rates and causes of false-positive atypia such as papillomas.

Finding malignant cells that could be repeatedly lavaged from a single ductal orifice with negative clinical and radiographic findings in the breast was quite disconcerting. After a number of imaging techniques such as galactograms, magnetic resonance imaging (MRI), ultrasound (US), etc. failed to identify routinely the occult source of the atypia, I applied the Oriental approach of duct endoscopy. The lavage experience had taught us how to relax the smooth muscle of the ducts and get maximal distension of the ductal system using local anaesthetic topically prior to saline distension. Using that major variation, I began to scope first those patients with concerning atypia where imaging had failed to identify the source. Rapidly the technique was successful at not only identifying the source of the atypia, but also in identifying multiple tumours and extensive intraductal component in early-stage breast cancer.[32] Papers from a number of American investigators now show the benefit of ductoscopy in investigation of symptomatic nipple discharge and discharge or ellicitable fluid from a cancerous breast.[33–37] New biopsy technologies to direct non-surgical minimal access biopsy either through the scope or in conjunction with other devices are being developed and tried in pilot settings.

The current technologies can identify a group of high-risk women with epithelial atypia. What percentage of atypia is missed? We cannot answer since this is really our first attempt to screen for atypia and we have nothing to compare with this technology. Ductoscopy appears to be a viable option for the identification of intraluminal defects which either cause symptomatic nipple discharge or give rise to severe cytological atypia on nipple aspiration or ductal lavage. Much is said of the power of MRI to screen for multifocal breast cancer. Unfortunately it sees primarily invasive cancer with increased blood flow and grossly underestimates low-grade ductal carcinoma in situ (DCIS), which is more often a problem in breast conservation in early-stage breast cancer. My personal series show that ductoscopy of breast cancer patients at lumpectomy yields far more evidence of widespread proliferative disease than any MRI protocol. Further, the assumption of most MRI studies is that multiple lesions make mastectomy necessary. In all cases so far of multifocality in my ductoscopy series, all tumours appear connected to the same duct orifice at the nipple. The operative surgeon can work out the anatomy of the ductal system and a cosmetically satisfactory lumpectomy with clear margins can be accomplished with the first operation in the vast majority of cases.[35]

Advances in the laboratory will drive the future of these technologies. For the first time we have the ability to multiply sample premalignant ductal epithelium and monitor its response to prevention strategies. We can obtain optimal samples for molecular investigations.[38] For the intraductal approach to have value beyond the highest risk patients we will need molecular markers that are identifiable in simple nipple aspirates. Then those with 'molecular risk' can be screened through lavage and endoscopy and intraductal biopsy of premalignant and early malignant lesions prior to radiographic image detection. We can then begin to merge prevention and treatment as we alter the development and progression of these lesions.

# Special technical considerations

The difficulty of all the intraductal technologies is achieving initial access to the lactiferous sinus without puncturing the ductal system. The key whether using the ductal lavage catheter or a prolene suture as a soft guidewire is timing. The sphincter of each duct in the papilla has a sort of 'anal wink' when expressing fluid. It is usually open for only fractions of a second when expressing fluid and successful cannulation of a duct occurs when the catheter or prolene is introduced during this brief relaxation of the sphincter. In women with symptomatic spontaneous discharge the sphincter stays open more widely for longer intervals and is therefore much easier to cannulate. Cannulating the minimally fluid-producing duct associated with a peripheral subcentimetre breast cancer is much more difficult. Initially, the nipple should be cleaned thoroughly with a facial exfollient until all keratin and sebaceous plugs are removed from its surface. Next, the breast should be lubricated with hand lotion and massaged deeply from periphery to centre to move any fluid into the lactiferous sinuses from the periphery. The kneading is similar to kneading bread and should always be done in this centripetal fashion. These first two steps are the most important and often the most neglected in achieving success with any of the intraductal technologies. Lastly, radial compression of each lactiferous sinus will identify the fluid-producing orifice. As soon as an orifice is identified, stop expressing fluid until you are ready to cannulate. With cannulating tool in hand, re-express fluid while slowly distracting the nipple upward. Cannulation should occur at the time fluid first appears on the nipple surface. If you fail then, do not empty the sinus of fluid before re-trying. I prefer using a tapered 2-0 prolene since it is much too soft to penetrate most duct walls and will not advance unless you meet minimal resistance. All harder objects must be approached with caution.

Once in the duct, you can use a 26- or 24-gauge angiocath and Seldinger technique using the prolene as a guidewire. Progressive dilation will allow up to 1-mm external diameter objects to be placed into the ductal system with ease. Injection of 3–5 mL of buffered local anaesthetic into the ducts comes next. It is important then to wait for 2–5 minutes to get relaxation of the ductal walls before starting saline distension. Success in cannulation technique can be measured readily by following the cellularity of ductal lavage samples. If the lactiferous sinus is perforated, then the samples will have few epithelial cells (<100). If the ducts are intact (and even if normal), the cell counts will be >1000.

When performing endoscopy, patients with spontaneous nipple discharge will be the easiest to cannulate and scope. Furthermore, because of chronic fluid production the ducts are often larger and it is easier to manipulate the scope in such patients. For the first several cases I would suggest getting preoperative galactograms. Until you learn how to manipulate through some of the lengthy papillomas, it can be very disconcerting to put in a scope and find yourself in a yellow kelp forest of papilloma without a central lumen. The best starter cases are the ones with 1–1.5 cm of normal duct before any lesion is found. This way you can get inside and get oriented before pathological findings distort landmarks. After success with spontaneous discharge patients, patients with central DCIS with or without invasive cancer can be tackled next. The spectrum of findings associated with malignant and premalignant breast disease can be visualised and the surgeon's expertise at recognition of differing pathological lesions rapidly improves (**Figs 3.1–3.4**).

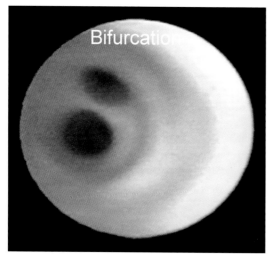

**Figure 3.1** • Bifurcation.

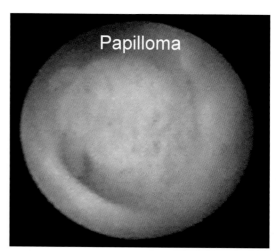

**Figure 3.2** • Papilloma.

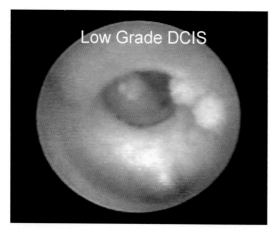

**Figure 3.3** • Low-grade ductal carcinoma in situ.

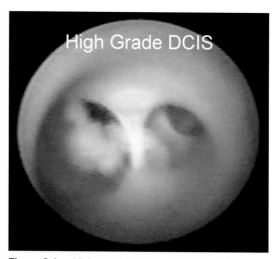

**Figure 3.4** • High-grade ductal carcinoma in situ.

## Key points

- The majority of non-obstructing malignant and premalignant breast diseases are associated with fluid production.
- Cytological analysis of fluid produced in high-risk women can identify subgroups at high short-term risk of breast cancer development. Molecular analysis offers opportunities to extend this to pre-cancerous detection as these technologies evolve.
- Direct ductal endoscopy with submillimetre endoscopes is now feasible and can offer value beyond simple investigation of symptomatic nipple discharge.
- Technical developments are rapidly innovating this field of submillimetre endoscopy – for both diagnostics and therapy.

# References

1. Jacobs VR, Paepke S, Ohlinger R et al. Breast ductoscopy; technical development from a diagnostic to an interventional procedure and its future perspective. Onkologie 2007; 11:545–9.

2. Hunerbein M, Raubach M, Gebauer B et al. Ductoscopy and intraductal vacuum assisted biopsy in women with pathologic nipple discharge. Breast Cancer Res Treat 2006, 3:301–7.

3. Hunerbein M, Dubowy A, Raubach M et al. Gradient index ductoscopy and intraductal biopsy of intraductal breast lesions. Am J Surg 2007; 4:511–14.

4. Jacobs VR, Paepke S, Schaaf H et al. Autofluorescence ductoscopy; a new imaging technique for intraductal breast endoscopy. Clin Breast Cancer 2007; 8:619–23.

5. Louie LD, Crowe JP, Dawson AE et al. Identification of breast cancer in patients with pathologic nipple discharge; does ductoscopy predict malignancy? Am J Surg 2006; 4:530–3.

6. Grunwald S, Heyer H, Paepke S et al. Diagnostic value of ductoscopy in the diagnosis of nipple discharge and intraductal proliferatons in comparison to standard methods. Onkologie 2007; 5:243–8.

7. Grunwald S, Bojahr B, Schwesinger G et al. Mammary ductoscopy for the evaluation of nipple discharge and comparison with standard diagnostic techniques. Minim Invasive Gynecol 2006; 5:418–23.

8. Makita M, Akiyama F, Gomi N et al. Endoscopic and histologic findings of intraductal lesions presenting with nipple discharge. Breast J 2006; 12(5, Suppl 2):S210–7.

9. Uchida K, Toriumi Y, Kawase K et al. Percutaneous endoscopy-guided biopsy of an intracystic tumor with a mammary ductoscopy. Breast Cancer 2007; 2:215–18.

10. Hunerbein M, Raubach M, Gebauer B et al. Intraoperative ductoscopy in women undergoing surgery for breast cancer. Surgery 2006; 6:833–8.

11. Valdes EK, Boolbol SK, Cohen JM et al Clinical experience with mammary ductoscopy. Ann Surg Oncol 2006 (Epub ahead of print).

12. Papanicolau GN, Holmquist DG, Bader GM et al. Exfoliative cytology of the human mammary gland and its value in the diagnosis of cancer and other diseases of the breast. Cancer 1958; 11:377–409.

13. Sartorius OW, Smith HS, Morris P et al. Cytologic evaluation of breast fluid in the detection of breast disease. J Natl Cancer Inst 1977; 59:1073–8.

14. Wrensch MR, Petrakis NL, King EB et al. Breast cancer incidence in women with abnormal cytology in nipple aspirates of breast fluid. Am J Epidemiol 1992; 135:130–41.

15. Fabian CJ, Kimler BF, Zalles CM et al. Short-term breast cancer prediction by random periareolar fine-needle aspiration cytology and the Gail risk model. J Natl Cancer Inst 2000; 92:1217–27.

16. Dupont WD, Page DL. Risk factors for breast cancer in women with proliferative breast disease. N Engl J Med 1985; 312:146–51.

17. Dupont WD, Parl FF, Hartmann WH et al. Breast cancer risk associated with proliferative breast disease and atypical hyperplasia. Cancer 1993; 71:1258–65.

18. Okazaki A, Okazaki M, Asaishi K et al. Fiberoptic ductoscopy of the breast: a new diagnostic procedure for nipple discharge. Jpn J Clin Oncol 1991, 21(3): 188–93.

19. Okazaki A, Okazaki M, Hirata K et al. Progress of ductoscopy of the breast [in Japanese]. Nippon Geka Gakkai Zasshi 1996; 97(5):357–62.

20. Okazaki A, Hirata K, Okazaki M et al. Nipple discharge disorders; current diagnostic management and the role of fiberductoscopy. Eur Radiol 1999; 9(4):583–90.

21. Shen KW, Wu J, Lu JS et al. Fiberoptic ductoscopy for patients with nipple discharge. Cancer 2000; 89(7):1512–19.

22. Shao ZM, Liu Y, Nguyen M. The role of the breast ductal system in the diagnosis of cancer (review). Oncol Rep 200; 8(1):153–6.

23. Matsunaga T, Ohta D, Misaka T et al. Mammary ductoscopy for diagnosis and treatment of

intraductal lesions of the breast. Breast Cancer 2001; 8(3):213–21.

24. Shen KW, Wu J, Lu JS et al. Fiberoptic ductoscopy for breast cancer patients with nipple discharge. Surg Endosc 2001; 15(11):1340–5.

25. Yamamoto D, Shoji T, Kawanishi H et al. A utility of ductography and fiberoptic ductoscopy for patients with nipple discharge. Breast Cancer Res Treat 2001; 70(2):103–8.

26. Yamamoto D, Ueda S, Senzaki H et al. New diagnostic approach to intracystic lesions of the breast by fiberoptic ductoscopy. Anticancer Res 2001; 21(6A):4113–6.

27. Makita, M, Akiyama F, Gomi N et al. Endoscopic classification of intraductal lesions and histological diagnosis. Breast Cancer 2002; 9(3):220–5.

28. Tamaki Y, Miyoshi Y, Noguchi S. Application of endoscopic surgery for breast cancer treatment [in Japanese]. Nippon Geka Gakkai Zasshi 2002; 103(11):835–8.

29. Love, SM, Barsky SH. Breast-duct endoscopy to study stages of cancerous breast disease. Lancet 1996; 348(9033):997–9.

30. Fisher B, Costantino JP, Wickerham DL et al. Tamoxifen for prevention of breast cancer: report of the National Surgical Adjuvant Breast and Bowel Project P-1 Study. J Natl Cancer Inst 1998; 90:1371–88.

31. Dooley WC, Ljung, B-M, Veronesi U et al. Ductal lavage for detection of cellular atypia in women at high risk for breast cancer. J Natl Cancer Inst 2001; 93(21):1624–32.

32. Dooley WC. Endoscopic visualization of breast tumors. JAMA 2000; 284(12):1518.

33. Khan SA, Baird C, Staradub VL et al. Ductal lavage and ductoscopy: the opportunities and the limitations. Clin Breast Cancer 2002; 3(3):185–91; discussion 192–5.

34. Dietz JR, Crowe JP, Grundfest S et al. Directed duct excision by using mammary ductoscopy in patients with pathologic nipple discharge. Surgery 2002; 132(4):582–7; discussion 587–8.

35. Dooley WC. Routine operative breast endoscopy during lumpectomy. Ann Surg Oncol 2003; 10(1):38–42.

36. Dooley WC. Routine operative breast endoscopy for bloody nipple discharge. Ann Surg Oncol 2002; 9(9):920–3.

37. Dooley WC. Ductal lavage, nipple aspiration, and ductoscopy for breast cancer diagnosis. Curr Oncol Rep 2003; 5(1):63–5.

38. Evron E, Dooley WC, Umbricht CB et al. Detection of breast cancer cells in ductal lavage fluid by methylation-specific PCR. Lancet 2001; 357: 1335–6.

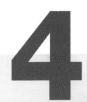

# 4

# Breast-conserving surgery: the balance between good cosmesis and local control

J. Michael Dixon

## Introduction

The aim of local treatment of breast cancer is to achieve long-term local disease control with the minimum of local morbidity. The majority of women presenting symptomatically to breast clinics or who are diagnosed with breast cancer through screening programmes have small breast cancers, which are suitable for breast-conserving surgery.

The major advantages of breast-conserving treatment are as follows:
- breast-conserving treatment produces an acceptable cosmetic appearance in the majority of women;[1]
- breast-conserving treatment results in lower levels of psychological morbidity, with less anxiety and depression and improved body image, sexuality and self-esteem, compared with mastectomy;[2,3]
- two systematic reviews have shown equivalence in terms of disease outcome for breast-conserving treatment and mastectomy.[4,5]

One of these reviews (search date 1995) analysed data from six randomised controlled trials that compared breast conservation treatment with mastectomy.[4] A meta-analysis of data from five of these six trials involving 3006 women found no significant difference in the risk of death at 10 years (odds ratio 0.91, 95% CI 0.78–1.05). The sixth randomised trial used different protocols. In the second systematic review, nine randomised controlled trials involving 4981 women randomised to mastectomy or breast-conserving treatment were included in the analysis.[5] A meta-analysis of these nine trials found no significant difference in the risk of death over 10 years: the relative risk reduction for breast-conserving surgery compared with mastectomy was 0.02 (95% CI –0.05 to +0.09).[5] There was also no difference in the rates of local recurrence in the six randomised controlled trials involving 3006 women where data were available: the relative risk reduction for mastectomy versus breast-conserving surgery was 0.04 (95% CI –0.04 to +0.12).[4]

Originally it was thought that local therapy had little influence on overall survival but it is becoming clear that local failure is responsible, at least in part, for some patients developing metastatic disease.[6–8]

It is thus important in those patients selected for breast-conserving surgery to minimise local recurrence and at the same time achieve a good cosmetic outcome.

## Selection of patients for breast conservation

Traditionally single cancers clinically measuring 4 cm or less, without signs of local advancement, have been managed by breast-conserving treatment (Box 4.1). Different units have different size criteria and many units have a tumour size cut-off for breast-conserving surgery of 3 cm or less clinically.

Box 4.1 • Indications and contraindications for breast-conserving surgery

**Indications**

T1, T2 (<4 cm), N0, N1, M0

T2 >4 cm in large breasts

Single clinical and mammographic lesion

**Contraindications**

T4, N2 or M1

Patients who prefer mastectomy

Clinically evident multifocal/multicentric disease

**Relative contraindications**

Collagen vascular disease

Large or central tumours in small breasts

Women with a strong family history of breast cancer or BRCA1 and BRCA2 mutation carriers

Increasing tumour size does not equate with increasing local recurrence rates and this approach is illogical.

Clinical tumour size overestimates actual tumour size. There is a much better correlation between pathological tumour size and the size measured on imaging, with ultrasound assessment being more accurate than mammographic measurements. There is some evidence that magnetic resonance imaging (MRI) might be even better than ultrasound in assessing disease extent, particularly in invasive lobular carcinoma. The problem with MRI is that it has low specificity and low positive predictive value in that not all lesions identified which are considered to be suspicious are subsequently confirmed as malignant. The role of MRI in assessing patients for breast-conserving surgery is therefore at present uncertain. It is the balance between tumour size as assessed by imaging and breast volume that determines whether a patient is suitable for breast-conserving surgery. Patients with tumours measuring clinically larger than 4 cm can be treated by breast-conserving surgery if the patient has large breasts. Conversely, in a patient with small breasts, excision of even a small tumour may produce an unacceptable cosmetic result. Options for patients with tumours considered too large, relative to the size of the breast, for breast-conserving treatment include neoadjuvant systemic therapy to shrink the tumour, an oncoplastic procedure (see Chapter 5) involving either transfer of tissue into the breast or remodelling of the breast with surgery to the opposite breast to obtain symmetry.[9,10]

Patients with multiple tumours in the same breast have not previously been considered good candidates for breast-conserving treatment because they have a high reported incidence of in-breast recurrence[11,12] and so are usually treated by mastectomy, combined in appropriate patients with immediate reconstruction. It is, however, feasible to excise two separate cancers in different parts of the breast and there is a definite move to challenge the current dogma that these patients require mastectomy. Part of the reason for this is that patients who have two cancers very close together on mammography, or those with multifocal disease identified by the pathologist, have satisfactory rates of local control following breast-conserving treatment, providing that all disease is excised to clear margins.[12] Patients with bilateral small cancers can be treated by bilateral breast conservation. The rates of breast-conserving surgery vary significantly between countries and within countries. These rates are more influenced by the views of the surgeon treating the patient than the availability of radiotherapy equipment. Failure to offer breast-conserving surgery to suitable and appropriate patients is now a medico-legal issue. If a patient who fulfils the criteria for breast-conserving surgery is treated by mastectomy then the exact reasons should be recorded legibly in the patient's notes.

Clinical and pathological factors have until recently influenced selection of patients for breast-conserving surgery because of their perceived impact on local recurrence. These include young age (under 35–39 years), the presence of an extensive in situ component associated with an invasive tumour, grade 3 histology and widespread lymphatic/vascular invasion.[13,14] These are considered in detail below.

# Breast-conserving surgery

Two surgical procedures have been studied extensively: quadrantectomy and wide local excision. Quadrantectomy is based on the belief that the breast is organised into segments, with each segment draining into its own major duct, and that invasive cancer spreads down the duct system towards the nipple.[15] The evidence is that both of these premises are incorrect.

A single major subareolar duct does not drain a localised segment of tissue but can drain widespread areas of the breast.

Studies have also shown that both invasive and non-invasive disease are no more likely to extend toward the nipple than in any other direction.[14] The effectiveness of quadrantectomy relates to the large amount of tissue excised around the tumour rather than to the removal of a cancer and its draining duct.[16] One of the early studies of breast-conserving treatment randomised patients to lumpectomy or quadrantectomy. A significantly greater number of patients who had lumpectomy had incomplete local excisions.[17] Not surprisingly, therefore, local recurrence was greater after lumpectomy than after quadrantectomy, although survival was no different.[15] Other non-randomised studies have shown similar rates of local recurrence in both quadrantectomy and wide local excision, providing margins of excision are clear.[16] Quadrantectomy is not advocated because it produces a significantly poorer cosmetic outcome than wide excision.[18]

The consensus view is that the majority of patients having breast-conserving surgery can be adequately treated by wide local excision and do not require either a segmental or quadrantic excision.[13,19]

## Special technical details: wide local excision

The aim of wide local excision is to remove all invasive and any ductal carcinoma in situ with a 1-cm macroscopic margin of normal surrounding breast tissue. Controversy has surrounded which incisions give the best cosmetic results. The predominant orientation of collagen fibres in the skin was described by Langer[20] and these skin crease lines around the breast are essentially circular (**Fig. 4.1**). Subsequent work by Kraissl[21] demonstrated that the lines of maximum resting skin tension run in a more transverse orientation across the breast (Fig. 4.1). In general, scars that are parallel both to the lines of maximum resting skin tension and to the orientation of collagen fibres are quickest to heal and produce the best cosmetic outcomes, with least hypertrophy and keloid formation.

Incisions at right angles to both the orientation of collagen fibres and to the lines of maximum resting skin tension, such as radial incisions in the upper outer quadrant, produce the most cosmetically unacceptable scars.

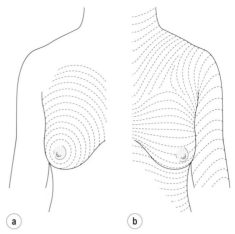

**Figure 4.1** • The direction of Langer's lines **(a)** and lines of maximum resting skin tension **(b)** in the breast (so-called dynamic lines of Kraissl).

A knowledge of Langer's lines and Kraissl's lines thus allows a surgeon to make incisions that enhance the cosmetic outcome of breast-conserving surgery. It has been tradition to place an incision to excise a cancer directly over the lesion, but this can result in unsightly scars, particularly if the cancer is high and medial. In such instances placing the scar some distance below in the skin crease lines and tunnelling up to the lesion produces a better cosmetic result. Cancers close to the nipple can be excised through circumareolar incisions. A cancer low in the breast close to the inframammary fold can similarly be excised through an incision placed in the fold. Excising skin directly overlying a cancer is only necessary if the carcinoma is very superficial and/or the skin is tethered. The cosmetic result after breast-conserving surgery is influenced by the amount of skin excised, with poor results being obtained in those patients who have most skin removed.[22]

Routine excision of skin when performing a wide excision is discouraged by current guidelines and cannot be justified.[13]

Limiting the length of incision is also important, as longer incisions produce significantly poorer cosmetic outcomes. In a patient who has previously had an incomplete excision, it is usual either to open the previous scar or to narrowly excise the previous scar. A knowledge of the depth of the cancer within the breast provided by preoperative or intraoperative breast ultrasound can be valuable when planning the extent of excision. For instance, if a cancer is 2 cm deep within the breast, then at least 1 cm of fat and subcutaneous tissue can be left on the skin flaps and leaving this tissue improves the cosmetic outcome. Whatever incision is used, it is important to have discussed the position of the scars with the patient prior to surgery.

Having made the skin incision, the skin and subcutaneous fat are dissected off the breast tissue. Care should be taken when elevating skin not to excise into the subcutaneous fat as thin skin flaps give a poor postoperative cosmetic result. Skin flaps 1–2 cm beyond the edge of the cancer are elevated and the fingers of the non-dominant hand are placed over the palpable cancer. The breast tissue is then divided beyond the fingertips. The line of incision through the breast should be approximately 1 cm beyond the limit of the palpable mass. Having incised through the breast plate, dissection then continues under the cancer. In the majority of patients it is necessary to continue dissection through the breast tissue down to the pectoral fascia to ensure that there is an adequate margin of tissue removed deep to the cancer. If the lesion is superficial, and there is a significant amount of breast tissue deep to the cancer, it is not necessary to remove the full thickness of breast tissue. Likewise if the lesion is deep, more tissue is left superficially on the skin flaps. Having reached the deep margin, which is usually the pectoral fascia, the breast tissue and cancer are dissected from this fascia. It is not necessary to excise pectoral fascia unless it is tethered to the tumour or the tumour is involving it. If a carcinoma is infiltrating one of the chest wall muscles, then a portion of the affected muscle should be removed beneath the tumour, the aim being to excise sufficient muscle to get beyond the limits of the cancer. Having dissected under the cancer, whether this is within the breast tissue or on the pectoral fascia, the cancer and surrounding tissue are grasped between the finger and thumb of the non-dominant hand and excision is completed at the other margins. The specimen is immediately orientated with Liga-clips, sutures or metal markers prior to submission to the pathologist. Metal markers or Liga-clips are preferred because they allow orientated anteroposterior intraoperative specimen radiography to be performed. This helps the surgeon assess whether the target lesion has been excised and also aids in assessing the completeness of excision at radial margins. If the specimen radiograph shows the cancer or any associated microcalcification as being close to a particular margin, then further tissue should be removed from the margin of concern, orientated and sent to pathology.

A number of studies have evaluated the use of cavity shavings and bed biopsies, but few have compared standard assessment of margins with cavity shavings or bed biopsies. There remain problems with their use. First, only a minority of surgeons take cavity shavings and bed biopsies routinely,[23,24] because neither have been shown to be reliable indicators of local recurrence. Second, the major concern of taking routine cavity shavings is that significant amounts of extra breast tissue are removed, particularly if the whole cavity is shaved; this adversely effects cosmetic outcome.[24] Third and most importantly, centres who do not use these techniques report excellent local control rates.[25] Wide excision with standard examination of margins thus provides sufficient information on margin status. Bed biopsies or cavity shavings are only of value where there is concern at operation that one particular margin is involved.

Having excised the cancer from the breast, suturing the defect in the breast without mobilisation of the breast tissue usually results in distortion of the breast contour. Small defects (<5% breast volume) can be left open and the final cosmetic outcome in such patients is usually good or excellent. Larger defects in the breast are best closed by mobilising surrounding breast tissue from both the overlying skin and subcutaneous tissue and the underlying chest wall. Large defects (>10% breast volume) that are left open fill with seroma which usually absorbs later, following which there is formation of scar tissue which contracts and results in an ugly distorted breast. Following large-volume excisions, with mobilisation it is usually possible to close the defect in the breast plate with a series of interrupted absorbable sutures. Larger defects require oncoplastic breast reshaping or a latissimus dorsi miniflap[9,10] (see Chapter 5). Drains are not necessary following wide local excision and should not be used routinely. They do not protect against haematoma formation and increase infection rates. Breast skin wounds should be closed in layers with absorbable sutures, finishing with a subcuticular suture.

Staples and interrupted sutures do not produce satisfactory results and are not an acceptable method of wound closure in the breast.

Complications of wide excision include haematoma, infection, incomplete excision and poor cosmetic results. Haematoma requiring evacuation should be rare and occur in less than 2% of patients. Infection requiring treatment affects 5–10% and is more common when combined with an axillary dissection. Incomplete excision rates should be in the range 10–25%. The most common problem following surgery by wide local excision is a poor cosmetic result. Factors influencing cosmetic outcome are considered in detail below.

## Excising impalpable cancers

Impalpable lesions can be localised prior to surgery using one of a number of different techniques, including skin marking, injection of blue dye, carbon or radioisotope, insertion of a hooked wire, or intraoperative ultrasound. Excising an impalpable cancer is easier if the skin incision is made directly over the cancer. The location of the lesion can be determined in three ways: (i) the surgeon calculates the position of the breast lesion from the mammogram; (ii) the radiologist marks the skin overlying the lesion; or (iii) the surgeon uses a gamma probe to localise the area of maximum radioactivity. An appropriately sized skin incision is made and deepened. If a wire is in place, then dissection continues towards the wire so that the wire can be located above where it enters the lesion. For instance, if a mammographic abnormality has been localised in the craniocaudal position, then dissection proceeds superiorly. Wires which are marked with beads or which change in diameter, or have a guide that can be placed over the wire, help the surgeon to determine exactly how far along the wire the lesion is situated. The direction of the wire on the preoperative mammogram is only a guide to the course of the wire through the breast. Once the wire is in place standard mammographic views are not always possible and thus a lesion that is apparently lateral to the entry point of the wire may not be lateral on the check craniocaudal film once the compression from the breast has been removed. The aim is to remove the mammographic lesion with a 1-cm clear radiological margin.

As for palpable lesions, all specimens should be orientated with Liga-clips or metal markers, or secured to an orientated grid so that specimen radiography can be performed. Radiography is performed following compression in a mammogram machine or non-compressed in a Faxitron. There have been conflicting reports about whether compressing the specimen affects the incidence of subsequent positive margins as reported by the pathologist. Orientated specimen radiography improves the rate of complete excision of impalpable cancers.[26] Cooperation between surgeon and pathologist is required to clarify the area of concern and assess the adequacy of excision.

The majority of wide excisions of palpable and impalpable cancers are performed under general anaesthesia, although it is possible to perform wide excision under local anaesthesia.

# Factors affecting breast-conserving surgery after breast conservation

Different centres have reported large variations in recurrence rates following breast-conserving surgery combined with radiotherapy for invasive breast carcinoma. Until recently the majority of these recurrences (approximately 80%) occurred adjacent to the site of initial excision. This is no longer true and now the majority of new events in the treated breast are actually second primaries.[25] Megavoltage radiation therapy to the whole breast in a dose of 4500–5000 cGy given over 3–5 weeks is used because radiotherapy reduces not only the rates of local recurrence but improves overall survival.[8] Ongoing studies are continuing to evaluate whether localised radiotherapy delivered either during or within a few days of surgery is as effective as whole-breast radiotherapy. As yet it has not been possible to identify groups of patients who do not require radiotherapy. However, there may be a group of older patients with low-risk cancers (completely excised, node negative and hormone receptor positive on hormone treatment) and women of any age whose cancers have an extremely good outcome (very well differentiated grade 1 or special type cancers that are completely excised, node negative and hormone receptor positive) whose rates of local recurrence without radiotherapy are acceptable. Following whole-breast radiotherapy, it is possible to increase the local dose of radiotherapy by boosting the tumour bed. This reduces local recurrence rates, particularly in younger women, although there are cosmetic penalties associated with the use of a boost.[27]

## Patient-related factors

Local recurrence following breast-conserving therapy is significantly more common in younger patients.[27,28]

In contrast, local recurrence is much less of a problem in older patients (>65 years). Ongoing randomised studies are examining whether older patients with hormone-sensitive tumours receiving adjuvant endocrine therapy, with limited factors for local recurrence, can safely avoid radiotherapy.

Recurrence is less frequent in women with large breasts but whether this relates to the larger excisions that can be performed in these patients or to alterations in steroid metabolism (fat is known to be an important site of conversion of androgens to estrogens) is uncertain.[29] A family history of breast cancer, particularly carriage of a mutation in one of the breast cancer genes, predisposes a patient to an increased rate of second primary cancers in both the treated and contralateral breast unless these women undergo a prophylactic oophorectomy, when local recurrence rates fall to that of the general population.[30]

## Tumour-related factors

Tumour location, tumour size, the presence of skin or nipple retraction, and the presence or absence of axillary node involvement have not been consistently shown to be factors predictive of local recurrence after breast-conserving surgery.[31–34] The hormone receptor status of a breast cancer does not seem to exert any influence on local control rates.

### Tumour size

There has been confusion with regard to tumour size. Only 3 of 28 series that have examined the relationship of tumour size and occurrence have shown a significant association between tumour size in breast recurrence.[35] A large study from Boston[36] demonstrated that cancers over 4 cm in size that were treated by breast conservation surgery had a rate of recurrence which was less than that of smaller cancers (Table 4.1).

**Table 4.1** • Size of tumour related to local recurrence

| Size (cm) | Local recurrence (%) |
|-----------|----------------------|
| 0–1       | 21                   |
| 1.1–2     | 8                    |
| 2.1–3     | 13                   |
| 3.1–4     | 17                   |
| 4.1–5     | 4                    |

Data from Eberlein TG, Connolly JN, Schnitt JS et al. Predictors of local recurrence following conservative breast surgery and radiation therapy. The influence of tumour size. Arch Surg 1990; 125:771–9.

### Tumour grade

A number of reports have analysed the relationship between tumour grade and local recurrence.

The lowest rates of local recurrence are reported in grade 1 tumours.

Although some series report a higher recurrence rate in grade 3 compared with grade 2 cancers, this is by no means universal.[37,38] The relative risk of local recurrence between grade 1 and grade 2/3 cancer is approximately 1.5. The British Association of Surgical Oncology undertook a trial that randomised patients with node-negative grade 1 or special-type cancers to no further treatment, tamoxifen alone, radiotherapy alone or both radiotherapy and tamoxifen. A recent presentation of this study reported no local recurrence in patients randomised to radiotherapy and tamoxifen, and acceptably low rates of annual recurrence in patients treated with either tamoxifen alone or radiotherapy alone. Higher rates of recurrence were seen in patients who received neither radiotherapy nor tamoxifen.

### Histological type

There are few data relating histological tumour type and recurrence. Invasive lobular cancer does not appear to be associated with a higher recurrence rate than so-called invasive 'ductal' carcinoma.[39–44] One study did suggest that patients with invasive lobular carcinoma who developed local recurrence were more likely to develop multifocal recurrence but this has not been confirmed by others. Patients with invasive lobular cancer appear more likely than patients with no special-type tumours to have incomplete excision. Patients with invasive lobular cancer on core biopsy should be warned of this and where the extent of disease is not assessable accurately on mammography and ultrasound, an MRI scan should has been reported to be valuable. A randomised study of pre-operative MRI however found no increase in the rates of complete excision in patients having an MRI compared to patients who did not have this investigation.

## Lymphatic/vascular invasion

Increased local failure rates have been reported in most, but not all, series in patients with histological evidence of lymphatic/vascular invasion (LVI).[28,31,36–38] Of concern, the percentage of tumours reported to have LVI varies widely between different series by up to a factor of four.

Carcinomas with LVI have approximately double the rate of local recurrence compared with tumours with no evidence of this feature.

LVI is more common in tumours of younger women (<35 years) than in those of older women (>50 years).

## Extensive in situ component

The histological factor that has been most frequently shown to be associated with an increased rate of local recurrence is the presence of an extensive in situ component (EIC) within and surrounding an invasive cancer. A tumour is defined as having EIC if 25% or more of the tumour mass is non-invasive *and* non-invasive carcinoma is also present in the breast tissue surrounding the invasive cancer.[45] EIC is a predictor not only of local recurrence but also of residual disease within the breast following an incomplete wide excision.[18] Early reports indicated that local recurrence rates were three to four times higher in cancers with EIC.[28,38,40,43,46] The majority of these studies did not, however, take account of margins and the authors did not perform multivariate analysis. Providing clear margins are obtained, then there is no increased rate of local recurrence in patients with EIC.[47,48] There is an interaction between age and EIC, with younger women being more likely to have EIC. It has been suggested that the higher frequency of EIC in younger women might explain some of the increased rate of local recurrence seen in younger women.[38]

## Multiple tumours

Patients with macroscopic multiple cancers have been reported to have an increased risk of local recurrence compared with a patient with a unifocal cancer but patient numbers in such reports have been small. If multifocality is identified by the pathologist or there are two cancers that are adjacent, then acceptable local recurrence rates can be obtained providing that all margins of excision are clear of disease.[40] This has led some to hypothesise that breast-conserving surgery can be offered to patients with two separate tumours in one breast providing the cancers are excised completely and a satisfactory cosmetic result obtained.

The most important surgical-related factor is completeness of excision. Current practice is to aim for at least microscopically disease-free margins. Ideally, there should be a clear rim of normal tissue (≥1 mm) around the carcinoma in all directions.[43]

# Treatment-related factors

Controversy has surrounded how much extra tissue should be removed and what constitutes an involved or positive margin. Some studies have defined a positive or involved margin as disease at the margin, others as disease within 1 mm or even disease within 2 mm of the margins. Conversely, negative margins or uninvolved margins have been variably defined as no tumour at the margin, 1 mm of normal tissue or greater than 1 mm of normal tissue beyond the edge of the invasive or in situ cancer. Whatever definition has been used, almost all studies have reported an increased rate of local recurrence in patients with positive, non-negative or involved margins. When comparing patients with involved margins to those with uninvolved or negative margins, the relative risk of local recurrence varies between 1.4- and 9-fold.[31,33,34,38–43,46–52] This is despite, in almost half of the series, patients with involved or close margins having received higher doses of radiotherapy than patients with clear margins. In the few studies which found that margins were not important predictors of local recurrence, the dose of radiotherapy delivered to the tumour bed ranged from 65 to 72 cGy, i.e. in the dose range that is effective without surgery.[41,48–50,53] In one study, patients with initially involved margins, who underwent re-excision to a negative margin, had a zero local recurrence rate compared with a 22% local recurrence rate in patients who had re-excision and still had non-negative margins ($P = 0.001$).[48] A recent survey in the UK demonstrated that approximately 50% of surgeons aim for a margin of more than 2 mm, whereas 50% of surgeons are happy with a margin of 2 mm or less.[23] This demonstrates that there is still no consensus about what is an adequate margin of excision for breast-conserving surgery. A systematic review of margins and local recurrence was conducted by Singletary, who reported that some of the lowest rates of local recurrence were in centres that had used narrow margins of excision (1 or 2 mm).

 From this review Singletary concluded that taking more surrounding tissue to obtain wider margins does not necessarily result in lower rates of local recurrence but that incomplete excision, i.e. tumour at a margin, does result in an unacceptable rate of local control.[25]

A recent large series of patients treated by breast-conserving surgery with a ≥1 mm margin reported rates of local recurrence of <0.5% per year[54]. The majority of these so-called recurrences were in fact second primaries and so the conclusion must be that a 1- or 2-mm margin is adequate and produces acceptable rates of long-term control. Based on this evidence and that from the systematic review, demanding margins wider than 1 or 2 mm is illogical and unnecessary.

Studies have looked at the presence of lobular carcinoma in situ[55] and atypical ductal hyperplasia[56] at the margins of excision. Neither of these features significantly increases local recurrence rates and so there is no need for the surgeon to re-excise if the pathologist reports these features alone at any of the margins of excision.

Age interacts with margins. Clear margins appear even more imperative in younger than in older women.[51]

There is a direct interaction between EIC and margins (Table 4.2). Patients with EIC and positive margins, who proceeded to radiotherapy without re-excision, had a 37% local recurrence rate in a series from Boston[47] and a 21% recurrence rate in a Stanford series.[48] In contrast, patients with EIC and negative margins, on primary or re-excision, had a zero local recurrence rate. These two studies demonstrate that patients with EIC do not have an increased rate of local recurrence providing the margins of excision are clear of invasive and in situ cancer.

Patients undergoing re-excision for close or involved margins have only a 30% incidence of residual cancer in re-excised tissue.[57] More than two foci of microscopic margin involvement in the original wide excision was associated with an incidence of residual cancer of 65% in one series, whereas patients with less than two foci had a much lower rate of residual cancer. This study showed that when there was no residual disease at re-excision there was a 4% local failure rate at 4.7 years compared with patients who had residual disease at re-excision who had a 13% failure rate. Patients younger than age 50 in this study were more likely to have disease in the re-excision specimen. The conclusion was that the majority of patients who undergo re-excision do not benefit from the procedure. Patients with lucent breasts and a well-defined lesion appeared particularly unlikely to benefit from re-excision if margins were close or focally positive, whereas younger women with dense breasts were much more likely to benefit from further surgery to obtain clear final margins.[57] Further studies in this area are required. If it were possible to identify a group of women who did not benefit from re-excision, this would have great clinical utility.

## Adjuvant systemic therapy

Aromatase inhibitors, tamoxifen and chemotherapy, in the presence of radiotherapy, reduce local recurrence after breast-conserving surgery.[58–61] In the absence of radiotherapy, aromatase inhibitors, tamoxifen or chemotherapy alone do not produce satisfactory rates of local control apart from in low-grade, node-negative cancers.[61,62] The interval between surgery and radiotherapy may be important and there are suggestions that the rates of local recurrence increase if radiotherapy is delayed. The sequencing of radiotherapy and chemotherapy is the subject of ongoing trials.

Table 4.2 • Local recurrence rates (%) at 5 years in patients from Boston[47] and Stanford[48] subdivided by margin status and the presence (EIC+) or absence (EIC−) of an extensive in situ component

| | Boston | | Stanford | |
|---|---|---|---|---|
| **Margins** | **EIC+** | **EIC−** | **EIC+** | **EIC−** |
| Positive/non-negative | 37 | 7 | 21 | 11 |
| Close | 0 | 5 | | |
| Negative | 0 | 2 | 0 | 1 |

# Factors influencing cosmetic outcome after breast-conserving surgery

There is a great variation in different series in the number of patients with good to excellent cosmetic results after breast-conserving surgery (**Fig. 4.2**).

 The importance of good cosmetic results is demonstrated in a study from Nottingham,[2] which showed that there is a significant correlation between poor cosmetic outcome and increased levels of anxiety, depression, poor body image, problems with sexuality and low self-esteem.

## Patient factors

There is conflicting evidence about whether age influences cosmetic outcome, with some studies claiming that older women have worse cosmetic results than younger women.[1] One problem in younger women is that as the patient ages, in contrast to the normal contralateral breast, the treated breast does not increase in size, so a treated breast

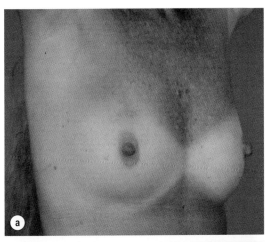

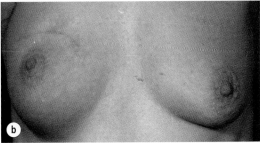

**Figure 4.2** • Examples of excellent **(a)** and poor **(b)** cosmetic results from breast-conserving surgery and radiotherapy.

which is symmetrical immediately following treatment becomes asymmetrical over time.

There is a trend towards increased fibrosis in large breasts, which leads to poor cosmetic results.[63] For this reason large-breasted women are sometimes best treated by an operation which excises their cancer and at the same time reduces the volume of the breast. Such procedures are usually bilateral and performed through reduction-type incisions. The best cosmetic results are obtained in medium- and moderate-sized breasts; achieving a good cosmetic outcome can be a problem in small breasts.[1]

## Tumour factors

Increasing tumour size means that increasingly large amounts of tissue have to be removed. The volume of tissue excised is the most important factor relating to cosmetic outcome and so not surprisingly patients with larger tumours tend to have worse cosmetic results than women with smaller cancers.[58,64] There are some data that have indicated that when tumours are small and impalpable, a disproportionately large amount of normal surrounding breast tissue is removed to ensure that all the affected tissue is excised. The role of the surgeon is to excise the cancer completely in as small a volume as possible and removing large volumes for small screen-detected cancers is not satisfactory surgical practice.

### Location of tumour

Cosmetic outcomes tend to be better if the tumour is localised in the upper outer quadrant.[65] Studies have shown that major nipple displacement occurs when surgery is performed on tumours located in the inferior half of the breast.[66] This can be corrected at the time of initial surgery by de-epithelialising a crescentic portion of skin above the nipple to re-centre it within the breast. If the tumour is central and the nipple–areola complex needs to be removed, then this can have a major effect on cosmetic outcomes.[1] This is why central tumours have been considered a relative contraindication to breast-conserving surgery. However, studies have suggested that excision of central cancers not directly involving the nipple–areola complex can be treated by wide excision and nipple preservation, and are not associated with a significantly increased rate of local recurrence compared with more peripherally situated cancers.[67] Good cosmetic outcomes are possible with this approach.[64] In women with moderate-sized breasts and cancers

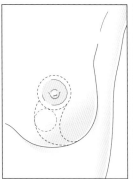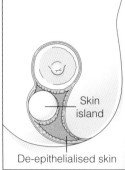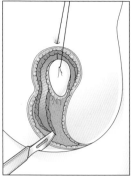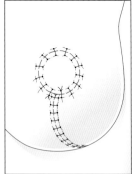

Skin island

De-epithelialised skin

**Figure 4.3** • How to excise a central cancer under the nipple and produce a satisfactory cosmetic outcome without major breast distortion. This procedure has been called central quadrantectomy. The nipple–areola complex is excised and a portion of skin inferior is marked out. An incision around the circular skin island is made and the remaining skin around the island is de-epithelialised. A full-thickness incision is then made in the breast and the skin island is rotated to fill the central defect. Staples are useful to position the flap. When the flap is deemed to be in an optimal position, the staples are removed and the wound closed in two layers with absorbable sutures.

directly involving or close to the nipple–areola complex, the nipple and areola can be excised in continuity with the cancer and the skin closed by a purse string and suture or by rotating a local flap from the lower part of the breast to fill the defect (**Fig. 4.3**). This so-called central quadrantectomy produces satisfactory long-term cosmetic outcomes and local control. In women with central superficial cancers in larger breasts, the nipple can be excised as part of a reduction-type procedure with direct closure, or the defect caused by excising the nipple and areola can be filled with a new island of skin developed on an inferior dermoglandular pedicle. This can only be performed if there is at least 9 cm of skin between the margin of skin excision and the inframammary fold (**Fig. 4.4**).

## Surgical factors

 The extent of surgical excision or the volume of resected breast tissue is the most important factor affecting cosmesis.[1,64]

The inferior cosmetic results obtained with quadrantectomy, even in the most experienced hands, compared with wide excision are well documented and are related to the much larger volumes of tissue removed by quadrantectomy.[18,66,68]

Even more critical is the percentage of the breast excised. There is a highly statistical correlation between cosmetic outcome and percentage of the breast excised (**Fig. 4.5**), with excisions of less than 10% of breast volume generally being associated with a good cosmetic outcome, whereas excisions over 10% usually produce a poor cosmetic result (**Fig. 4.6**). Where it is clear that more than 10% of breast volume needs to be excised in order to remove the cancer, then consideration should be given to volume replacement with a latissimus dorsi miniflap,[9,10] an oncoplastic reduction procedure, neoadjuvant drug therapy or a mastectomy with or without immediate reconstruction.

## Re-excision and number of procedures

Re-excision of the tumour bed has a negative impact on cosmesis.[1,64] This is mainly as a consequence of the increased total volume of tissue excised from the breast. There is no limit to the number of re-excisions that a patient can have to achieve complete removal of all invasive and in situ disease, but with the greater number of re-excisions the more tissue is removed, so cosmetic outcomes are more frequently poor in patients having two or more re-excisions.

## Axillary surgery

Axillary clearance seems to be associated with a worse cosmetic outcome than sentinel node biopsy or axillary sampling procedures, primarily because of an increasing risk of breast oedema.[1]

## Postoperative complications

Development of a seroma, haematoma or postoperative infection is associated with a worse cosmetic result.[1]

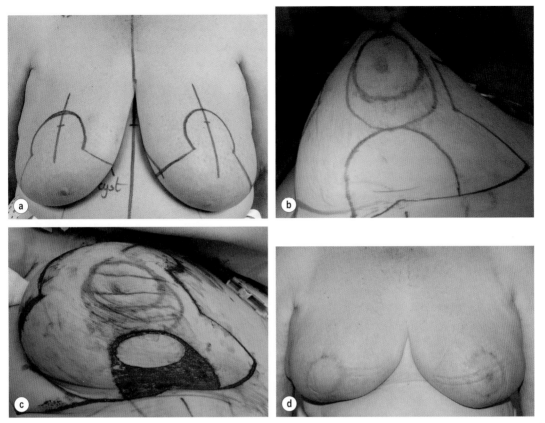

**Figure 4.4** • **(a)** Patient prior to operation – cancer under right nipple evident by asymmetry with right nipple flatter and right nipple higher than left. **(b)** Preoperative markings showing the area around the nipple which will be excised. **(c)** Operative view of the island of skin which is mobilised on a de-epithelialised inferior dermoglandular flap. **(d)** Final result after radiotherapy prior to nipple reconstruction.

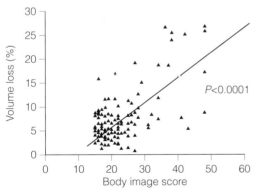

**Figure 4.5** • Percentage of breast excised compared with body image score. Percentage of breast excised calculated by measuring total weight of excision and estimating breast volume (from initial diagnostic craniocaudal mammogram). Body image score based on patient-administered questionnaire of 15 questions (score runs from 15, the best possible score, to 60, the worst and highest possible score). Data from a series of 120 patients treated in the Edinburgh Breast Unit.

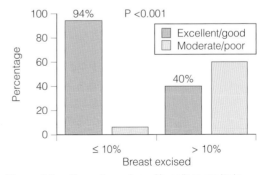

**Figure 4.6** • Percentage of good/excellent results in patients subdivided according to whether 10% or less or more than 10% of breast volume was excised by breast-conserving surgery.

## Breast-conserving surgery after neoadjuvant therapy

Significant numbers of patients are diagnosed with large or locally advanced breast cancer, many of whom are best treated by neoadjuvant chemotherapy or endocrine therapy. Up to a half of these patients will subsequently become candidates for breast-conserving surgery. To improve complete excision rates and minimise cosmetic deformity in these patients there are some guiding principles when performing breast conservation after completion of neoadjuvant therapy. First, it is important to know the exact site of the tumour within the breast, as some (10–15%) patients after chemotherapy will have a complete pathological response. All patients undergoing neoadjuvant chemotherapy who might be candidates for subsequent breast-conserving surgery should therefore have a tumour marker placed before or early during treatment. Second, the pattern of response to neoadjuvant chemotherapy and neoadjuvant endocrine therapy differs. The most common form of pathological change in patients undergoing neoadjuvant endocrine therapy is central scar formation.[69] It is thought this central scar results in concentric reduction in tumour size and tumour volume. Breast-conserving surgery following neoadjuvant endocrine therapy is therefore usually successful and few patients have involved margins. In contrast, a significant number of patients after neoadjuvant chemotherapy have a diffuse pattern of response with reduction in tumour cellularity but without significant shrinkage of volume. Much of this diffuse tumour is impalpable and approximately 25% of patients undergoing breast-conserving surgery after neoadjuvant chemotherapy will have incomplete excision of disease because of this pattern of histological response.

 MRI following neoadjuvant chemotherapy is the best of the currently available imaging methods to assess extent of disease and thus the likely success of breast-conserving surgery.[70]

All patients undergoing breast-conserving surgery after neoadjuvant chemotherapy should be warned of this possibility.

## Radiotherapy

Increasing doses of radiotherapy, particularly with the use of boost, have a detrimental effect on cosmetic outcomes.[38,71–74] Long-term follow-up is necessary to assess cosmetic outcome; 3 years after treatment, radiotherapy effects tend to stabilise. Fibrosis is a late effect of radiotherapy and produces breast retraction and contour distortion. Over time a treated breast loses tissue faster than the opposite breast and some patients develop increasing asymmetry over many years. The treated breast will not increase in size to the same extent as the opposite untreated breast, so patients who put on weight develop asymmetry even when the initial cosmetic result was excellent. The main reason boost has a negative impact on cosmesis is that it produces intense fibrosis and unsightly skin changes including telangiectasia.[38,64,72–74]

## Other treatment effects

Studies have suggested that tamoxifen and aromatase inhibitors have little if any effect on cosmetic outcome, whereas a few studies have shown that chemotherapy has a negative impact on cosmesis.[1]

## Treatment of poor cosmetic results after breast-conserving surgery

Options include augmentation of one or both breasts if the main problem is loss of volume without significant radiation fibrosis. Swelling following implant insertion in a radiotherapy-treated breast is often marked and takes many months to settle. Some patients develop marked capsular contraction after implant placement following radiotherapy but there are no data on whether the incidence is greater in this population than women having augmentation with no previous radiotherapy. If the problem is simply one of asymmetry and the treated breast is a satisfactory shape but smaller than the normal contralateral breast, then the contralateral breast can be reduced. If the treated breast is shrunken, misshapen and scarred, then either the whole or part of the treated breast can be removed and reconstructed. Pedicled myocutaneous latissimus dorsi or tram flaps offer an opportunity to excise unsightly skin and areas of breast distortion and scarring, and provide one option to regain symmetry (**Fig. 4.7**).

# Significance and treatment of local recurrence

Local recurrence rates vary widely in the literature but rates of 0.5% or less per year after breast-conserving treatment are now achievable. If local recurrence rates for any surgeon or any unit are consistently higher than 1% per annum, then a thorough audit of the practice of the surgeon or the unit is indicated.

 While an isolated local breast recurrence does not appear to be a threat to survival, breast recurrence is a predictor of distant disease;[6,7] the aim of primary treatment is thus to avoid local recurrence.

Isolated recurrences of the breast can be treated by re-excision or mastectomy.[75] Re-excision alone is associated with a high rate of subsequent local recurrence if the initial recurrence occurs within the first 5 years of treatment.[76] Until recently 80% of local recurrences in the conserved breast occurred at the site of the original breast cancer, with 90% of these local recurrences following breast-conserving surgery being invasive. This is no longer true and the majority of the 'recurrences' in treated breasts are now second primary cancers. Local recurrence within the first 5 years is associated with a worse long-term outlook than recurrence thereafter.[6,7] The role of systemic therapy following mastectomy for an apparently localised breast recurrence is not clear.[75] Uncontrollable local recurrence is uncommon after breast conservation, but when it does occur it is difficult to treat.

 A recent study has shown that extended hormonal treatment with letrozole following completion of 5 years of tamoxifen reduces so-called local recurrences by almost two-thirds (Table 4.3) and also reduces the rate of contralateral breast cancer development.[77]

Prolonging adjuvant hormonal therapy beyond 5 years thus has an impact on the rate of subsequent local relapse.

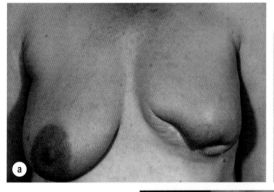
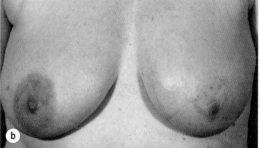
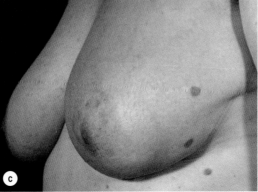

**Figure 4.7** • Patient with a poor cosmetic result after breast-conserving surgery before **(a)** and after **(b,c)** partial breast reconstruction with a pedicled latissimus dorsi myocutaneous flap.

Table 4.3 • Efficacy end-points in 4922 patients enrolled into the MA17 trials

| | Letrozole (*n* = 2463) | | Tamoxifen (*n* = 2459) | |
|---|---|---|---|---|
| | No. of patients | % | No. of patients | % |
| **Disease-free survival events** | 352 | 14.3 | 418 | 17.0 |
| Local | 19 | 0.8 | 38 | 1.6 |
| Contralateral breast | 14 | 0.6 | 26 | 1.1 |
| Regional | 13 | 0.5 | 11 | 0.5 |
| Distant | 182 | 7.4 | 212 | 8.6 |
| Deaths without cancer | 60 | 2.4 | 48 | 2.0 |
| **Deaths (overall survival events)** | 194 | 7.9 | 211 | 8.6 |
| **Systemic failures** | 331 | 13.4 | 374 | 15.2 |

Modified from Coates AS, Keshaviah A, Thurlimann B et al. Five years of letrozole compared with tamoxifen as initial adjuvant therapy for postmenopausal women with endocrine-responsive early breast cancer: update of study BIG 1-98. J Clin Oncol 2007; 25(5):486–92. With permission from the American Society of Clinical Oncology.

## Key points

- For patients with single small breast cancers, survival outcomes from breast-conserving treatment are equivalent to that of mastectomy.
- Radiotherapy (after breast-conserving surgery) reduces the rate of local recurrence and appears to improve overall survival. No subgroup of patients has yet been identified that can avoid radiotherapy.
- The major surgical factor influencing local recurrence is completeness of excision, and clear margins must be obtained when performing breast-conserving surgery.
- Wide margins do not appear to achieve better local control rates than margins ≥1 mm.
- Younger patients have an increased rate of local recurrence after breast-conserving surgery and, conversely, older patients have a lower rate of local recurrence.
- Tumour grade, EIC and LVI have only a small influence on the rate of local recurrence. Patients with these factors should not be denied breast-conserving surgery, providing the cancer can be excised with clear margins.
- There is a direct correlation between cosmetic outcome after breast-conserving surgery and psychological morbidity, with better cosmetic outcomes being associated with less anxiety and depression and better body image and self-esteem.
- The most important factor influencing cosmetic outcome after breast-conserving surgery is the percentage volume of breast excised. Removing more than 10% of breast volume results in the majority of women having a poor cosmetic outcome.
- Patients who develop local recurrence after breast-conserving surgery, particularly in the first 5 years, are at increased risk of having systemic relapse.
- Isolated local recurrences after breast-conserving surgery are usually treated by mastectomy, although re-excision is possible, particularly if the recurrence develops more than 5 years after treatment or the patient has not received radiotherapy to the breast.
- Prolonged hormonal therapy beyond 5 years reduces the rate of subsequent 'in-breast recurrence' and the rate of contralateral breast cancer.

# References

1. Sharif K, Al-Ghazal SK, Blamey RW. Cosmetic assessment of breast-conserving surgery for primary breast cancer. Breast 1999; 8:162–8.

2. Al-Ghazal SK, Fallowfield L, Blamey, RW. Comparison of psychological aspects and patient satisfaction following breast conserving surgery, simple mastectomy and breast reconstruction. Eur J Cancer 2000; 36:1938–43.

3. Shain WS, d'Angelo TM, Dunn ME et al. Mastectomy versus conservative surgery and radiation therapy: psychological consequences. Cancer 1994; 73:1221–8.

4. Early Breast Cancer Trialists' Collaborative Group. Effects of radiotherapy and surgery in early breast cancer: an overview of the randomised trials. N Engl J Med 1995; 333:1444–55.

   This review analyses data on 10-year survival from six randomised controlled trails comparing breast conservation with mastectomy. Meta-analysis of data from five of the randomised trials (3006 women) found no difference in the risk of death at 10 years. Where more than half of node-positive patients in both the mastectomy and breast-conserving groups received adjuvant nodal radiotherapy, both groups had similar survival rates. In contrast, where less than half of node-positive women in both groups received adjuvant nodal radiotherapy, survival was better for the breast-conserving surgery group (overall risk vs. mastectomy 0.69, 95% CO 0.5, 90% 0.57). Level I evidence.

5. Morris AD, Morris RD, Wilson JF et al. Breast conserving therapy versus mastectomy in early stage breast cancer: a meta-analysis of 10 year survival. Cancer J Sci Am 1997; 3:6–12.

   In this review nine randomised controlled trials involving 4981 women potentially suitable for breast-conserving surgery were analysed. Meta-analysis found no significant difference in the risk of death over 10 years for patients treated by mastectomy or breast-conserving surgery. The authors also found no significant difference in the rates of local recurrence in the six trials where data were available. Level I evidence.

6. Fortin A, Larochelle M, Laverdière J et al. Local failure is responsible for the decrease in survival for patients with breast cancer treated with conservative surgery and postoperative radiotherapy. J Clin Oncol 1999; 17:101–9.

7. Fisher B, Anderson S, Fisher E et al. Significance of ipsilateral breast tumour recurrence after lumpectomy. Lancet 1991; 338:327–31.

8. Dixon JM, Gregory K, Johnston S et al. Breast cancer: non-metastatic. Clin Evid Concise 2002; 8:355–9.

9. Dixon JM, Venizelos B, Chan P. Latissimus dorsi mini-flap: a technique for extending breast conservation. Breast 2002; 11:58–65.

10. Raja MAK, Straker VF, Rainsbury RM. Extending the role of breast-conserving surgery by immediate volume replacement. Br J Surg 1997; 84:101–5.

11. Fisher ER, Sass R, Fisher B et al. Pathologic findings from the national surgical adjuvant breast project (protocol 6): relation of local breast recurrence to multicentricity. Cancer 1986; 57:1717–24.

12. Kurtz JM, Jacquemier G, Amalaric R et al. Breast-conserving therapy for macroscopically multiple cancers. Ann Surg 1990; 212:38–44.

13. NIH Consensus Conference. Treatment of early-stage breast cancer. JAMA 1991; 265:391–5.

14. Holland DR, Connolly JL, Gelman R et al. The presence of an extensive intraductal component (EIC) following a limited excision predicts for prominent residual disease in the remainder of the breast. J Clin Oncol 1990; 8:113–18.

15. Veronesi U, Banfi A, Salvadore B et al. Breast conservation is the treatment of choice in small breast cancer: long term results of a randomised trial. Eur J Cancer 1990; 26:668–70.

16. Ghossein NA, Alpert S, Barba J et al. Importance of adequate surgical excision prior to radiotherapy in the local control of breast cancer in patients treated conservatively. Arch Surg 1992; 127:411–15.

17. Veronesi U, Volterrani F, Luini A et al. Quadrantectomy versus lumpectomy for small size breast cancer. Eur J Cancer 1990; 16:671–3.

18. Sacchini V, Luini A, Tana S et al. Quantitive and qualitative cosmetic evaluation after conservation treatment for breast cancer. Eur J Cancer 1991; 27:1395–400.

19. Fisher B, Wolmark N, Fisher ER. Lumpectomy and axillary dissection for breast cancer: surgical, pathological and radiation considerations. World J Surg 1985; 96:692–8.

20. Langer K. Zur anatomie and physiologie der Haut. Huber Die Spaltbarkiet Der Cutis. S-b-Akad Wiss Wein 1861; 44:19–46.

21. Kraissl CJ. The selection of appropriate lines for elective surgical incisions. Plast Reconstr Surg 1951; 8:1–28.

22. Osteen RT. Partial mastectomy, lumpectomy, quandrantectomy. In: Daly JM, Cady B (eds) Atlas of surgical oncology. St Louis: Mosby Year Book, 1993; pp. 113–21.

23. Vallasiadou K, Young OE, Dixon JM. Current practices in breast conservation surgery: results of a questionnaire. Br J Surg 2003; 90:44.

24. Beck NE, Bradburn MJ, Vincenti AC et al. Detection of residual disease following breast-conserving surgery. Br J Surg 1998; 85:1273–6.

25. Singletary SE. Surgical margins in patients with early-stage breast cancer treated with breast conservation therapy. Am J Surg 2002; 184:383–93.

   Ten-year follow-up of a cohort of patients treated by breast conservation reporting patterns of local, regional and systemic recurrence. Study reports low annual rate of breast tumour recurrence with a ≥1 mm margin.

26. Nedelman R, Dixon JM. Marking of specimens in patients undergoing stereotactic wide local excision for breast cancer. Br J Surg 1992; 79:55.

27. Bartelink H, Horiot JC, Poortmans P et al. Recurrence rates after treatment of breast cancer with standard radiotherapy with or without additional radiation. N Engl J Med 2001; 345:1378–87.

28. Kurtz JM. Factors influencing the risk of local recurrence in the breast. Eur J Cancer 1992; 28: 660–6.

29. Chauvet B, Simon JM, Reynaud-Bougnoux A et al. Récidives mammares après traitement conservateur des cancers du sein: facteurs prédictifs et signi-fication pornostique. Bull Cancer 1990; 77:1193–205.

30. Pierce L, Levin A, Rebbeck T et al. Ten-year outcome of breast-conserving surgery (BCS) and radiotherapy (RT) in women with breast cancer (BC) and germline BRCA 1/2 mutations: results from an international collaboration. Breast Cancer Res Treat 2003; 82:S7.

31. Calle R, Vilcoq JR, Zafrani B. Local control and survival of breast cancer treated by limited surgery followed by irradiation. Int J Radiat Oncol Biol Phys 1986; 12:873–8.

32. Fisher B, Anderson S, Bryant J et al. Twenty-year follow-up of a randomised trial comparing total mastectomy, lumpectomy, and lumpectomy plus irradiation for the treatment of invasive breast cancer. N Engl J Med 2002; 347:1233–41.

33. Fowble BL, Solin LJ, Schultz DJ et al. 10 year results of conservative surgery and irradiation for stage I and II breast cancer. Int J Radiat Oncol Biol Phys 1991; 21:269–77.

34. Haffty BG, Fischer D, Rose M et al. Prognostic factors for local recurrence in the conservatively treated breast cancer patient: a cautious interpretation of the data. J Clin Oncol 1991; 6:997–1003.

35. Asgiersson KS, McCulley SJ, Pinder SE et al. Size of invasive breast cancer and risk of local recurrence after breast-conservation therapy. Eur J Cancer 2003; 39:2462–9.

36. Eberlein TG, Connolly JN, Schnitt JS et al. Predictors of local recurrence following conservative breast surgery and radiation therapy. The influence of tumour size. Arch Surg 1990; 125:771–9.

37. Locker AP, Ellis IO, Morgan DAL et al. Factors influencing local recurrence after excision and radiotherapy for primary breast cancer. Br J Surg 1989; 76.890–4.

38. Kurtz JM, Jacquemier G, Amalric R et al. Risk factors for breast recurrence in premenopausal and postmenopausal patients with ductal cancers treated by conservation therapy. Cancer 1990; 65:1867–78.

39. Mate TP, Carter D, Fischer DB et al. A clinical and histopathological analysis of the results of conservation surgery and radiation therapy in stage I and stage II breast carcinoma. Cancer 1986; 58:1995–2002.

40. Zafrani B, Viehl P, Fourqhet A et al. Conservative treatment of early breast cancer: prognostic value of the ductal in situ component and other pathological variables on local control and survival. Long term results. Eur J Cancer Clin Oncol 1989; 25:1645–50.

41. Ryoo MC, Kagan AR, Wollin M. Prognostic factors for recurrence and cosmesis in 393 patients after radiation therapy for early mammary carcinoma. Radiology 1989; 172:555–9.

42. Jacquemier RG, Kurtz JM, Amalric R et al. An assessment of extensive intraductal component as a risk factor for local recurrence after breast-conserving surgery. Br J Cancer 1990; 61:873–6.

43. Fourquet A, Campan F, Zafrani B et al. Prognostic factors of breast recurrence in the conservative management of early breast cancer: a 25 year follow up. Int J Radiat Oncol Biol Phys 1989; 17:719–25.

44. du Toit RS, Locker AP, Ellis IO et al. An evaluation of differences in prognosis, recurrence patterns and receptor status between invasive lobular and other invasive carcinomas of the breast. Eur J Surg Oncol 1991; 17:251–7.

45. Schnitt SJ, Connolly JL, Kettry U. Pathologic find-ings on re-excision of the primary site in breast cancer patients considered for treatment by primary radiation therapy. Cancer 1987; 59:675–81.

46. Recht A, Danoff BS, Solin LJ et al. Intraductal carcinoma of the breast: results of treatment with excisional biopsy and irradiation. J Clin Oncol 1985; 313:39–43.

47. Gage I, Schnitt SJ, Nixon AJ et al. Pathologic margin involvement and the risk of recurrence in patients treated with breast-conserving therapy. Cancer 1996; 78:1921–8.

48. Smitt MC, Nowels KW, Zdeblick MJ et al. The importance of the lumpectomy surgical margin status in long term results of breast conservation. Cancer 1995; 76:259-67.

49. Solin LJ, Fowble BL, Schultz DJ et al. The significance of the pathology margins of the tumour excision on the outcome of patients treated with definitive irradiation for early stage breast cancer. Int J Radiat Oncol Biol Phys 1991; 21:279–87.

50. Spivack B, Khanna MM, Tafra L et al. Margin status and local recurrence after breast-conserving surgery. Arch Surg 1994; 129:952–7.

51. Wazer DE, Jabro G, Ruthazer R et al. Extent of margin positivity as a predictor for local recurrence after breast conserving irradiation. Radiat Oncol Invest 1999; 7:111–17.

52. Borger J, Kemperman, H, Hart A et al. Risk factors in breast-conservation therapy. J Clin Oncol 1994; 12:653–60.

53. Schmidt-Ullrich R, Wazer DE, DiPetrillo T et al. Breast conservation therapy for early stage breast carcinoma with outstanding ten year locoregional control rates: a case for aggressive therapy to the tumour bearing quadrant. Int J Radiat Oncol Biol Phys 1993; 27:545–52.

54. Montgomery DA, Krupa K, Jack WJL et al. Changing pattern of the detection of locoregional relapse in breast cancer: the Edinburgh experience. Br J Cancer 2007; 96:1802-7.

55. Abner AL, Connolly JL, Recht A et al. The relation between the presence and extent of lobular carcinoma in situ and the risk of local recurrence for patients with infiltrating carcinoma of the breast treated with conservative surgery and radiation therapy. Cancer 2000; 88:1072-7.

56. Fowble B, Hanlon AL, Patchefsky A et al. The presence of proliferative breast disease with atypia does significantly influence outcome in early-stage invasive breast cancer treated with conservative surgery and radiation. Int J Radiat Oncol Biol Phys 1998; 42:105-15.

57. Swanson GP, Rynearson K, Symmonds R. Significance of margins of excision on breast cancer recurrence. Am J Clin Oncol 2002; 25:438-41.

58. Wazer DE, DiPetrillo T, Schmidt-Ullrich R et al. Factors influencing cosmetic outcome and complication risk after conservative surgery and radiotherapy for early-stage breast carcinoma. J Clin Oncol 1992; 10:356-63.

59. Fisher B, Redmond C, Poisson R et al. Eight year results of a randomised clinical trial comparing total mastectomy and lumpectomy with or without irradiation in the treatment of breast cancer. N Engl J Med 1989; 320:822-8.

60. Rose MA, Henderson IC, Gellman R et al. Premenopausal breast cancer patients treated with conservative surgery, radiotherapy and adjuvant chemotherapy have a low risk of local failure. Int J Radiat Oncol Biol Phys 1989; 17:717-21.

61. Haffty BG, Fischer D, Beinfield M et al. Prognosis following local recurrence in the conservatively treated breast cancer patient. Int J Radiat Oncol Biol Phys 1991; 21:293-8.

62. Forrest P, Stewart HJ, Everington D et al. Randomised controlled trial of conservative therapy for breast cancer: 6-year analysis of the Scottish trial. Lancet 1996; 348:708-13.

63. Prosnitz LR, Goldenberg IS, Packard RA et al. Radiation therapy as initial treatment for early stage cancer of the breast without mastectomy. Cancer 1977; 39:917-23.

64. Dewar JA, Benhamou S, Benhamou E et al. Cosmetic results following lumpectomy, axillary dissection and radiotherapy for small breast cancers. Radiother Oncol 1988; 12:273-80.

65. Liljegren G, Holmberg L, Westman G et al. The cosmetic outcome in early breast cancer treated with sector resection with or without radiotherapy. Eur J Cancer 1993; 29A:2083-9.

66. Greco M, Sacchiai V, Agresti R et al. Quadrantectomy is not a disfiguring operation for small breast cancer. Breast 1994; 3:3-7.

67. Haffty BG, Wilson LD, Smith R et al. Subareolar breast cancer: long-term results with conservative surgery and radiation therapy. Int J Radiat Oncol Biol Phys 1995; 33:53-7.

68. Amichetti M, Busana L, Caffo O. Long-term cosmetic outcome and toxicity in patients treated with quandrantectomy and radiation therapy for early-stage breast cancer. Oncology 1995; 52:177-81.

69. Thomas JStJ, Julian HS, Green RV et al. Histopathology of breast carcinoma following neoadjuvant systemic therapy: a common association between letrozole therapy and central scarring. Histopathology 2007; 51:219-26.

70. Manton DJ, Chaturvedi A, Hubbard A et al. Neoadjuvant chemotherapy in breast cancer: early response prediction with quantitative MR imaging and spectroscopy. Br J Cancer 2006; 94:427-35.

71. Sneeuw KA, Aaronson N, Yarnould J et al. Cosmetic and functional outcomes of breast conserving treatment for early stage breast cancer. 1. Comparison of patients' ratings, observers' ratings and objective assessments. Radiother Oncol 1992; 25:153-9.

72. Christie DRH, O'Brien MY, Christie JA et al. A comparison of methods of cosmetic assessment in breast conservation treatment. Breast 1996; 5:358-67.

73. Hamilton CS, Nield JM, Alder GF et al. Breast appearance and function after breast conserving surgery and radiotherapy. Acta Oncol 1990; 29:291-5.

74. Kurtz JM. Impact of radiotherapy on breast cosmesis. Breast 1995; 4:163-9.

75. Anderson EDC. Treatment of breast recurrence after breast conservation. In: Dixon JM (ed.) Breast cancer: diagnosis and management. London: Elsevier, 2000; pp. 1-5.

76. Kurtz JM, Jacquemier G, Amalric R. Is breast conservation after local recurrence feasible. Eur J Cancer 1991; 27:240-4.

77. Goss PE, Ingle JN, Martino S et al. A randomized trial of letrozole in postmenopausal women after five years of tamoxifen therapy for early-stage breast cancer. N Engl J Med 2003; 349:1793-802.

# 5

# Techniques of mastectomy: tips and pitfalls

R. Douglas Macmillan

## Introduction

Mastectomy is used to treat approximately 35% of all breast cancers. The procedure can be accomplished using one of a wide variety of techniques depending on the clinical setting. Any mastectomy should be performed sensitive to the aims and principles of oncoplastic breast surgery. These are that optimal treatment of the malignancy should be achieved with minimal impact on quality of life.

Techniques of mastectomy are largely not evidence based. A few small trials exist but much of what is described in this chapter is based on reports of case series, expert opinion and personal preference. It is not intended to be prescriptive or dogmatic but merely a description of an approach to a commonly performed operation.

## General considerations

The patient may have risk factors for poor wound healing, which include:

- smoking;
- obesity;
- diabetes;
- poor skin quality;
- previous radiotherapy;
- severe comorbidities.

Of these, smoking is the most commonly encountered factor that can be improved to optimise outcome within the timescale of the urgent case. This and other factors may affect technique selection.

Other factors such as breast size, physical activities, preference for certain clothes (necklines) and expectations are all important discussion points that will influence choice of technique in many situations.

## Considerations for simple mastectomy

In addition to general considerations, four questions should be answered:

1. Is it necessary/desirable to excise skin overlying the cancer?

   In principle skin only requires to be excised if the cancer is involving the skin or is so close that a margin cannot clearly be achieved around it without skin resection.

2. Is there likely to be a lateral dog ear/redundant tissue?

   The all too frequently seen but completely avoidable complication of simple mastectomy is redundant tissue, also know as a dog ear, which is unsightly, causes difficulty with bra fitting and often chaffs on the prosthesis, arm or bra (**Fig. 5.1**).

3. Would the patient benefit from a contralateral reduction?

   This is a simple and very effective option to enable women with a heavy breast to wear a lighter prosthesis and feel less unbalanced (**Fig. 5.2a**). In some cases a woman may choose a bilateral mastectomy to achieve better overall symmetry.

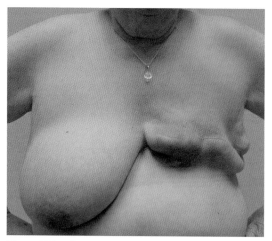

**Figure 5.1 •** Poor result from mastectomy.

4. Is a delayed breast reconstruction planned?

The scar should be sympathetic to the method of delayed reconstruction planned. In most cases a low scar is best if this is being achieved (as in Fig. 5.2a). It allows a flap-based reconstruction to be set at the inframammary fold with the upper scar low enough to be hidden in low-neckline clothes (**Fig. 5.2b**).

## Planning a simple mastectomy

- Examine the patient sitting up to assess lateral tissue and plan the likely lateral end of scar. The predicted lateral extent of the incision can be marked.
- Mark any skin that needs to be removed over the cancer.

- Decide if a second incision is required for sentinel node biopsy (usually not necessary in this setting).

### Technique

Most scars can be based around the inframammary fold (IMF). The incision pattern is drawn in theatre initially with a line at or just below the IMF (in women with any intertrigo the scar should be placed below this). Then with repeated upward and downward movement of the breast the planned transposition of this line on the breast skin can be marked (**Fig. 5.3**). In most cases the upper incision line passes a little above the areola. Attention should be paid to the degree of tension applied to the upward or downward breast movement as this represents the tension that will be exerted on the wound on closure. The upper and lower incision lines should be planned so that they comfortably meet but without excess laxity. The incisions should be planned to avoid any dog ear. To achieve this it is often best to continue the incision along the bra line laterally, curving up slightly until the upper and lower lines meet (**Fig. 5.4**) or, if there is doubt about how to fashion the lateral end, stop the incision at the lateral edge of the breast and fashion it once the mastectomy is complete, before closure (see comments regarding dog ear below).

Inferior broad-based flaps can be designed to allow skin excisions in the upper pole. In breasts with a high nipple position or in cases where skin excision in the upper pole is desired, the lower incision line can be adjusted to preserve skin on the lower flap. Such modifications to the inferior skin

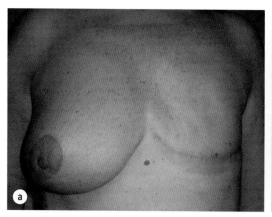
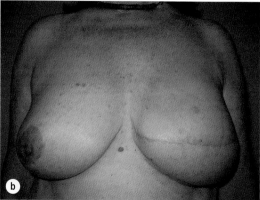

**Figure 5.2 • (a)** A low mastectomy scar with contralateral reduction. **(b)** Delayed reconstruction with LD flap.

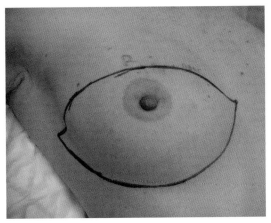

**Figure 5.3** • Drawing of IMF-based incision.

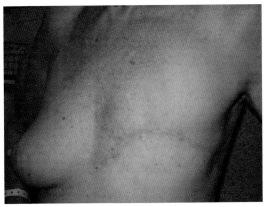

**Figure 5.5** • Dome-type mastectomy scar to allow excision of upper pole skin.

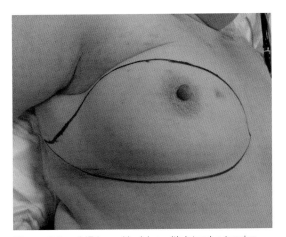

**Figure 5.4** • IMF-based incision with lateral extension.

flap should be broad based. Other scar patterns to consider in such situations are the Wise pattern or dome-shaped scar (**Fig. 5.5**).

### Lighting

A headlight is valuable and should be part of the equipment available for any breast operation.

### Retraction

Care should be taken with the edges of the mastectomy flaps. Sharp hooks or tissue forceps applied to dermis cause less trauma to mastectomy flaps than blunt retractors.

### Identifying the 'plane'

Some would contest its existence, but there is a readily identifiable plane between the breast and subcutaneous fat that defines the dissection. That is not to say

that it is obvious in every case and it may be quite irregular. Importantly, however, the subcutaneous vessels (extensions of the intercostal perforators) lie superficial to this plane. It is identified as a white line after performing a skin incision before the flaps are lifted and retracted. With opposing retraction on skin and breast and light initial dissection, tissues are seen to separate at the level of the plane. Dissection then chases this white line with continued opposing retraction (with skin hook retraction on the upper flap, skin kept as straight as possible), cutting on its superficial surface. This produces a flap of uniform thickness that will be thicker in fatter women and thinner in others.

### Surgical tools

My preference is to use a hand-held diathermy on a fulgurate setting throughout. Different surgeons have different preferences. Blood loss should be less than 100 mL if diathermy is used. Some prefer scissors or the knife because of concern of the 'burn' which results from diathermy dissection. Some use hydrodissection to identify the plane with a mixture of adrenaline (1:409 000) injected between the breast and subcutaneous fat. Following hydrodissection the plane of dissection can be identified with blunt instruments such as Hagar's dilators – dividing residual Cooper's ligaments with diathermy.

### Preserving the intercostal perforators

These represent the main blood supply to the mastectomy flaps once the breast tissue is removed. Their preservation is important not just for the prevention of flap necrosis and wound problems, but also to maximise the longer-term quality of the skin. The largest tends to originate at the second or third intercostal space. These are usually encountered early in the dissection just superior to the areola and can be seen (especially in thin women) and preserved during dissection upwards and medially.

### Issues regarding posterior margin

Strong opinions are often expressed regarding whether or not to excise the pectoral fascia and when to excise some muscle. The posterior plane or breast plate is very well defined, certainly in the middle and upper part of the breast. In these areas there is no need and no clinical evidence to support removal of the pectoral fascia. For simple mastectomy, preservation of the fascia is only an issue if the cancer lies posterior in the breast. If this is the case and there is any doubt about adherence to muscle then a section of pectoral muscle should also be taken. In such situations a wide margin of muscle excision avoids the situation where a margin is reported as histologically close (due to its contraction following fixation), at no additional cost in terms of morbidity.

### Inframammary fold

With a simple mastectomy this is normally excised, avoiding a ridge and enabling a flat surface.

### The anterior fat over the shoulder

This is often prominent and yet not part of the breast. If not contoured, it can produce a bulge in the upper outer aspect of the mastectomy site. Undermining the upper flap towards the shoulder often releases this fat pad so that it is more evenly distributed. Where it is particularly prominent and unsightly, at the end of the mastectomy it can be contoured with liposuction.

### A flat surface

After mastectomy, before closure, the chest wall should be palpated with the flat of the hand to make sure there are no ridges or prominent irregularities. If so these can be contoured prior to closure. There is some evidence that suturing the mastectomy flaps to the chest wall, so-called 'quilting', reduces seroma formation.

### Suturing

Interrupted deep dermal sutures to approximate skin edges and gather any discrepancy between upper and lower flaps is advisable prior to a subcuticular suture. My preference is to use 3-0 absorbable suture throughout.

### Managing the potential dog ear

Several techniques have been described for this. One approach is as follows. If the patient is fairly

thin, a flat lateral chest wall can be achieved by using an IMF scar as described above. In women with excess lateral tissue, it is often useful to complete the mastectomy with minimal extension of the scar laterally and then plan this part of the scar. The easiest way to do this is with temporary placement of skin staples. This then allows variations of lateral scar closure to be visualised before commitment to any particular one. They can be removed and replaced as many times as necessary to get the best scar. Final wound closure is with two layers of absorbable deep and superficial subcuticular absorbable sutures. Some lateral laxity can be accommodated by gathering the upper flap.

The two most useful techniques for lateral scar design in my experience are vertical extensions in the posterior axillary line or the fishtail technique (**Fig. 5.6**). When performing fishtailing use staples to approximate the wound edges and take the lateral edge of the transverse incision and staple it medially to flatten out the lateral end of the wound to leave two dog ears. Mark out these dog ears and then excisie or de-epithelialise these (this preserves the blood supply and stops the wound problems that some experience at the 'T' where the three wounds meet) to produce the fishtail pattern. Ensure that the wound is flat, if necessary by using liposuction. Liposuction can be a useful adjunctive technique in selected cases.

Cases in which difficulty with the lateral tissue is predicted preoperatively can be performed either with the patient on their side (ideally) or with some degree of rotation. Women with excess lateral tissue can be challenging cases, and should be managed by those familiar with a range of flap-based surgery as well as liposuction, and be planned preoperatively.

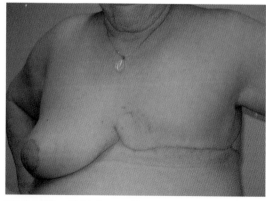

**Figure 5.6** • Fishtail scar with contralateral reduction (correction of case in Fig. 5.1).

Dressing

Glue provides a dressing that does not need to be changed, is waterproof (so patients can shower next day) and rarely produces skin reaction, so minimising further trauma to the skin surface around the flap edges.

## Bilateral simple mastectomy

Ideally these should be symmetrical. Bilateral IMF-based scars work well (**Fig. 5.7**). It is important to leave a skin bridge in the midline and not have a continuous scar across the chest.

## Undesirable scar patterns

High transverse and most diagonal scars should be historical other than in salvage situations, likewise any scar that does not leave a flat surface with a

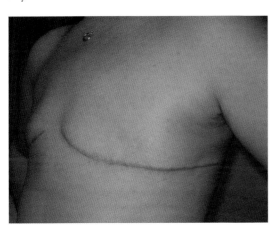

**Figure 5.7** • Bilateral IMF-based scars.

contoured lateral chest wall. Transverse scars rarely leave a satisfactory result without fishtailing at the lateral end and are not recommended.

## Considerations for mastectomy with immediate reconstruction

Of the general issues listed above, smoking is a particular concern and the major risk factor for flap necrosis and wound problems with skin-sparing mastectomy.[1]

The following questions should be considered:

- Is it necessary/desirable to excise skin overlying the cancer?

In general terms the same principles apply as described above. Skin-sparing mastectomy performed for reconstruction does, however, deserve discussion. Studies assessing the safety of this procedure relative to rates of local recurrence are summarised in Table 5.1. Although there are several that report acceptable recurrence rates, no large randomised trial data are available. It seems sensible to apply the same principles as one would for simple mastectomy. In other words, if the cancer is close to skin such that a healthy margin of normal tissue cannot easily be excised around it, then the overlying skin should be resected. An important principle of oncoplastic surgery is that treatment must not be compromised for the sake of cosmesis. Different designs of skin-sparing mastectomy can allow skin excisions at any site.

**Table 5.1** • Case series of over 100 patients reporting local recurrence rates after skin-sparing mastectomy

| Authors | Year of publication | Number of patients | Local recurrence rate/annum (%) | Follow-up (months) |
|---|---|---|---|---|
| Newman et al.[2] | 1998 | 372 | 1.5 | 50 |
| Kroll et al.[3] | 1999 | 114 | 1.2 | 72 |
| Medina-Franco et al.[4] | 2002 | 173 | 0.7 | 73 |
| Spiegel and Butler[5] | 2003 | 221 | 0.5 | 118 |
| Carlson et al.[6] | 2003 | 565 | 1.0 | 65 |
| Gerber et al.[7] | 2003 | 112 | 1.0 | 65 |
| Greenway et al.[8] | 2005 | 225 | 0.4 | 49 |
| Meretoja et al.[9] | 2007 | 146 | 0.6 | 51 |

# Chapter 5

- Is overall reduction or augmentation planned?

This will obviously influence the scar pattern planned to facilitate the adjustment and obtain optimal symmetry of scars.

- What scar design will give the optimum aesthetic result?

Familiarity with a range of different options will enable the best outcome. Designs will vary according to method of reconstruction as described below.

- Is scar position important for maintaining integrity of an implant pocket?

This consideration can arise if a partially submuscular implant placement is planned (see below).

- Is the nipple–areola complex to be excised?

This applies particularly to prophylactic mastectomy in small breasts but is sometimes considered and has been described in small series of cancer cases.[2–9] Scar placement in this setting should allow good access to the breast and the nipple itself.

## Planning a mastectomy with reconstruction

Examine and mark-up with the patient standing. Different techniques are best described according to whether tissue-based or implant-based reconstruction is being performed.

### Tissue-based reconstruction
#### Circumareolar

This is perhaps the most commonly employed technique. It gives excellent access to all but very large breasts. It can be extended easily by a lateral or inferior extension or by widening the circular skin excision. The resulting defect is replaced with skin from the flap, often with nipple reconstruction at the same time (**Fig. 5.8**).

#### Wise pattern

This is another commonly employed technique that can be used for any ptotic breast. The design is more conservative than would be used for a standard breast reduction, and is often best planned as very conservative with adjustment of the vertical limbs at the time of closure according to viability and tension. A vulnerable part of this design is the lateral part of the inverted 'T'. With division of the

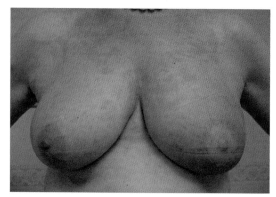

**Figure 5.8** • Circumareolar mastectomy with immediate LD flap and nipple reconstruction.

lateral thoracic vessels as part of the mastectomy, this often ends up as the most ischaemic part of the mastectomy flap. Designing an inverted 'V' component to the lower incision that will release tension at the 'T' junction is often prudent and this can always be excised if all skin edges look very healthy at the time of closure (**Fig. 5.9**). Likewise preservation of a larger section of lower flap skin until the time of closure enables the option of wider skin excision if viability is a concern.

#### Dome

This allows excision of an aesthetic unit of the breast of variable size. It also allows the flap to be inserted directly into the IMF. It is a very 'safe' design for higher risk cases.

#### Vertical

This is only really suitable for small breasts.

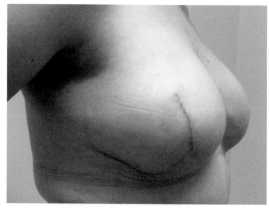

**Figure 5.9** • Preservation of inverted 'V' on lower flap in Wise pattern mastectomy with implant reconstruction.

## Implant reconstruction

### Wise pattern

This is probably the best option for the large breast and possibly any breast with some ptosis. It gives excellent access to the breast. It is particularly useful when a lower de-epithelialised flap is being used to create a partial submuscular/partial subdermal pocket (**Fig. 5.10a,b**). This has become a standard approach when available.

### Vertical

This is a good option in small breasts when a total submuscular pocket is planned. Shortening of the scar is rarely possible to any significant degree.

### Short transverse

This is sometimes a good option when a patient has a small areola that can be excised as a circumareolar incision but closed transversely.

## Is a second incision required for sentinel lymph node biopsy?

This is often prudent with skin-sparing mastectomy to allow a timely search for blue nodes and limit the degree with which skin flaps are retracted with small distal incisions to access the axilla.

## Subcutaneous mastectomy

A variety of incisions are possible. My own preference is for a skin crease incision starting just below and lateral to the areola and heading laterally as much as is required for access in a skin tension line (drawn with the patient standing). This gives good access to the entire breast envelope and particularly good access to the nipple. It is not visible to the patient as she looks down, seems to cross hardly any skin blood vessels and heals well (**Fig. 5.11**). An alternative in a small-breasted patient is an infero-lateral incision at the edge of the breast.

Other scar patterns to consider are as follows:

- **Hemicircumareolar.** This allows very restricted and in my opinion difficult access to the breast in all but very small breasts.
- **IMF.** This leaves a very long upper flap consisting of the entire breast envelope. Access is difficult in all but very small breasts.
- **Moire's curve.** This has similar restrictions to the IMF scar but the advantage of maintaining

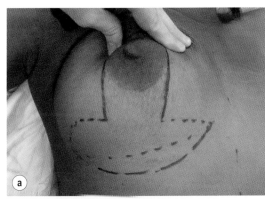

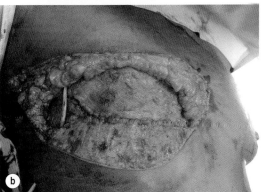

**Figure 5.10 • (a)** Drawing of a Wise pattern mastectomy. **(b)** Intraoperative demonstration of partial submuscular (pectoralis major and serratus anterior)/ partial subdermal pocket before skin closure.

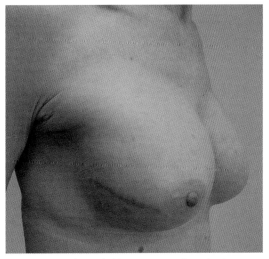

**Figure 5.11 •** Lateral skin crease scar for subcutaneous mastectomy.

the IMF. It can result in lateral deviation of nipple (although this can be a problem with all subcutaneous mastectomies).

- **Purse-string.** This is intuitive, but creates ischaemia at the skin edge, can result in a central sinus, stretches to produce an unsightly scar and results in a scar that presents difficulties for nipple reconstruction and tattooing.

Undesirable scar patterns are long transverse/oblique. These really have no role in immediate reconstruction.

## Technique

### Pre-operating marking

Mark with the patient standing. Put a mark on the midline and draw a dashed line around the circumference of the breast. For the periphery above the IMF take the weight of the breast and move it towards each periphery to enable the edge of the breast to be seen and marked. In practice this becomes most useful when a mastectomy is performed with the patient on their side simultaneous to raising a latissimus dorsi (LD) flap. Other markings will depend on the scar pattern to be used.

Circumareolar incisions can be marked pre- or intraoperatively. In women with a large areola some areola can be preserved.

For Wise and vertical patterns the breast meridian is drawn and patients marked up as for a reduction or mastopexy but with more conservative vertical incision lines (Fig. 5.11a). In Wise pattern mastectomy the vertical components are usually 10 cm in length from apex to horizontal incision. They often hug the areola margin. They can always be trimmed if necessary on closure. As described above, an inverted 'V' above the meridian at the IMF is prudent. In high-risk cases (smokers, larger breast, thin skin, concomitant axillary clearance), preservation of a lower skin flap allows judicious modification of the 'T' junction if required.

Dome-shaped incisions are based just above the IMF. The base width can be varied. The apex of the dome is on the breast meridian and can be extended to the required height.

### Lighting

A headlight is essential.

### Retraction

Sharp retractors such as skin hooks or sutures limit trauma to the skin edges.

### Identifying the plane

In a similar fashion to simple mastectomy, the plane is often best identified using opposing traction on the wound before skin hooks or similar retractors are applied.

### Dissection with limited access

A bloodless field is essential to allow visualisation of the plane of dissection throughout and preservation of the perforators. If access is really felt to be compromising the dissection, then the incision should be extended.

### Intercostal perforators

See the section above. Preservation becomes essential for good-quality skin-sparing mastectomy.

### Inframammary fold

This should be preserved.

### Pectoral fascia

It is an advantage to preserve this if an implant reconstruction is being performed as it adds reinforcement to a submuscular pocket.

### Suturing

The use of deep dermal interrupted sutures before subcuticular closure maximises wound quality.

### Skin stapler

This is particularly useful in Wise pattern mastectomy or any mastectomy where a skin-bearing flap is being inserted. The shape can be visualised and flaps trimmed as appropriate.

### Glue

Again, this produces a waterproof dressing that does not need re-dressing.

### Over-dressing

If a support over-dressing (e.g. gauze and Elastoplast) is used this should be lightly applied so as not to compromise mastectomy flap blood flow.

# Flap necrosis

Using the principles and techniques described this should be a rarity (1% or 2% of cases). The main reasons for it are smoking, technique selection, failure to preserve the intercostal perforators and too much tension of wound edges. In the circumstances

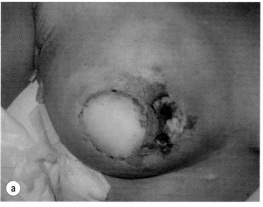
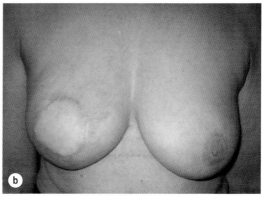

**Figure 5.12 •** **(a)** Skin necrosis after circumareolar mastectomy and LD flap in a heavy smoker. **(b)** Appearance a few weeks after early (next day) debridement and primary re-closure.

where flap necrosis is encountered, early surgical debridement may allow direct re-closure and usually results in a satisfactory outcome (**Fig. 5.12a,b**). Occasionally a small skin graft is required.

# Radical mastectomy

This still has a role to control locally advanced disease. In escalating order the following options for wound closure should be considered:

- abdominal advancement flap;
- split-skin graft;
- abdominal transposition flap;
- LD flap;
- deep inferior epigastric perforator/transverse rectus abdominis myocutaneous flap.

All have a potential role depending on size of defect, patient fitness and suitability of donor sites.

## Key points

### Simple mastectomy

- A flat, even chest wall should be achievable in all patients.
- The technique should be sympathetic if a delayed reconstruction is planned.

### Mastectomy with reconstruction

- Many techniques are available.
- The technique should be appropriate to the method of reconstruction.
- The technique should not compromise on access or cancer excision.

# References

1. Woerdeman LAE, Hage JJ, Hofland MMI et al. A prospective assessment of surgical risk factors in 400 cases of skin-sparing mastectomy and immediate breast reconstruction with implants to establish selection criteria. Plast Reconstr Surg 2007; 119:455–63.

2. Newman LA, Kuerer HM, Hunt KK et al. Presentation, treatment, and outcome of local recurrence after skin-sparing mastectomy and immediate breast reconstruction. Ann Surg Oncol 1998; 5:620–6.

3. Kroll SS, Khoo A, Singletary SE et al. Local recurrence risk after skin-sparing and conventional mastectomy: a 6-year follow-up. Plast Reconstr Surg 1999; 104:421–5.

4. Medina-Franco H, Vasconez LO, Fix RJ et al. Factors associated with local recurrence after skin-sparing mastectomy and immediate breast

reconstruction for invasive breast cancer. Ann Surg 2002; 235:814–19.

5. Spiegel AJ, Butler CE. Recurrence following treatment of ductal carcinoma in situ with skin-sparing mastectomy and immediate breast reconstruction. Plast Reconstr Surg 2003; 111:706–11.

6. Carlson GW, Styblo TM, Lyles RH et al. Local recurrence after skin-sparing mastectomy: tumor biology or surgical conservatism? Ann Surg Oncol 2003; 10:108–12.

7. Gerber B, Krause A, Reimer T et al. Skin-sparing mastectomy with conservation of the nipple–areola complex and autologous reconstruction is an oncologically safe procedure. Ann Surg 2003; 238:120–7.

8. Greenway RM, Schlossberg L, Dooley WC. Fifteen-year series of skin-sparing mastectomy for stage 0 to 2 breast cancer. Am J Surg 2005; 190: 933–8.

9. Meretoja TJ, von Smitten KAJ, Leidenius MHK et al. Local recurrence of stage 1 and 2 breast cancer after skin-sparing mastectomy and immediate breast reconstruction in a 15 year series. Eur J Surg Oncol 2007; 33:1142–5.

# 6

# Oncoplastic procedures to allow breast conservation and a satisfactory cosmetic outcome

Richard M. Rainsbury
Krishna B. Clough
Gabriel J. Kaufman
Claude Nos

## Part 1
### Volume replacement techniques to improve cosmetic outcomes after breast-conserving surgery

Richard M. Rainsbury
Krishna B. Clough

## Introduction

Breast-conserving surgery (BCS) combined with radiotherapy has become the treatment of choice for the majority of women presenting with primary breast cancer over the last 20 years.

 A number of prospective randomised trials have compared BCS with mastectomy, showing a survival rate that is unrelated to the type of surgery performed,[1–4] although local recurrence (LR) rates may be higher when the breast is conserved.[1]

The risk of LR is related to a number of factors, including positive margins, tumour grade, extensive in situ component, lymphovascular invasion and age. Whole-breast section analysis techniques have been used to show the likelihood of complete excision of unicentric carcinomas using different margins of excision (see Chapters 4 and 15).

 Holland et al.[5] showed that a margin of 2 cm would eradicate all microscopic disease in about 60% of cases compared with a margin of 4 cm, which increases this figure to about 90%.

## Local recurrence and cosmetic outcome

The margins of clearance and to a lesser degree the extent of local excision during BCS are strong predictors of subsequent LR.[6]

The extent of local excision remains a controversial issue in BCS. The wider the margin of clearance, the less the risk of incomplete excision and thus potentially of LR (Table 6.1), but the greater the amount of tissue removed, the higher the risk of visible deformity leading to an unacceptable cosmetic result. This clash of interests[8] is most evident when attempting BCS in patients with smaller breast-tumour ratios, for example when planning BCS for a 10-mm tumour in a 200-g breast or a 5-cm tumour in a 700-g breast.

The chances of a poor cosmetic outcome are increased still further when the tumour is in a central, medial or inferior location.[9,10] Cosmetic failure is

**Table 6.1 •** Technique-related outcomes of breast-conserving surgery

|  | Quadran-tectomy | Wide local excision |
|---|---|---|
| Margin (cm) | 2–4 | 1–2 |
| Clearance (%)* | <90 | <58 |
| Recurrence (%)† | 2 | 7 |
| Cosmesis | Fair | Good |

* Holland et al.[5]

† Veronesi et al.[7]

more common than generally appreciated, occurring in up to 50% of patients after BCS.[11–15] A number of factors are responsible, including volume loss of more than 10–20% leading to retraction and asymmetry, nipple–areola displacement or distortion, ugly and inappropriate incisions, and the local effects of radiotherapy. Volume loss underlies many of the most visible and distressing examples of poor cosmetic outcome and the effects may be compounded by associated displacement of the nipple–areola complex (NAC). Poor surgical technique leading to postoperative haematoma, infection or necrosis will increase the amount of scarring and retraction, and will add to the risks of deformity. Moreover, the use of suction drains, inappropriate incisions and en bloc resections can worsen the cosmetic result still further.

# Role of oncoplastic surgery

The interrelationship between breast-tumour ratio, volume loss, cosmetic outcome and margins of clearance is complex, and the widespread popularity of BCS has focused attention on new oncoplastic techniques that can avoid unacceptable cosmetic results. Until now, surgical options have been limited to BCS or mastectomy, the choice depending on fairly well-defined indications and factors. Oncoplastic techniques provide a 'third option' that avoids the need for mastectomy in selected patients and can influence the outcome of BCS in three respects:

1. Oncoplastic techniques allow very wide excision of breast tissue without risking major local deformity.
2. The use of oncoplastic techniques to prevent deformity can extend the scope of BCS to include patients with 3–5 cm tumours, without compromising the adequacy of resection or the cosmetic outcome.

3. Volume replacement can be used after previous BCS and radiotherapy to correct unacceptable deformity[16] and may prevent the need for mastectomy in some cases of LR when further local excision will result in considerable volume loss.

# Choice of oncoplastic technique

The choice of technique depends on a number of factors, including the extent of resection, position of the tumour, timing of surgery, experience of the surgeon and expectations of the patient. Reconstruction at the same time as resection (breast-sparing reconstruction) is gaining in popularity. As a general rule, it is much easier to prevent than to correct a deformity, as the sequelae of previous surgery do not have to be addressed. Immediate reconstruction at the time of mastectomy is associated with clear surgical,[17] financial[18, 19] and psychological[20] benefits, and similar benefits are seen in patients undergoing immediate breast-sparing reconstruction after partial mastectomy.

Resection defects can be reconstructed in one of two ways: (i) by volume replacement, importing volume from elsewhere to replace the amount of tissue resected; or (ii) by volume displacement, recruiting and transposing local dermoglandular flaps into the resection site. Volume replacement techniques can restore the shape and size of the breast, achieving symmetry and excellent cosmetic results without the need for contralateral surgery. However, these techniques require additional theatre time and may be complicated by donor-site morbidity, flap loss and an extended convalescence. In contrast, volume displacement techniques require less extensive surgery, limiting scars to the breast and avoiding donor-site problems. These procedures may be complicated by necrosis of the dermoglandular flaps and contralateral surgery is usually required to restore symmetry as volume loss is inevitable (Table 6.2).

A number of factors need to be considered when making the choice between volume replacement and volume displacement. Volume replacement is particularly suitable for patients who wish to avoid volume loss and contralateral surgery after extensive local resections. They must be prepared to accept a donor-site scar and be made aware of the possibility of major complications that may result in prolonged convalescence. Volume replacement is equally well

Table 6.2 • Comparison of techniques for breast-conserving reconstruction

| | Volume replacement | Volume displacement |
|---|---|---|
| Symmetry | Good | Variable |
| Scars | Breast+back | Periareolar inverted-T |
| Problems | Donor scar Seroma flap loss | Parenchymal necrosis Nipple necrosis Volume loss |
| Theatre time (hours) | 2–3 | 1–2 (per side) |
| Convalescence (weeks) | 4–6 | 1–2 |
| Timing | Immediate or delayed | Immediate > delayed |
| Mammographic surveillance | Possibly enhanced | Unaffected |

suited to immediate and delayed reconstruction and is the method of choice for correcting severe deformity after previous breast irradiation.

Volume displacement techniques are particularly useful for patients with large ptotic breasts who gain benefit from a 'therapeutic' reduction mammoplasty that incorporates wide removal of the tumour. Volume displacement is less reliable in irradiated breasts, and patients need to be warned about the risk of asymmetry that may require simultaneous or subsequent contralateral surgery.

# Volume replacement techniques

Several different approaches to volume replacement have been developed over the last 10 years, including myocutaneous, myosubcutaneous and adipose flaps, and implants. Autologous latissimus dorsi (LD) flaps are the most popular option because of their versatility and reliability.

The myocutaneous LD flap carries a skin paddle that can be used to replace skin which has been resected at the time of BCS or as a result of contracture and scarring following previous resection and radiotherapy[16] (**Fig. 6.1**). Although the skin paddle adds to the replacement volume, it can lead to an ugly 'patch' effect because of the difference in colour between the donor skin and the skin of the native breast.

 A myosubcutaneous LD miniflap[21] circumvents this problem by harvesting the flap in a plane deep to Scarpa's fascia. This produces a bulky flap without a skin island and carrying a layer of fat on its superficial surface that is used to reconstruct defects following wide excision with preservation of the overlying skin (**Fig. 6.2**).

Transverse rectus abdominis myocutaneous (TRAM) flaps provide a third alternative, but the bulk of these flaps renders them a less attractive choice than LD flaps in this particular situation. Moreover, fat necrosis is a more common

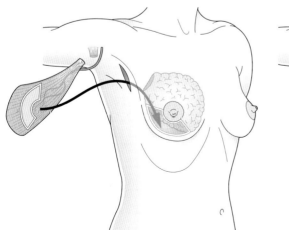
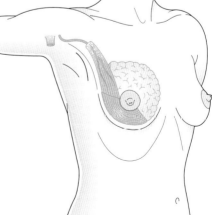

**Figure 6.1** • Latissimus dorsi myocutaneous miniflap.

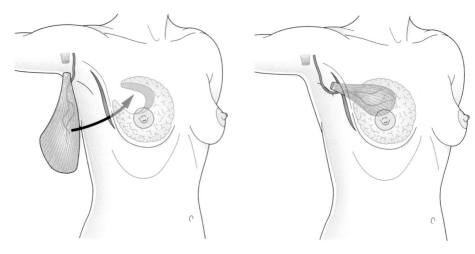

**Figure 6.2** • Latissimus dorsi myosubcutaneous miniflap.

complication of TRAM flaps, creating the potential for diagnostic confusion on follow-up. Other flaps, such as the lateral thoracic adipose tissue flap, have been described[22] but their clinical utility is unclear.

Non-autologous volume replacement with saline or silicone implants has been tried with very mixed success.[23, 24] Implants can be placed directly into the resection defect or under pectoralis major. They cannot be moulded to fit the resection defect and they form localised capsules, particularly in irradiated tissues. This interferes with not only clinical examination, but also mammographic surveillance. Autologous tissue transfer circumvents these problems, and results in a life-like breast of normal shape and size.

A number of innovative surgical procedures have evolved that facilitate volume replacement at the time of BCS or at a later date:

1. Resection through a radial incision and LD harvest through an axillary incision.[25]

 This was the original description by Noguchi et al. of the use of LD myocutaneous flaps to reconstruct resection defects during BCS in small-breasted Japanese patients.

2. Conventional LD myocutaneous flap harvest for correction of major resection defects.[16]
3. Resection through a circumferential incision and endoscopic LD flap harvest and reconstruction through an axillary incision.[26]
4. Resection, LD harvest and reconstruction through a single lateral incision.[22]

## Indications for volume replacement

Volume replacement should always be considered when adequate local tumour excision leads to an unacceptable degree of local deformity in those patients who wish to avoid mastectomy or contralateral surgery. Typically, this will occur after loss of 10–20% or more of the breast volume, particularly when this is resected from the central zone, lower pole or medial quadrants of the breast.

Breast conservation with or without reconstruction should be reserved for patients with unicentric tumours and is inappropriate in those with more widespread disease or locally advanced T4 tumours. Likewise, LD volume replacement is hazardous in patients with a history suggesting damage to the thoracodorsal pedicle or to the LD muscle, and alternative methods should be considered (Box 6.1). Patients should be informed that using LD for breast conservation precludes its subsequent use for full breast reconstruction. If a mastectomy is required to treat recurrent disease, the options are limited to TRAM flap or subpectoral reconstruction.

## Timing of procedures

Ideally, reconstruction of the partial mastectomy defect should be performed alongside tumour resection in order to prevent deformity rather than to correct deformity months or years later. The emergence of the multiskilled 'oncoplastic' breast surgeon will

Box 6.1 • Selection of patients for volume replacement

**Indications**

Breast of any size

Resection of 10–50% breast volume

Specimen weight typically 150–350 g

Correcting deformity after breast-conserving surgery

When mastectomy declined

When full reconstruction declined

When contralateral surgery declined

When radiotherapy planned after mastectomy

**Contraindications**

Multicentric tumours

T4 tumours

Diffuse malignant microcalcification

Comorbidity

Previous division of vascular pedicle

Previous ipsilateral thoracotomy

in future help to circumvent the current problems encountered when organising a 'two-team' approach involving breast and plastic surgeons. Moreover, immediate reconstruction is associated with fewer technical problems and complications than delayed procedures. Delayed reconstruction may be compromised by previous radiotherapy, leading to reduced tissue viability and an increased risk of fat necrosis, infection and delayed wound healing.

Immediate reconstruction can be carried out as a one-stage procedure,[22,27] which involves simultaneous resection and correction of the resulting defect. This requires perioperative confirmation of complete tumour excision using frozen-section techniques. As an alternative, the procedure can be split into two steps.[28] The first step involves the partial mastectomy and the second step includes axillary dissection, flap harvest and reconstruction, and is carried out a few days later after confirmation of clear tumour resection margins. Patients undergoing a one-stage procedure must be informed that a mastectomy with or without reconstruction may be required if subsequent histopathological analysis confirms incomplete tumour excision.

## Volume replacement with latissimus dorsi miniflaps

There are many similarities between the different surgical approaches used in breast-conserving reconstruction and these can be best illustrated by summarising

the main steps involved in LD miniflap reconstruction, which has been described in detail elsewhere.[29] This procedure involves the use of a myosubcutaneous flap of LD for immediate reconstruction of a partial mastectomy defect, most commonly in the central zone but also in the upper outer and upper inner quadrants of the breast. The term 'miniflap' is somewhat misleading, as the flap needs to be of sufficient volume to replace resection defects resulting from the excision of 150–350 g of breast tissue. Moreover, the miniflap needs to be bulky enough to allow for a small degree of postoperative flap atrophy.

When planning immediate volume replacement, the patient needs to be fully informed about the nature of the procedure and the possibility that a subsequent total mastectomy may be required if partial mastectomy results in incomplete excision. Careful preoperative mark-up of the tumour, the margins of resection and the line of incision are essential. The operation allows simultaneous partial mastectomy, axillary dissection, mobilisation of part of LD (the miniflap) and reconstruction of the resection defect through a single lateral incision. The procedure is greatly simplified by high-quality equipment, which is essential when developing the narrow optical spaces behind the breast and on the superficial and deep surfaces of the miniflap.

The operation involves tumour resection, axillary dissection, flap harvest and reconstruction. First, the tumour is resected in a subcutaneous plane by separating the skin envelope overlying the tumour-bearing quadrant from the underlying breast disc by sharp dissection, using the preoperative skin marks to determine the exact extent of dissection. By developing a mirror-image retromammary space deep to pectoralis fascia, the mobilised tumour-bearing quadrant is gripped firmly between fingers and thumb and resected with a generous margin of normal breast tissue. Four biopsies taken from opposite poles of the resection defect are sent for frozen-section analysis to allow intraoperative assessment of completeness of excision. The cavity wall is inked in situ with methylene blue to identify the inner surface, and then can be re-excised in its entirety if considered necessary. Further bed biopsies can also be examined after re-excising the cavity wall if frozen-section examination of the initial biopsies shows incomplete excision. A mastectomy is performed if these further bed biopsies fail to confirm complete excision. Next, appropriate axillary surgery (sentinel node or axillary dissection) is carried out and the vascular pedicle is prepared.

The third step involves mobilisation of the LD mini-flap by developing superficial and deep perimuscular spaces that mirror each other. The myosubcutaneous flap carries a layer of fat on its superficial surface to increase its volume and this is achieved by developing the superficial pocket just deep to Scarpa's fascia. Division of the miniflap around the perimeter of the dissection pocket and division of the tendon of LD near its insertion ensures unrestricted transposition of the miniflap into the resection defect. Finally, reconstruction of the resection defect is completed by careful use of sutures to model the flap, before fixing it to the cavity walls.

## Perioperative outcomes

The time required for breast-conserving immediate reconstruction with a miniflap lies somewhere between BCS alone and total mastectomy combined with immediate LD reconstruction. Early postoperative complications include infection, flap necrosis, haematoma formation and transient brachial plexopathy,[27] although postoperative stay and disability are similar to other types of BCS. Breast oedema is common, particularly after extensive segmental resection, and usually settles within 6–8 weeks. It may be caused by division of multiple afferent lymphatic pathways during retromammary dissection. Donor-site seroma formation occurs in almost all patients, and can be reduced by quilting or delaying drain removal. Flap necrosis is rare, and can be avoided by gentle resection and handling of the pedicle and by taking care to prevent traction and twisting injuries during transposition and fixation of the flap after tendon division.

Late sequelae of volume replacement include lateral retraction of the flap, leading to distortion and hollowing of the resection site, and flap atrophy. Flap retraction can be avoided by division and fixation of the tendon and careful suture of the flap into the resection defect. Detectable flap atrophy occurs in a minority of patients followed for up to 10 years.[30] It can be counteracted by over-replacement of the resected volume with a fully innervated flap that has been harvested with a generous layer of subcutaneous fat, or by using a myocutaneous flap.[16]

Frozen-section analysis of bed biopsies has been found to correlate closely with the adequacy of excision determined by formal histopathology (unpublished data). Moreover, the use of LD miniflap reconstruction leads to a significant fall in the number of incomplete excisions compared with BCS alone[22] without compromising the cosmetic outcome. Sensory loss following miniflap reconstruction is minimal compared with the loss following total mastectomy.[31] The sensory innervation of the breast and NAC is largely intact, except over the resected quadrant. Finally, volume replacement preserves symmetry, avoiding the need for alterations to the contralateral breast in almost all patients (**Fig. 6.3**).

## Mammographic surveillance

The mammographic appearance of the partially reconstructed breast compares favourably with the appearances after routine BCS. Symmetry is preserved and the fibres of the isodense flap may be detectable, often associated with a variable zone of radiolucency that corresponds to the layer of surface fat. Flaps may be indistinguishable from the surrounding breast

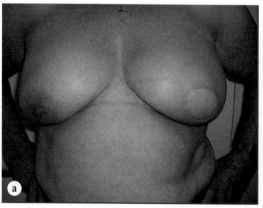
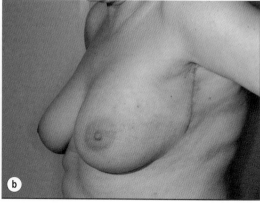

**Figure 6.3** • **(a)** Latissimus dorsi myocutaneous miniflap. **(b)** Latissimus dorsi myosubcutaneous miniflap.

tissue, and important radiological characteristics such as skin thickening, stellate lesions and microcalcifications are easily visualised after flap transfer. Volume replacement does not compromise the early detection of LR,[32] which typically develops at the junctional zone between muscle and breast parenchyma. The appearance of miniflap on mammograms contrasts with the radiodense distorting stellate scars that are a common source of diagnostic confusion following conventional BCS. Lastly, very few patients develop clinically detectable flap atrophy, with the majority of flaps remaining bulky and functional throughout the period of follow-up.

## Future prospects

The role of breast-conserving volume replacement is set to increase as more precise, image-guided resection of specific zones of breast tissue becomes possible. Increasingly sophisticated imaging techniques, such as high-frequency ultrasound and contrast-enhanced dynamic magnetic resonance imaging,[33] may in future enable exact delineation and excision of all malignant and premalignant changes. Endoscopically assisted techniques[34] may increase the ability to harvest more bulky myosubcutaneous flaps, allowing the reconstruction of more extensive resection defects. This will require the further development of novel techniques for endoscopic dissection,[26] including the use of balloon-assisted techniques[34,35] and carbon dioxide insufflation to maintain the epimuscular optical cavities. Current progress is hampered by the use of non-flexible straight endoscopes to carry out dissection over the rigid convex surface of the chest wall

## Deformities following breast-conserving surgery

Until recently, little attention has been paid to the cosmetic sequelae of BCS, as most patients are relieved not to lose their breast and many surgeons are unfamiliar with the plastic surgery techniques that can eliminate postoperative deformities. Moreover, there has been a tendency to recommend delayed reconstructive surgery some time after completion of radiotherapy. Although this is possible, partial reconstruction of the breast after surgery and radiotherapy is technically challenging and requires sophisticated techniques, with cosmetic results that are often disappointing.

In order to better assess the surgical approach for these patients, a classification of the cosmetic sequelae after BCS has been published by Clough et al.[36,37] This simple classification defines three groups of patients based on clinical examination (**Fig. 6.4**). The advantage of this classification is

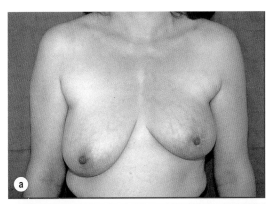

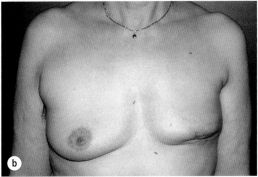

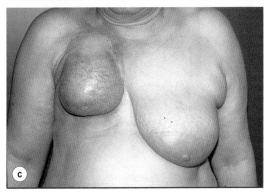

**Figure 6.4** • Deformities after conservative treatment of breast cancer. **(a)** Type I: a symmetrical breast with no deformity of the treated breast. **(b)** Type II: deformity of the treated breast, compatible with partial reconstruction and breast conservation. **(c)** Type III: major deformity of the breast requiring mastectomy. Reproduced from Klough KB, Claude N, Fitoussi A et al. Oncoplastic conservative surgery for breast cancer. In: Operative techniques in plastic and reconstructive surgery. Philadelphia: WB Saunders, 1999; pp. 50–60. With permission from Elsevier.

that it is a valuable guide for choosing the optimal reconstructive technique, but it is also a good predictor of the final cosmetic result after surgery.

- Type I deformities: patients have a treated breast with a normal appearance but there is asymmetry between the two breasts.
- Type II deformities: patients have a deformity of the treated breast. This deformity can be corrected by partial breast reconstruction and breast conservation, with the irradiated breast tissue being spared in the reconstruction.

Type III deformities: patients have a major distortion of the treated breast, or diffuse painful fibrosis. These sequelae are so severe that only a mastectomy can be considered.[36]

For type I deformities, a contralateral mammoplasty is performed to restore symmetry, avoiding any surgery on the irradiated breast. This is a simple and reliable approach, the irradiated breast serving as the model for a contralateral breast lift or breast reduction. Type II sequelae are almost always postoperative and are the most difficult to treat. A wide range of techniques can be used to repair these defects, from recentralisation of the nipple to the insetting of a flap to reconstruct a missing quadrant. Type III sequelae require treatment by mastectomy and immediate reconstruction with a myocutaneous flap.

Poor remodelling is one of the reasons for an ugly deformity after lumpectomy or quadrantectomy.[38,39] Some surgeons perform no remodelling at all, leaving an empty defect and relying on a postoperative haematoma to fill the dead space. This may produce acceptable results in the short term but breast retraction of larger defects invariably occurs with longer follow-up, leading to major deformities that are increased by postoperative radiotherapy.[10,36,40,41]

Reshaping of the breast is required after any tumour excision in order to recreate a normal breast shape in one operative procedure. In most cases this can be achieved with a simple unilateral approach, mobilising glandular flaps to close the defect or by recentralising the NAC. In other cases, a bilateral approach incorporating a bilateral mammoplasty will be the only way to perform a wide excision with no deformity.[42] This graded approach to breast reshaping is discussed below.

# Conclusion

Breast-conserving reconstruction extends the role of BCS by enabling complete excision of a greater range of tumours without compromising cosmesis, postoperative surveillance or symmetry. Volume replacement and displacement techniques are likely to become increasingly popular as an alternative to mastectomy in patients with small breast-tumour ratios and localised disease who wish to avoid more major surgery and the use of implants. Further experience of these techniques will lead to a better understanding of their role in the surgical management of primary breast cancer and in the management of local relapse and cosmetic deformity after previous breast-conserving procedures.

## Key points

- Local recurrence following BCS can be minimised by extensive local excision.
- Deformity following extensive local excision can be avoided by breast-sparing reconstruction using volume replacement or volume displacement.
- Volume replacement is most suitable for patients with small or medium-sized breasts who wish to avoid contralateral surgery. It can also be used for the correction of deformity following previous BCS.
- Breast-conserving reconstruction may be carried out as a one-stage or two-stage procedure.
- The type of breast-sparing reconstruction selected will be determined by the site and extent of resection, and by the patient's size, morphology and personal preference.

# References

1. Fisher B, Redmond C, Posson R et al. Eight-year results of a randomised clinical trial comparing total mastectomy and lumpectomy with or without irradiation in the treatment of breast cancer. N Engl J Med 1989; 320:822–8.

   A seminal trial (NSABP B-06) showing equivalent overall survival in patients with breast cancer treated either by mastectomy or by lumpectomy and radiotherapy.

2. Veronesi U, Saccozzi R, Del Vecchio M et al. Comparing radical mastectomy with quadrantectomy, axillary dissection and radiotherapy in patients with small cancers of the breast. N Engl J Med 1981; 305:6–11.

   A seminal trial comparing the treatment of patients with breast cancer by radical mastectomy or quadrantectomy, showing equivalent overall survival in each group.

3. Veronesi U, Banfi A, Del Vecchio M et al. Comparison of Halsted mastectomy with quadrantectomy, axillary dissection, and radiotherapy in early breast cancer: long-term results. Eur J Cancer Clin Oncol 1986; 22:1085–9.

   A seminal trial comparing the treatment of patients with breast cancer by radical mastectomy or quadrantectomy, showing equivalent overall survival in each group after long-term follow-up.

4. Abrams J, Chen T, Giusti R. Survival after breast-sparing surgery versus mastectomy. J Natl Cancer Inst 1994; 86:1672–3.

5. Holland R, Veling SH, Mravunac M et al. Histologic multifocality of Tis, $T_{1-2}$ breast-carcinomas: implications for clinical trials of breast-conserving surgery. Cancer 1985; 56:979–90.

   A detailed study using serial whole-breast sections to establish the distribution of breast malignancy in relation to the margin of the reference tumour.

6. Dixon J. Histological factors predicting breast recurrence following breast-conserving therapy. Breast 1993; 2:197.

7. Veronesi U, Voltarrani F, Luini A et al. Quadrantectomy versus lumpectomy for small size breast cancer. Eur J Cancer 1990; 26:671–3.

   A seminal trial comparing very wide local excision (quadrantectomy) with limited excision of breast carcinoma (lumpectomy). Quadrantectomy was associated with significantly lower rates of local recurrence when compared with lumpectomy.

8. Audretsch WP. Reconstruction of the partial mastectomy defect: classification and method. In: Spear SL (ed.) Surgery of the breast: principles and art. Philadelphia: Lippincott-Raven, 1998; pp. 155–95.

9. Pearl RM, Wisnicki J. Breast reconstruction following lumpectomy and irradiation. Plast Reconstr Surg 1985; 76:83–6.

10. Berrino P, Campora E, Sauti P. Postquadrantectomy breast deformities: classification and techniques of surgical correction. Plast Reconstr Surg 1987; 79:567–72.

11. Borger JH, Keijser AH. Conservative breast cancer treatment: analysis of cosmetic role and the role of concomitant adjuvant chemotherapy. Int J Radiat Oncol Biol Phys 1987; 13:1173–7.

12. Van Limbergen E, Rijnders A, van der Schueren E et al. Cosmetic evaluation of conserving treatment for mammary cancer. 2. A quantitative analysis of the influence of radiation dose, fractionation schedules and surgical treatment techniques on cosmetic results. Radiother Oncol 1989; 16:253–67.

13. Van Limbergen E, Van der Schueren E, Van Tongelen K. Cosmetic evaluation of breast conserving treatment for mammary cancer. 1. Proposal of quantitative scoring system. Radiother Oncol 1989; 16:159–67.

14. Olivotto IA, Rose MA, Osteen RJ et al. Late cosmetic outcome after conservative surgery and radiotherapy: analysis of causes of cosmetic failure. Int J Radiat Oncol Biol Phys 1989; 17:747–53.

15. Ray GR, Fish BJ, Marmor JB et al. Impact of adjuvant chemotherapy on cosmesis and complications in stages 1 and 2 carcinoma of the breast treated by biopsy and radiation therapy. Int J Radiat Oncol Biol Phys 1984; 10:837–41.

16. Slavin SA, Love SM, Sadowsky NL. Reconstruction of the irradiated partial mastectomy defect with autogenous tissues. Plast Reconstr Surg 1992; 90:854–65.

17. O'Brien W, Hasselgren P-O, Hummel RP et al. Comparison of postoperative wound complications in early cancer recurrence between patients undergoing mastectomy with or without immediate breast reconstruction. Am J Surg 1993; 116:1–5.

18. Eberlein TJ, Crespo LD, Smith BL et al. Prospective evaluation of immediate reconstruction after mastectomy. Ann Surg 1993; 218:29–36.

19. Elkowitz A, Colen S, Slavin S et al. Various methods of breast reconstruction after mastectomy: an economic comparison. Plast Reconstr Surg 1993; 92:77–83.

20. Dean C, Chetty U, Forrest APM. Effect of immediate breast reconstruction on psychosocial morbidity after mastectomy. Lancet 1983; i:459–62.

21. Raja MAK, Straker VF, Rainsbury RM. Extending the role of breast-conserving surgery by immediate volume replacement. Br J Surg 1997; 84:101–5.

22. Ohuchi N, Harada Y, Ishida T et al. Breast-conserving surgery for primary breast cancer; immediate volume replacement using lateral tissue flap. Breast Cancer 1997; 4:135–41.

23. Thomas PRS, Ford HT, Gazet JC. Use of silicone implants after wide local excision of the breast. Br J Surg 1993; 80:868–70.

24. Elton C, Jones PA. Initial experience of intramammary prostheses in breast conserving surgery. Eur J Surg Oncol 1999; 25:138–41.

25. Noguchi M, Taniya T, Miyasaki I et al. Immediate transposition of a latissimus dorsi muscle for correcting a post quadrantectomy breast deformity in Japanese patients. Int Surg 1990; 75:166–70.

26. Eaves FF, Bostwick J, Nahai F et al. Endoscopic techniques in aesthetic breast surgery. Clin Plast Surg 1995; 22:683–95.

27. Rainsbury RM, Paramanathan N. Recent progress with breast-conserving volume replacement using latissimus dorsi miniflaps in UK patients. Breast Cancer 1998; 5:139–47.

28. Dixon JM, Venizelos B, Chan P. Latissimus dorsi mini-flap: a technique for extending breast conservation. Breast 2002; 11:58–65.

29. Rainsbury RM. Breast-sparing reconstruction with latissimus dorsi miniflaps. Eur J Surg Oncol 2002; 28:891–5.

30. Laws SAM, Cheetham JE, Rainsbury RM. Temporal changes in breast volume after surgery for breast cancer and the implications for volume replacement with the latissimus dorsi miniflap. Eur J Surg Oncol 2001; 27:790.

31. Gendy RK, Able JA, Rainsbury RM. Impact of skin-sparing mastectomy with immediate reconstruction and breast-sparing reconstruction with miniflaps on the outcomes of oncoplastic breast surgery. Br J Surg 2003; 90:433–9.

32. Monticciolo DL, Ross D, Bostwick J et al. Autogenous breast reconstruction with endoscopic latissimus dorsi with musculo-subcutaneous flaps in patients choosing breast-conserving therapy: mammographic appearance. Am J Radiol 1996; 167:385–9.

33. Gilles R, Guinebretiere J-M. Magnetic resonance imaging. In: Silverstein MJ (ed.) Ductal carcinoma in situ of the breast. Baltimore: Williams & Wilkins, 1997; pp. 159–66.

34. Bass LS, Karp NS, Benacquista T et al. Endoscopic harvest of the rectus abdominus free flap: balloon dissection in the fascial plain. Ann Plast Surg 1995; 34:274–9.

35. Van Buskark ER, Krehnke RD, Montgomery RL et al. Endoscopic harvest of the latissimus dorsi muscle using balloon dissection technique. Plast Reconstr Surg 1997; 99:899–903.

36. Clough KB, Cuminet J, Fitoussi A et al. Cosmetic sequelae after conservative treatment for breast cancer: classification and results of surgical correction. Ann Plast Surg 1998; 41:471–81.

   The original classification of types of deformity following partial mastectomy and the use of therapeutic mammoplasty to avoid rather than correct deformity.

37. Clough KB, Thomas SS, Fitoussi AD et al. Reconstruction after conservative treatment for breast cancer: cosmetic sequelae classification revisited. Plast Reconstr Surg 2004; 114(7):1743–53.

38. Petit J-Y, Rigault L, Zekri A et al. Poor esthetic results after conservative treatment of breast cancer. Techniques of partial breast reconstruction. Ann Chir Plast Esthet 1989; 34:103–8.

39. Rose MA, Olivotto IA, Cady B et al. Conservative surgery and radiation therapy for early breast cancer. Long-term cosmetic results. Arch Surg 1989; 124:153–7.

40. Berrino P, Campora E, Leone S et al. Correction of type II breast deformities following conservative cancer surgery. Plast Reconstr Surg 1992; 90:846–53.

41. Petit J-Y, Rietjens M. Deformities following tumourectomy and partial mastectomy. In: Noone B (ed.) Plastic and reconstruction surgery of the breast. Philadelphia: BC Decker, 1991.

42. Clough KB, Kroll S, Audretsch W. An approach to the repair of partial mastectomy defects. Plast Reconstr Surg 1999; 104:409–20.

   Pooled experience of breast-conserving reconstruction from France, USA and Germany using volume replacement and volume displacement techniques.

# Part 2
# Breast displacement techniques to increase resection volumes for breast-conserving surgery

Krishna B. Clough
Gabriel J. Kaufman
Claude Nos

## Introduction

Breast-conserving surgery (BCS) combined with postoperative radiotherapy has become the preferred locoregional treatment for the majority of patients with early-stage breast cancer, with equivalent survival to that of mastectomy and improved body image and lifestyle score. The success of BCS for breast cancer is based on the tenet of complete removal of the cancer with adequate surgical margins while preserving the natural shape and appearance of the breast. Achieving both goals together in the same operation can be challenging, and BCS has not always produced good cosmetic results in all patients. The limiting factor is the amount of tissue removed, not only in absolute volume, but also in relation to tumour location and relative size of breast. If either of these two goals is not achievable, mastectomy is often chosen as an alternative to BCS. The failure of classical BCS techniques to offer solutions for challenging scenarios has stimulated the growth and advancement of new techniques in breast surgery during the past decade.

The dichotomy between extent of excision and cosmetic outcome has made it evident that new surgical techniques need to be developed to address the problems and shortfalls of BCS, and accommodate the expanding indications for BCS.

Oncoplastic surgery (OPS) has emerged as a new approach to allow wide excisions for BCS without compromising the natural shape of the breast. It is based upon integration of plastic surgery techniques for immediate reshaping of the breast after a wide excision for breast cancer. The conceptual idea of OPS is not new and its oncological efficacy in terms of margin status and recurrence compare favourably to traditional BCS.[1,2]

The difference in the level of difficulty in performing various oncoplastic procedures has created a dichotomy in oncoplastic surgery. Complexity of oncoplastic techniques ranges from simple reshaping and mobilisation of breast tissue to more advanced mammoplasty techniques that allow resection of up to 50% of the breast volume. Variations in difficulty and the need for advanced training for some OPS techniques requires a clear classification system of oncoplastic techniques which provides a systematic approach that all breast surgeons can follow when undertaking BCS.

# Oncoplastic considerations

## Selection criteria for oncoplasty

There are three elements that are important in the identification of patients that would benefit from an oncoplastic approach. The two factors already recognised as major indications for OPS are excision volume and tumour location.[3] The third additional element is glandular density, a new concept in the determination of the safest OPS approach required for breast reshaping. When considered together, these three major elements provide a sound basis for determining when and what type of OPS to perform and more importantly in reducing the guesswork when performing BCS.

### Volume

The first element is excision volume, which is the single most predictive factor of surgical outcome and potential for breast deformity. Studies have suggested that once 20% of the breast volume is excised there is a clear risk of deformity.[4]

Excision volume compared to the total breast volume is estimated preoperatively. Through systematic correlation of specimen weights compared with tumour size, an accurate preoperative estimation of excision volume can be achieved, once the tumour size is known from preoperative imaging. The average specimen from BCS should weigh between 20 and 40 g, and as a general rule 80 g of breast tissue is the maximum weight that can be removed from a medium-sized breast without resulting in deformity (see Chapter 4).

OPS techniques allow for significantly greater excision volumes while preserving the natural breast shape. Reshaping of the breast is based upon rearrangement of breast parenchyma to create a homogeneous redistribution of volume loss. This redistribution can be achieved easily though either the advancement or rotation of breast tissue into excision defects. Another option is to harvest a latissimus dorsi 'miniflap' to fill in the lumpectomy cavity (see Part 1 of this chapter).[3]

### Tumour location

High-risk zones in the breast are more likely to be followed by deformity after BCS when compared to more forgiving locations.

The upper outer quadrant of the breast is a favourable location for large-volume excisions. In this location, defects can readily be corrected by the mobilisation of adjacent tissue. Excision from less favourable locations such as the lower pole or upper inner quadrants of the breast often results in breast deformity.

For example, the 'bird's beak' deformity is classically seen during excision of tumours from the lower pole of the breast (**Fig. 6.5a**). Other examples of poor results are seen with excision of a central tumour (**Fig. 6.5b**) and upper inner quadrant (**Fig. 6.5c**). Therefore, a basic tool used in planning the appropriate surgical approach is evaluating the tumour location and the likely level of associated deformity. With this knowledge, an oncoplastic atlas of surgical techniques has been based on tumour location. The atlas provides a specific surgical technique for each possible tumour location in the breast.

### Glandular characteristics and breast density

Glandular density is evaluated both clinically and radiographically. Although clinical examination provides reliable information on density, mammographic evaluation is a more reproducible approach

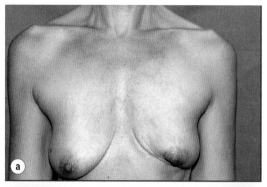

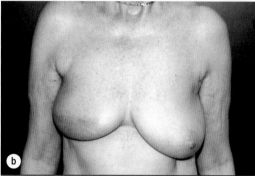

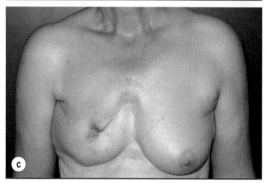

**Figure 6.5** • Deformities after breast-conserving surgery. **(a)** Lower pole: bird's beak deformity. **(b)** Central tumour. **(c)** Upper inner quadrant.

for breast density determination. Breast density predicts the amount of fat in the breast and determines the ability to perform extensive breast undermining and reshaping without complications. Breast density can be classified into four categories based on the Breast Imaging Reporting and Data System (BI-RADS). The four categories comprise: (1) fatty; (2) scattered fibroglandular; (3) heterogeneously dense; or (4) extremely dense breast tissue.[5]

A dense glandular breast (BI-RADS 3/4) can be mobilised easily with undermining and advancement of breast tissue into the excision cavity with-

out risk of necrosis. Low-density breast tissue with a major fatty component (BI-RADS 1/2) has a much higher risk of fat necrosis if extensive undermining is required. Undermining the breast from both the skin and pectoralis fascia is a major requirement to perform level I OPS. A low breast density means that either the amount of undermining from the breast and skin during level I OPS should be limited, or a decision made to proceed with a level II option that requires limited skin undermining. Level II procedures that require extensive skin undermining such as the round-block procedure are likewise not suitable for the patient with a predominantly fatty breast.

# Classification system

## Complexity of surgical procedure: a bi-level system

A new classification of OPS techniques is proposed that is based upon the relative level of surgical difficulty. Level I techniques should be able to be performed by all breast surgeons without specific training in OPS. A level I approach includes skin and glandular undermining, including the nipple–areola complex (NAC), and NAC recentralisation if nipple deviation is anticipated. Level II techniques encompass more complex procedures that involve skin excision and glandular mobilisation to allow major volume resection. Level II techniques are derived from breast reduction techniques and require additional training.

The bi-level classification system lends itself to the creation of a practical guide to OPS and provides the necessary framework during surgical planning to correctly select the most appropriate surgical procedure for the patient (Table 6.3).

If less than 20% of the breast volume is excised then a level II approach is not usually required and a level I procedure is usually adequate. Anticipation that 20–50% of breast volume excision is to be

**Table 6.3** • Oncoplastic decision guide

| Criteria | Level I | Level II |
|---|---|---|
| Maximum excision volume ratio | 20% | 20–50% |
| Requirement of skin excision for reshaping | No | Yes |
| Specific training in reduction and mammoplasty techniques | No | Yes |
| Glandular characteristics | Dense | Dense or fatty |

excised will require a level II procedure to produce a satisfactory cosmetic outcome. Large-volume excisions require concurrent skin excision to adequately reshape the skin envelope. Another important consideration is glandular density. If the breast parenchyma is fatty in composition, it may be risky to employ a level I technique if excising more than 10% of the breast volume. A superior outcome is likely to be obtained in such patients by selecting an appropriate level II procedure.

## General considerations for all OPS techniques

The approach to OPS includes careful patient selection and starts with patient counselling. It is important to stress to the patient that although oncoplastic procedures can provide greater satisfaction with a better final breast shape and in some situations will avoid the need for mastectomy, outcomes do vary. During the consultation period patients need to be informed that OPS will result in longer and multiple scars. The position of each incision should be described in detail. The patient should also be made aware of the possible asymmetry that will follow from a level II OPS. Asymmetry in volume is expected, but necessary to limit breast distortion and deformity. The patient must be informed that in such circumstances to achieve symmetry an immediate reduction of the contralateral side can be performed at the same time or later as a second-stage procedure.

All oncoplastic procedures begin with preoperative marking of the patient sitting upright or standing prior to the induction of anaesthesia. Once marked, the patient is carefully centred on the operating room table and secured so that she can be moved from the supine to the upright position during the operation. The arms can be extended if any axillary surgery is planned, or secured by the side if no axillary surgery is required. Movement between these positions allows optimisation of contralateral breast symmetry and allows for optimal reshaping.

## Level I oncoplastic techniques

### The step-by-step approach for level I OPS

The driving force behind level I OPS is the ability of all surgeons to adopt the following steps into their surgical practice. There are six general steps for level

I OPS that begin with the skin incision (1) followed by undermining of the skin (2) and NAC (3). After completion of undermining, a full-thickness glandular excision incorporating the cancer and a surrounding rim of normal breast tissue is performed from subcutaneous fat down to pectoralis fascia (4). The glandular defect is subsequently closed following specimen X-ray to demonstrate complete radiological excision with tissue re-approximation (5). If required, an area in the shape of a crescent bordering the areola can be de-epithelialised to reposition the NAC (6). If this is not performed the NAC displaces towards the site of excision and is no longer positioned in the centre of the breast mound.

## Incisions

The concepts of oncoplastic surgery are not based on minimising incision length. Short incision lengths limit mobilisation of the gland and do not allow creation of adequate glandular flaps to fill excision defects.

 Effective mobilisation of the gland is a key component in achieving a natural breast shape.

In our experience, OPS is not minimally invasive surgery. The location of the incision is at the discretion of the operating surgeon. In general, incisions should allow for both en bloc excision of the cancer, without causing fragmentation of the specimen, and also allow undermining of the surrounding breast tissue to facilitate reshaping. The general principle for placing incisions is to follow Kraissl's lines of maximum resting skin tension to limit visible scaring[6] (see Chapter 4). However, in many cases an incision away from the cancer is possible such as along the areola border with radial extension towards the tumour or in the inframammary fold for cancers in the lower half of the breast.

## Skin undermining

Extensive subcutaneous undermining ranging from one-half to two-thirds of the breast envelope may be required to facilitate glandular redistribution after removal of the tumour (**Fig. 6.6a**). Aggressive undermining can free an entire quadrant from the overlying skin envelope. In terms of technique, it is easier to undermine a large area of skin before excising the lesion.

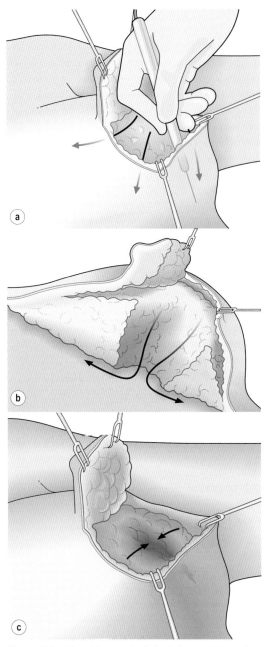

Figure 6.6 • Level I oncoplastic techniques: skin and NAC undermining. **(a)** Extensive skin undermining. **(b)** Wide excision from subcutaneous fat to muscle, then NAC undermining. **(c)** Glandular flap re-approximation.

Risk factors for vascular compromise should be evaluated prior to performing extensive undermining. Smoking, diabetes mellitus and connective tissue disease should be taken into consideration prior to planning the surgery to be performed.

Although smoking does not prevent the completion of a safe level I oncoplasty, it decreases the total area of skin that can be safely undermined. Patients who smoke should be warned of the greater risk of complications and advised to reduce or stop smoking for as long as possible before and immediately after surgery.

The area of undermining should be inversely proportional to the number of risk factors present, but the final factor in determining the amount of undermining that is safe is the fat composition of the breast. Division of the perforating blood vessels in a fatty breast is much more of a problem, and to maintain tissue vascularity and reduce the risk of postoperative necrosis, a level II procedure, which involves direct glandular excision and less skin undermining, should be considered if extensive undermining is considered necessary to close the defect.

## Nipple–areola complex undermining

Major NAC distortion is a common cause of breast deformity.

Fibrosis after surgery creates tension on adjacent tissue, which results in NAC deviation towards the area of excision. Fortunately, NAC repositioning can be performed easily with simple undermining and this is a key component of both level I and II OPS. The first step is to completely transect the terminal ducts under the nipple and separate the NAC from the underlying breast tissue. A width of 0.5–1 cm of glandular tissue is generally left attached to the nipple to ensure the integrity of its vascular supply. This amount of subareolar tissue prevents NAC necrosis and limits venous congestion. The level of NAC sensitivity is reduced by extensive mobilisation and undermining and patients should be warned of this.[7]

## Tissue excision

The standard approach is to perform a full-thickness excision from the subcutaneous fat underlying the skin down to the pectoral fascia.

Full-thickness excision ensures free anterior and posterior margins, leaving only the lateral margins in question (**Fig. 6.6b**).

The breast parenchyma itself can be excised in a fusiform pattern oriented towards the NAC to facilitate re-approximation of the remaining gland. Before closing the defect, metal clips are placed on the lateral edges of the tissue defect in the breast to guide future radiotherapy. For superficial or deep cancers in breasts with an anterior posterior distance of >4 cm then full-thickness excisions are not always required. Preoperative imaging is valuable in planning such excisions.

## Re-approximation of the glandular defect

During BCS, breast tissue is either re-approximated or left open allowing for the eventual formation of a haematoma or seroma. Seroma formation, however, does not always result in predictable long-term cosmetic results for larger volume excisions. Once reabsorption of the seroma occurs, the excision cavity becomes prominent due to fibrosis and retraction of the surrounding tissue, creating a noticeable defect and causing NAC displacement. For this reason, where there has been an extensive resection redistribution of the volume loss is required. Tissue mobilised from lateral portions of the remaining gland or recruited from the central part of the breast allows the creation of glandular flaps that can be sutured together to close the defect (**Fig. 6.6c**).

## De-epithelialisation and NAC repositioning

A major source of patient dissatisfaction after BCS is the unnatural position of the NAC because it is deviated towards the excision site. This is likely to happen after all extensive volume resections. NAC repositioning is difficult to attempt later after radiotherapy, so immediate recentralisation is preferred and the need to recentralise the NAC should be anticipated during initial resection.

Avoiding NAC displacement is a key element for both level I and II OPS. The NAC is repositioned to adjust for both the anticipated deviation and the new shape of the breast. An area of periareolar skin opposite the excision defect is de-epithelialised in the shape of a crescent (**Fig. 6.7a–c**). De-epithelialisation should be achieved sharply, using a scalpel blade or fine scissors. This technique is simple and safe and used systematically in aesthetic surgery of the breast. The vascular supply of the NAC after its separation from the gland and de-epithelialisation is based on the vasculature from the dermal plexure and this is not compromised by careful de-epithelialisation.[8]

# Level II oncoplastic surgery

## Introduction

The major consideration when choosing between OPS levels is the extent of excision volume. A level I approach is suitable for excision volumes less than 20% of the entire gland. The resulting glandular defect can usually be filled by advancement of adjacent tissue. Level II techniques are generally reserved for situations that require major volume excisions between 20% and 50%.

To simplify the selection of a level II OPS technique, an atlas has been devised based on tumour location. This atlas does not contain an exhaustive list of options, but provides one or two options for each location.

## Atlas principles

The concept of this oncoplastic atlas is based primarily on tumour location. Initially used only for lower pole tumours, OPS has evolved to allow resection of breast lesions located almost anywhere in the breast. Different mammoplasty techniques have been adapted for specific locations in the breast.[9]

The superior pedicle reduction mammoplasty is a model for the description of all mammoplasty techniques. Schematically rotating the NAC on a pedicle based directly opposite the site of tumour excision allows the application of this technique for a variety of tumour locations. These procedures are listed in an anticlockwise direction and described for the left breast.

Level II OPS will generally result in a smaller breast which is rounder and higher on the chest wall than the contralateral breast, thus the need for a contralateral symmetrisation and the necessity to discuss this with the patient prior to the excision. Either immediate or delayed symmetrisation can be performed depending on the amount of tissue resected and the desire of the patient.

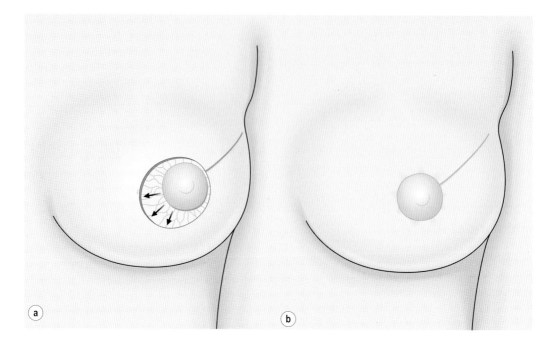

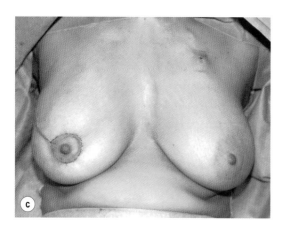

**Figure 6.7** • Level I oncoplastic techniques: NAC recentralisation. **(a)** De-epithelialisation opposite the tumour bed. **(b)** NAC recentralisation. **(c)** Intraoperative result (upper outer quadrant resection).

## Lower pole location (4–7 o'clock)

### General principles

The lower pole of the breast was the first location recognised to be at high risk of deformity following BCS.[1] Removal of tissue from the 6 o'clock position results in retraction of the skin and downward deviation of the NAC, producing what is known as the 'bird's beak' deformity, which results in a low level of patient satisfaction. A superior pedicle mammoplasty can allow for large-volume excision of the lower pole without causing NAC deviation and has the added benefit of breast reshaping and elevation.

### Techniques

'Standard' superior pedicle mammoplasty with inverted-T scar **(Fig. 6.8a–e)**

The superior pedicle mammoplasty technique that is in routine use involves using the inverted-T and

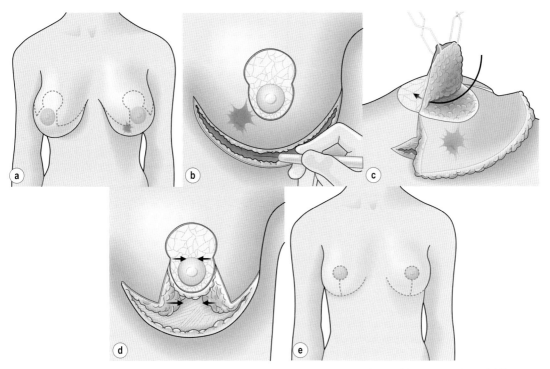

**Figure 6.8** • Level II oncoplastic techniques for lower pole breast cancers: superior pedicle mammoplasty. **(a)** Treatment planning: superior pedicle mammoplasty and contralateral symmetrisation. **(b)** Superior pedicle de-epithelialised. Submammary fold incision. **(c)** Superior pedicle elevated. Wide excision of tumour and surrounding tissues. **(d)** Breast reshaping. **(e)** Result.

periareolar scars as utilised in most breast reductions.[10] The procedure begins with the de-epithelialisation of the area surrounding the NAC. Once completed, the NAC is dissected away from the underlying breast tissue. A superior pedicle of dermoglandular tissue is preserved to provide the NAC with a blood supply.

The inframammary incision is then completed, followed by wide undermining of the breast tissue from the pectoral fascia. The undermining starts inferiorly and proceeds superiorly beneath the tumour while encompassing the medial and lateral aspects of the breast as well as the NAC. The tumour is removed en bloc with a wide margin of normal breast tissue and overlying skin as determined by the preoperative marking.

As for all BCS, the goal of the excision is to obtain at least a 1-cm macroscopic margin of normal tissue in order to ensure free microscopic margin. Mobilisation of the breast tissue from the pectoralis fascia allows for palpation of both the deep and superficial surfaces of the tumour, which improves the ability of the surgeon to obtain clear margins.

The breast tissue is remodelled after the resection is completed. Remodelling incorporates the re-approximation of the medial and lateral glandular columns towards the midline to fill in the defect, followed by NAC recentralisation. All tissues excised are weighed and this provides a guide to the amount of tissue to be excised in any contralateral reduction procedure. As a general rule the resection of the cancer-bearing breast should be less than the opposite breast to allow for shrinkage of the treated breast following whole-breast radiotherapy. Results from excision of ductal carcinoma in situ at the lower pole of the left breast are shown in **Fig. 6.9a** and **b**. The result 2 years postoperation is shown in **Fig. 6.9c**.

Vertical mammoplasty (Lejour/Lassus)

One modification to the technique to excise lower quadrant tumours is to use the vertical-scar mammoplasty described by Lejour[11] and Lassus.[12] The site and volume of excision are identical to the inverted-T scar, but this approach avoids the submammary scar.

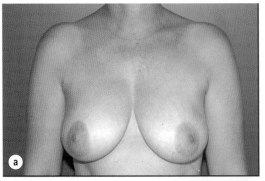

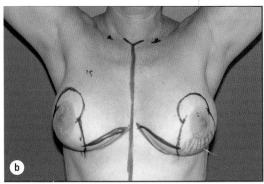

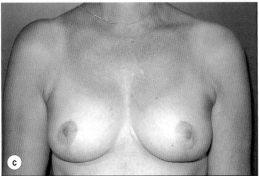

**Figure 6.9** • Level II technique for a 6-cm ductal carcinoma in situ of the lower pole of the left breast. Wide excision and postoperative radiotherapy. **(a,b)** Preoperative. **(c)** Two years postoperation.

## Lower inner quadrant (7–9 o'clock)

### General principles

Standard superior pedicle mammoplasty described for tumours located at the 6 o'clock position can be extended to 7 o'clock. However, adaptation for tumours located more medially, between 7 and 8 o'clock, is more difficult and requires a novel level II technique.

### Technique

#### V mammoplasty

This procedure involves excising a pyramidal section of gland with the base located in the submammary fold and apex at the border of the areola. This skin and underlying breast tissue are removed en bloc down to the pectoralis fascia. An incision is then made along the inframammary fold and developed starting at the medial aspect of the base of resection moving towards the anterior axillary line and taken as far as necessary to perform adequate mobilisation and rotation of the remaining gland into the defect. The lower pole of the breast is mobilised off the pectoralis fascia for use as an advancement flap to fill the defect. Volume replacement is

thus achieved through the advancement of the gland from the remaining lower medial and lateral aspects of the breast. The NAC is then recentralised on a de-epithelialised superior lateral pedicle.[13]

## Upper inner quadrant (10–11 o'clock)

### General principles

Special caution is needed when considering BCS for lesions in the upper inner aspect of the breast. A wide excision in this location can have a significant impact on the overall quality of the breast shape by distorting the visible breast line known as the 'décolleté'. This represents the visible area of the breast.

For moderate resections, level I techniques can be utilised safely. For more extensive excisions, the ability and likelihood of being able to preserve the natural breast shape should be discussed with the patient. Standard level II oncoplastic procedures that reliably address the specific limitations of BCS at this troublesome location are limited. Silverstein and colleagues have described an effective OPS procedure to address the upper inner quadrant. Their approach utilises a batwing excision pattern.[14] Silverstein et al.'s OPS solution is innovative and reproducible; however, more research is needed for excisions exceeding 20%.

## Upper pole (11–1 o'clock)

### General principles

Lesions located at the 12 o'clock position can be excised widely followed by volume redistribution of tissue from a central location. Access to lesions in this location of the breast is accomplished either using an inferior pedicle or round-block mammoplasty approach. The inferior pedicle mammoplasty is commonly performed in the USA as a breast reduction technique and utilises an inverted-T scar pattern.[15] A round-block approach, on the other hand, is more technically challenging when trying to achieve the desired breast shape. These two techniques are used extensively for breast reduction with low complication rates and durable results. They can be applied for wide excision of upper pole tumours while preserving a patient's natural breast shape.

### Techniques
#### Inferior pedicle mammoplasty

The skin markings are identical to those described for the superior pedicle. The resection, however, is located in the upper pole, hence the vascular supply of the NAC is based on its inferior and posterior glandular attachments. The excision of the cancer is performed through an incision placed within the skin to be removed. Once the cancer has been excised and the specimen X-ray shows complete radiological excision, the inferior pedicle is de-epithelialised and advanced upwards towards the excision defect to achieve volume redistribution. Resection of the breast tissue is performed in the inner and outer lower quadrants to optimise the breast shape.

#### Round-block mammoplasty

The round-block mammoplasty utilises a periareolar incision and was originally described by Benelli.[16,17] The procedure starts by making two concentric periareolar incisions, followed by de-epithelialisation of the intervening skin. The outer edge of de-epithelialised skin is incised and the entire skin envelope can then be undermined to allow access to the tumour. The NAC remains vascularised through its posterior glandular base. Resection of the lesion from the subcutaneous tissue down to the pectoralis fascia is performed and this results in the formation of an external and internal glandular flap. The flaps are then mobilised off the pectoralis fascia and advanced towards each other to eliminate the excision defect. The two incisions are then approximated, resulting in a periareolar scar.

Although the round-block mammoplasty has been used mainly for upper pole tumours, it is a versatile technique that can be easily adapted for tumours in any location of the breast.

## Upper outer quadrant (1–3 o'clock; Fig. 6.10a–c)

### General principles

In the upper outer quadrant, large lesions can often be excised with standard BCS without causing deformity. However, resection of greater than 20% of the breast volume will result in retraction of the overlying skin with NAC displacement towards the excision site. A result of a patient with a T3 cancer treated by neoadjuvant chemotherapy and wide excision with mammoplasty is shown in **Fig. 6.11a–d**. Level II OPS can be utilised to increase resection possibilities while limiting deformity risk in this forgiving region of the breast.

### Technique
#### Fusiform mammoplasty

A large portion of the upper outer quadrant can be excised utilising a fusiform skin excision pattern oriented in a radial direction from the NAC towards the axilla, similar to a quadrantectomy.[18,19] After wide excision, the reshaping is performed by mobilising the lateral and central gland into the cavity and suturing it together. Central gland advancement is accomplished easily following NAC undermining. Complete detachment of the retroareolar gland from the NAC enables the central part of the gland for volume redistribution without compromise of NAC vascularity. Once the defect is eliminated, the NAC is placed in its optimal position, at the centre of the new breast mound. The area of glandular excision directly follows the skin excision. Additional glandular excision can be accomplished to remove almost the entire quadrant depending on tumour size and the amount of tissue required to be removed to obtain clear margins.

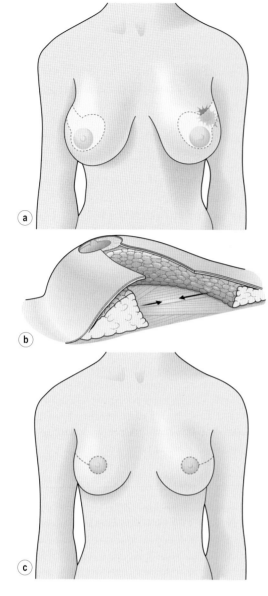

**Figure 6.10** • Level II oncoplastic techniques for upper outer quadrant breast cancers. **(a)** Treatment planning: wide resection and NAC de-epithelialisation. **(b)** Resection. **(c)** Breast reshaping and contralateral symmetrisation.

## Lower outer quadrant (4–5 o'clock)

### General principles

A large-volume resection of the lower outer quadrant leaves a deformity similar to the bird's beak. As for lower inner pole lesions, the inverted-T mammoplasty does not 'fit' well for excisions within this quadrant. The optimal procedure is a J-type mammoplasty described by Gasperoni et al.[20]

### Technique

J mammoplasty (Gasperoni)

The first incision begins at the medial edge of the de-epithelialised periareolar area and then gently curves upwards with a concavity to the inframammary crease. The second incision starts at the lateral border of the de-epithelialised zone and follows a similar pattern. The parenchymal excision then follows the skin pattern in the shape of the letter J. The NAC remains vascularised on a de-epithelialised superior pedicle and is detached from the retroareolar gland. Lateral and central breast tissue can then be recruited into the excision defect to achieve an equitable redistribution of remaining breast volume.

## Retroareolar location

### General principles

Subareolar breast cancers are candidates for BCS. However, superficial subareolar tumours are associated with a risk of NAC involvement approaching 50%.[21] Such cases require en bloc removal of the NAC with the tumour. This often results in a 'flattened breast' or 'shark-bite' deformity and poor cosmetic outcome. If the patient has a glandular breast allowing wide undermining for reshaping, a level I OPS is a reasonable option.

Level II mammoplasty techniques are reserved for patients with ptosis or fatty breasts or for patients for which excision of more then 20% of the breast volume is required. There are a number of mammoplasty approaches that can be chosen for the centrally located lesion. They include the inverted-T mammoplasty with resection of the NAC, a modified Lejour or J pattern with NAC excision or a Grisotti flap (see Chapter 4). The latter offers the advantage of allowing for immediate NAC reconstruction through preservation of a skin island on an advancement flap.[22]

### Technique

Modified inverted-T mammoplasty

Oncoplastic techniques for centrally located tumours have recently been outlined by Huemer et al.[23] An inverted-T incision is preferred, similar to that used in a superior pedicle mammoplasty. The only modification is that the two vertical incisions encompass the NAC, which is removed together with the tumour. The breast shape is reconstructed as already

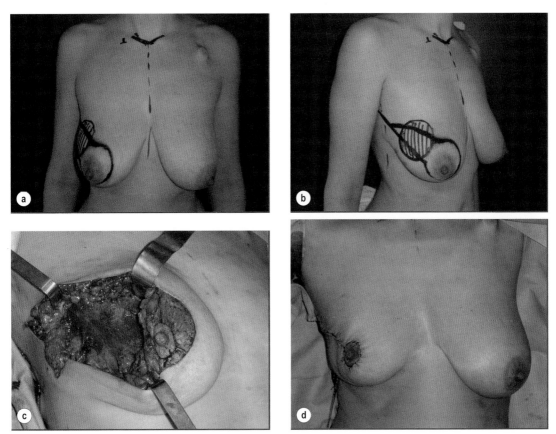

**Figure 6.11** • Level II technique for a T3N0 cancer of the upper outer quadrant of the right breast. Preoperative chemotherapy: partial response. Wide excision and mammoplasty. **(a,b)** Preoperative. **(c)** Resection weight 215 g. **(d)** Result prior to contralateral symmetrisation.

demonstrated for the superior pedicle approach. The NAC is usually reconstructed at a later stage, after completion of radiotherapy, although it can be reconstructed during the same procedure. A modification of this technique is to leave a circular island of skin or an inferior dermoglandular flap, which is relocated in the position of the new NAC and produces symmetry with the opposite NAC.

## Discussion

### General

Until recently, the breast surgeon has been able to provide only two options for patients with breast cancer: either a modified radical mastectomy or a wide local excision followed by radiation. BCS indications have expanded, but only moderate surgical advancements have been made since its introduction.

The integration of plastic surgery techniques at the time of tumour excision has delivered a third pathway, enabling surgeons to perform major resections involving more then 20% of breast volume without causing breast deformity. This new combination of oncological and reconstructive surgery is commonly referred to as oncoplastic surgery. This 'third pathway' has allowed surgeons to extend the indications for BCS without compromising oncological goals or aesthetic outcomes. It is a logical extension of the quadrantectomy technique described by Veronesi et al.[18] The innovation of the quadrantectomy provided women with a safe oncological option for conserving their breast.

 The recurrence rates of quadrantectomy compared favourably with that of lumpectomy, but cosmetic outcomes were unpredictable with more poor cosmetic outcomes than or a wide excision alone.[24–26]

With immediate reshaping employing OPS, large resections can now be achieved with satisfactory cosmetic outcomes.

The second advantage of OPS is avoiding the need for secondary reconstruction by preventing major breast deformities.[27] Prior to the development of OPS, patients with major deformities were subsequently referred to plastic surgeons.[28] A classification system of these deformities has been described and reconstructive techniques for breast deformity after BCS have been developed.[29,30] Despite continued efforts to treat these deformities, the results of postoperative repair of BCS defects in irradiated tissue were found to be poor, regardless of the surgical procedure or team.[31,32] Immediate reshaping of the breast will eliminate the need for complex reconstruction.

Advances in OPS have been restricted by the diversity of techniques, the lack of uniformity in classifying oncoplastic techniques and few guidelines of the optimum OPS procedures in the surgical literature. This has generated confusion and difficulty in patient and technique selection. The foundation of OPS starts with simple techniques that are easily incorporated into everyday practice (level I techniques), followed by acquiring the experience to perform the various mammoplasty techniques utilised for more extensive resections (level II techniques).

## Indications for oncoplastic surgery

The main indication for OPS is the need to excise large lesions or a significant percentage of the breast, so permitting BCS for large lesions for which a standard excision with safe margins would be either impossible or lead to major deformity. Extensive ductal carcinoma in situ, invasive lobular carcinoma, multifocality, and partial or poor responses to neoadjuvant therapy are areas where there may be benefits for OPS intervention. Standard BCS that results in positive margins and where re-excision is being considered as an additional category of patients for whom to consider using OPS.[33]

## Oncoplastic and oncological safety

Large randomised prospective clinical trials have not validated the efficacy and safety of oncoplastic techniques, but there is growing evidence, through prospective series, that the techniques offer patients safe and effective surgical treatment. Our prospective analysis of over 100 patients undergoing OPS at our institution demonstrated 5-year overall and disease-free survival rates of 95.7% and 82.8% respectively.[10] Delay in adjuvant treatment was related to slow wound healing in four patients, but all patients received the appropriate postoperative radiotherapy and chemotherapy during the study. The cosmetic results at 5 years were favourable in 82% of patients. Final cosmetic outcomes and complication rates are not altered in patients undergoing neoadjuvant chemotherapy. A more recent retrospective review of 298 patients treated with OPS demonstrated a 5-year recurrence-free rate of 93.7% and 94.6% overall survival. This larger review confirms the equivalent outcomes of OPS and standard BCS.[34] Rietjens et al. have reported long-term results from the European Institute of Oncology indicating no local relapse in the pT1 cohort. The pT2 and pT3 combined group had a 5-year local recurrence rate of 8% and a mortality rate of 15%. The overall local recurrence rate was determined to be 3%.[35]

## Integration into multidisciplinary treatment

Clinical management is enhanced by OPS and does not change the need for or adherence to the guidelines for preoperative chemotherapy. Our surgical approach using OPS is fully integrated into the multidisciplinary environment. Radiation treatment is not disturbed by the extensive undermining during OPS and complication rates remain comparable to BCS. There is no increase in treatment delays with the more extensive level II techniques, and the remodelling process does not affect continued screening and radiographic follow-up of patients.[36]

## Complications of oncoplastic surgery

Mammoplasty techniques for cosmetic breast reduction have low complication rates of 1–2%. Early common complications include seroma, haematoma, infection, and skin or NAC necrosis leading to delayed healing. Late complications during the postoperative course may involve fat necrosis, loss of nipple sensitivity and NAC necrosis.[37,38]

Extensive data are not available on complication rates for oncoplastic procedures. Our prospective evaluation of complications in an initial oncoplastic surgery series demonstrated low seroma rates (1%), but a higher overall incidence of delayed wound healing (9%). A delay in postoperative treatment was observed in only 4% of patients.[10] This complication rate is higher than that for cosmetic mammoplasty but can be explained by the need for greater glandular undermining in OPS compared to cosmetic breast reduction to achieve volume redistribution to less favourable tumour locations.

Surgeons embarking on OPS should be aware of complications, their frequency and the factors that increase this risk. Glandular necrosis is the most challenging complication.

 Aggressive undermining of the skin envelope and gland from the pectoralis fascia can lead to glandular necrosis if the breast is fatty, as such breasts have less vascularity compared to glandular breasts.

Areas of fat necrosis can become infected and cause wound dehiscence resulting in postoperative treatment delay. Our rates of delayed wound healing have been reduced considerably since we have incorporated the third key element of breast density into our decision-making process. Our complication rate is now less than 5%, with no delay in postoperative treatment over the last 150 cases.

## Limitations of oncoplastic surgery

We can identify four different categories which limit the use of OPS: patient characteristics, tumour size, surgical level of difficulty and increased operative time.

Patient considerations including breast size and comorbidities are integrated into the initial evaluation. Although level I procedures can be applied to all patients, level II OPS is of limited value in women with small breast size, either A or smaller B cups. For these patients with small breasts who require excision of greater than 20% of the breast volume, either a latissimus dorsi miniflap or a total mastectomy with immediate reconstruction should be considered. Comorbidities that increase the risk of tissue necrosis, such as history of smoking, diabetes and obesity, must also be evaluated prior to surgical planning.

Once an acceptable risk is established for the patient, then tumour characteristics are used to decide the appropriate procedure and the best approach. Excision of tumours too large to redistribute volume into the index quadrant may require a volume replacement procedure such as a latissimus dorsi miniflap.[3] Location of the tumour is also critical, as upper inner quadrant tumours have few volume redistribution solutions.

Difficulty in performing advanced level II techniques comprises another category of limitation. However, training for OPS can be acquired gradually and level I techniques do not require any advanced training. Another solution for the more complex cases is to incorporate a dual team approach with a plastic surgeon. This may be the best option for most breast surgeons that do not wish to or do not have the time to invest in specific training for complex level II techniques. As this can be difficult to arrange logistically, dual training of breast surgeons is the best long-term solution.

Finally, can the additional time required for advanced procedures be justified? The increased length of the initial operation does translate into major benefits for both the patient and the surgeon. OPS leads to an overall reduction in operation time for many patients because it is more likely to achieve free margins at one procedure. The reduction in re-excision rates improves resource management for the whole cohort of patients. The greater amount of time utilised during the initial procedure also has the added benefit of reducing deformity rates, thus eliminating the need for repair of partial mastectomy defects. It also reduces the numbers who require mastectomy and breast reconstruction.

## Oncoplastic evolution and revolution

As surgical practice guidelines continue to evolve in the field of breast surgery, the training of future breast surgeons should include OPS techniques that rely on the experience and methodology gained from the fields of both surgical oncology and plastic and reconstructive surgery. Growth and acceptance of OPS as an alternative to BCS has seen an active collaboration between the divisions of breast and plastic surgery in the UK and much of Western Europe.

The pathway for obtaining the necessary training differs throughout the surgical world. In the UK, a formal oncoplastic training programme has already been established. Participants in this programme obtain both plastic and reconstructive training, as well as experience in the surgical oncological management of breast cancer. France has also witnessed the creation of a formal certification programme for breast surgeons interested in OPS. The programme involves clinical mentoring, technical lectures and a standardised written examination. The interest in OPS continues to expand, with courses on offer at the major breast surgery conferences in the USA and Europe. These courses provide the necessary background to complete level I procedures, but do not allow for application of level II OPS.

## Conclusions

The proliferation of oncoplastic publications in the surgical literature is a direct result of the awareness of the advantages of OPS.

 Oncoplastic surgery allows for wide resections with favourable cosmesis and integrates easily into the standard multidisciplinary approach for BCS.

The ultimate goal is to allow large-volume resections with free margins and fewer mastectomies than is currently obtainable with standard BCS.

OPS is best stratified into two levels. Three key factors have been defined – excision volume, tumour location and glandular density – and these form the basis of a cohesive set of surgical principles and teaching guidelines. The goal for developing an OPS classification and a quadrant-by-quadrant atlas is to improve communication between surgeons and their patients. Even though there is no clear-cut division between standard BCS and oncoplasty, and a crossover between levels I and II exists, the adoption of a standardised OPS classification system is advocated.

One benefit of this standardisation is the impact it will have for training in OPS. Surgeons will be able to select appropriate courses and training experience based on the distinct goals they wish to attain. The OPS classification and atlas are intended to assist surgeons to choose the optimal approach for each individual patient to avoid complications and obtain the best oncological and cosmetic results.

### Key points

- Volume displacement is most suitable for patients with medium or large breasts who are willing to undergo bilateral breast reduction, avoiding more major reconstructive surgery.
- Volume displacement allows massive resection of tissue without cosmetic penalty.
- Volume displacement can be designed around modifications of the superior pedicle, inferior pedicle and round-block techniques.

## References

1. Clough KB, Nos C, Salmon RJ et al. Conservative treatment of breast cancers by mammaplasty and irradiation: a new approach to lower quadrant tumours. Plast Reconstr Surg 1995; 96(2):363–70.

2. Cothier-Savey I, Otmezquine Y, Calitchi E et al. Value of reduction mammoplasty in the conservative treatment of breast neoplasm. Apropos of 70 cases. Ann Chir Plast Esthet 1996; 41(4): 346–53.

3. Rainsbury R. Surgery insight: oncoplastic breast-conserving reconstruction – indications, benefits, choices and outcomes. Nature Clin Pract Oncol 2007; 4(11):657–64.

4. Bulstrode NW, Shortri S. Prediction of cosmetic outcome following conservative breast surgery using breast volume measurements. Breast 2001; 10:124–6.

5. American College of Radiology. Breast imaging reporting and data systems (BI-RADS). Reston, VA: American College of Radiology, 2003.

6. Kraissl CJ. The selection of appropriate lines for elective surgical incisions. Plast Reconstr Surg 1951; 8(1):1–28.

7. Schlenz I, Rigel S, Schemper M et al. Alteration of nipple and areola sensitivity by reduction mammaplasty: a prospective comparison of five techniques. Plast Reconstr Surg 2005; 115(3):743–51.

8. O'Dey D, Prescher A, Pallua N. Vascular reliability of the nipple–areola complex-bearing pedicles: an anatomical microdissection study. Plast Reconstr Surg 2007; 119(4):1167–77.

9. Smith ML, Evans GR, Gurlek A et al. Reduction mammaplasty: its role in breast conservation surgery

for early-stage breast cancer. Ann Plast Surg 1998; 41(3):234–9.

10. Clough KB, Lewis J, Couturaud B et al. Oncoplastic techniques allow extensive resections for breast-conserving therapy of breast carcinomas. Ann Surg 2003; 237(1):26–34.

11. Lejour M. Reduction of mammaplasty scars: from a short inframammary scar to a vertical scar. Ann Chir Plast Esthet 1990; 35(5):369–79.

12. Lassus C. A 30-year experience with vertical mammaplasty. Plast Recontr Surg 1996; 97(2):373–80.

13. Clough KB, Kroll S, Audretsch W. An approach to the repair of partial mastectomy defects. Plast Reconstr Surg 1999; 104(2):409–20.

14. Anderson BO, Masetti R, Silverstein MJ. Oncoplastic approaches to partial mastectomy: an overview of volume-displacement techniques. Lancet Oncol 2005; 6:145–57.

15. Spear SL, Pelletiere CV, Wolfe AJ et al. Experience with reduction mammoplasty combined with breast conservation therapy in the treatment of cancer. Plast Reconstr Surg 2003; 111(3):1102–9.

16. Benelli L. A new periareolar mammaplasty: the "round block" technique. Aesth Plast Surg 1990; 14(2):93–100.

17. Hammon DC. Short scar periareolar inferior pedicle reduction (SPAIR) mammoplasty. Plast Reconstr Surg 1999; 103(3):890–901.

18. Veronesi U, Banfi A, Saccozzi R et al. Conservative treatment of breast cancer. A trial in progress at the cancer institute of Milan. Cancer 1977; 39(6):2822–6.

19. Veronesi U, Banfi A, del Vecchio M et al. Comparision of Halsted mastectomy with quadrantectomy, axillary dissection, and radiotherapy in early breast cancer: long term results. Eur J Cancer Clin Oncol 1986; 22:1085–9.

20. Gasperoni C, Salgarello M, Gasperoni P. A personal technique: mammaplasty with J scar. Ann Plast Surg 2002; 48(2):124–30.

21. Gerber B, Krause A, Reimer T et al. Skin-sparing mastectomy with conservation of the nipple–areolar complex and autologous reconstruction is an oncologically safe procedure. Ann Surg 2003; 238(1):120–7.

22. Galimberti V, Zurrida S, Grisotti A et al Central small size breast cancer: how to overcome the problem of nipple and areola involvement. Eur J Cancer 1993; 29A(8):1093–6.

23. Huemer G, Schrenk P, Moser F et al. Oncoplastic techniques allow breast-conserving treatment in centrally located breast cancers. Plast Reconstr Surg 2007; 120(2):390–X.

24. Veronesi U, Lunini A, Galimberti V et al. Conservation approaches for the management of

stage I/II carcinoma of the breast: Milan cancer institute trials. World J Surg 1994; 18(1):70–5.

25. Mariani L, Salvadori B, Veronesi U et al. Ten year results of a randomized trial comparing two conservative strategies for small size breast cancer. Eur J Cancer 1998; 149(3):219–25.

26. Amichetti M, Busana L, Caffo O. Long term cosmetic outcome and toxicity in patients treated with quadrantectomy and radiation therapy for early-stage breast cancer. Oncology 1995; 52:177–81.

27. Dewar JA, Benhamou E, Arrigada R et al. Cosmetic results following lumpectomy, axillary dissection and radiotherapy for small breast cancer. Radiother Oncol 1998; 12(4):273–80.

28. Petit J-Y, Regault L, Zekri A et al. Poor aesthetic results after conservative treatment of breast cancer. Techniques of partial breast reconstruction. Ann Chir Plast Esthet 1989; 34:103–8.

29. Clough KB, Cuminet JC, Fitoussi A et al. Cosmetic sequelae after conservative treatment for breast cancer: classification and results of surgical correction. Ann Plast Surg 1998; 41(8):471–81.

30. Clough KB, Thomas S, Fitoussi A et al. Reconstruction after conservative treatment for breast cancer. Cosmetic sequelae: classification revisited. Plast Reconstr Surg 2004; 114(7):1743–53.

31. Berrino P, Campora E, Leone S et al. Correction of type II breast deformities following conservative cancer surgery. Plast Reconstr Surg 1992; 90:846–53.

32. Bostwick J, Paletta C, Hartampf CR. Conservative treatment for breast cancer: complications requiring reconstructive surgery. Ann Surg 1986; 203:481–90.

33. Schwartz GF, Veronesi U, Clough KB et al. Proceedings of the consensus conference on breast conservation, April 28 to May 1, 2005, Milan, Italy. Cancer 2006; 107(2):242–50.

34. Staub G, Fitoussi A, Falcou MC et al. Breast cancer surgery: use of mammaplasty. Results from a series of 298 cases. Ann Chir Plast Esthet 2007; 53(2):124–34.

35. Rietjens M, Urban CA, Petit JY et al. Long term oncologic results of breast conservation treatment with oncoplastic surgery. Breast 2007; 16(4):387–95.

36. Brown FE, Sargernt SK, Cohen SR et al. Mammographic changes following reduction mammoplasty. Plast Reconstr Surg 1987; 80(5):691–8.

37. Spear SL, Evans KK. Complications and secondary corrections after breast reduction and mastopexy. Surg Breast 2006; 2:1220–34.

38. Munhoz AM, Montag E, Arruda EG et al. Critical analysis of reduction mammaplasty techniques in combination with conservative breast surgery for early breast cancer treatment. Plast Reconstr Surg 2006; 117(4):1091–103.

# 7

# The axilla: current management including sentinel node and lymphoedema

Massimiliano Cariati
Arnie D. Purushotham

## Introduction

Approximately 30–40% of symptomatic patients with early breast cancer have axillary nodal involvement. Node-positive breast cancers have a worse prognosis than node-negative cases.[1] However, the significance of nodal metastasis is incompletely understood and the management of the axilla in breast cancer has been a long-standing topic of significant controversy and debate. Most of this controversy has arisen from the evolving consensus on how breast cancer spreads. Late in the 19th century, Halsted[2] proposed that breast cancer spreads first to the axillary lymph nodes and then to distant sites. Thus, nodal metastasis was viewed as an indicator of tumour chronology. The better prognosis of node-negative tumours was attributed to timely resection, before distant metastasis via the axillary lymphatics had occurred.[3] This theory resulted in the introduction of radical mastectomy. However, subsequent large randomised trials showed that neither the extent of surgery nor delay in the treatment of the axilla had any influence on the prognosis of patients with operable breast cancer.[1 6] In addition, long-term follow-up of node-negative patients revealed that 30% eventually die of metastatic breast cancer.[7] Thus, axillary lymph nodes do not appear to be the sole mode of spread of breast cancer, as postulated by Halsted. Yet, nodal status is still considered an indicator of tumour chronology, and the better prognosis of node-negative patients is generally attributed to lead-time bias.[8] Nodal status is, however, also a marker of tumour biology, with node-positive tumours possessing a more aggressive phenotype. New models were suggested which challenged the Halstedian model of centrifugal spread. Both the systemic and the spectrum models acknowledge the role of the bloodstream in tumour dissemination independent of lymphatic invasion, but they differ conceptually.

The systemic theory, introduced by Bernard Fisher in the 1970s, describes a model in which breast cancer is a systemic disease from its inception or at least from the time that it is clinically detectable, and considers variations in local treatment as unlikely to have any impact on survival.[9] The spectrum model as described by Hellman[10] views breast cancer as a progressive disease in which invasion and metastasis are a function of tumour growth and biological transformation. In addition, this model acknowledges that the disease may manifest a spectrum of biological behaviour, with some tumours that are metastatic from the beginning and others that may reach a large size without dissemination.

## Anatomy of the axilla (Fig. 7.1)

### Introduction

The axilla is a conical space containing the soft tissue situated between the superolateral aspect of the thoracic wall and the scapulohumeral joint.

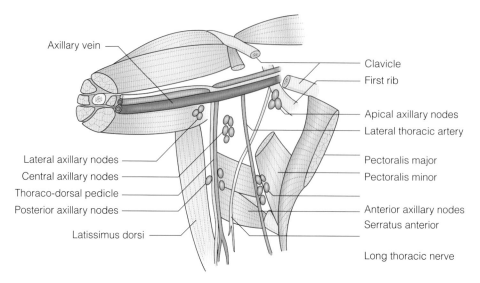

Axillary vein

Clavicle

First rib

Apical axillary nodes

Lateral thoracic artery

Lateral axillary nodes

Central axillary nodes

Thoraco-dorsal pedicle

Posterior axillary nodes

Pectoralis major

Pectoralis minor

Latissimus dorsi

Anterior axillary nodes

Serratus anterior

Long thoracic nerve

**Figure 7.1** • Anatomy of the axilla.

Its apex is directed upwards and is defined by the space existing between the first rib medially, the superior border of the scapula laterally, and the clavicle and subclavius muscle anteriorly. Its base has four margins, the anterior one constituted by the inferior margin of the pectoralis major muscle, the posterior one by the inferior border of the latissimus dorsi muscle, the medial and lateral ones by the lateral aspect of the chest wall and the medial aspect of the arm respectively. Its anterior boundary is defined by the pectoralis major and pectoralis minor muscles, the latter contained within the clavipectoral fascia. Its posterior boundary is defined by the anterior surface of the scapula, the subscapularis muscle and the latissimus dorsi muscle. The medial wall of the cavity is delineated by the first four ribs, the corresponding intercostal and serratus anterior muscles. The lateral boundary is defined by the narrow space contained between the insertion of pectoralis major and latissimus dorsi. This space is occupied by the tendons of the coracobrachialis and biceps muscles.

The axillary space contains the axillary vessels (artery and vein) and their branches, the brachial plexus, with its collateral branches, some branches of the intercostal nerves and a variable number of lymphatic glands, all surrounded by an amount of loose fatty areolar tissue.

## Topographic anatomy

The axillary artery and vein, along with the brachial plexus, extend obliquely along the lateral margin of

the axillary space, from its apex to its base, with the vein lying anteromedially to the artery and concealing it. The thoracic branches of the axillary vessels run within the anterior part of the axillary space. At the posterior part of the axillary space are the subscapularis vessels and nerves, from which the thoracodorsal pedicle originates.

The medial part of the space is free of vessels of any importance; however, important nerves are located medially such as the long thoracic nerve, innervation to the serratus anterior muscle.

The cavity of the axilla is filled by a variable amount of loose areolar tissue containing a number of small arteries and veins and numerous lymph nodes.

The topographic anatomy of the axillary lymph nodes has been widely studied in relation to their identification as the major route of regional spread of primary breast carcinoma. The anatomical arrangement of these glands has been subject to many different classifications, the most detailed of which, by Pickren,[11] divided the axillary lymphatic nodes into five groups (lateral thoracic, brachial, subscapular (apical), central and subclavicular groups respectively). An alternative way of dividing the axillary nodes, with the purpose of determining pathological anatomy and metastatic spread, is to split them arbitrarily into three levels: level I nodes, which lie lateral to the lateral border of the pectoralis minor muscle; level II nodes, which lie behind the pectoralis minor muscle; and level III nodes, which lie medial to the medial border of the pectoralis minor muscle.

## Internal mammary lymph nodes

The internal mammary nodes lie in the intercostal spaces in the parasternal region, close to the internal mammary vessels in extrapleural fat, and their described number varies between studies. Lymphatic drainage from the breast to the internal mammary nodes was first described in 1786 by Cruikshank.[12]

# Physiology of lymphatic drainage of the breast

Lymphatic drainage from the breast was initially studied, by means of injection of mercury directly into the lymphatic vessels of cadavers, in the 1780s by two different authors.[12,13] Nearly 100 years after these two studies, Sappey described two discrete lymphatic drainage systems for the breast: superficial lymphatics which drain the skin overlying the breast and deep lymphatics which drain the mammary tissue itself. The two systems were described as having frequent anastomoses. All these vessels were thought to empty into a subareolar lymphatic plexus from which two large collecting vessels passed to the axilla.

We now know that the plexus of the lymphatics found within the breast is confluent with the subepithelial lymphatics over the surface of the body. These lymphatics communicate with subdermal vessels and merge with the Sappey subareolar plexus. Lymph flows unidirectionally from the superficial to deep plexus and from the subareolar plexus to the deep subcutaneous plexus. From here lymph flow moves centrifugally toward the axillary (>85% of the flow) and internal mammary nodes (<15% of the flow).

# Axillary lymph node involvement in invasive breast cancer

Axillary nodes receive lymph from all quadrants of the breast. The likelihood of axillary nodal involvement is directly related to the size of the tumour.[14] Reported rates of nodal positivity in tumours smaller than 1 cm vary significantly, but may be as high as 12%.[15,16] Other factors influencing the risk of nodal positivity are higher histological grade and presence of lymphovascular invasion. Patients with grade I tumours have significantly lower rates of nodal positivity (10%) than patients with grade II and grade III tumours (up to 39%).[15] The age of the patient

and breast quadrant involved by a tumour are also predictors of axillary lymph node involvement, with tumours located in the upper outer quadrant and tumours in younger patients having a greater incidence of lymph node involvement. On the basis of these clinico-pathological variables, a scoring system has recently been developed to identify patients at high or low risk of nodal involvement, with 25% of patients in the low-score group displaying nodal positivity, versus 65% of patients in the high-score group.[16]

# Internal mammary node involvement

Internal mammary nodes (IMNs) receive between 3% and 15% of the lymphatic drainage of the breast. The overall frequency of IMN metastasis in historical studies of breast cancer is 22.5%, and correlates strongly with axillary lymph node (ALN) status, with 36% of ALN-positive patients having IMN positivity versus only 9% positivity in ALN-negative patients. Recent evidence has shown that even patients with early breast cancer display IMN positivity in 17–27% of cases. Factors increasing IMN positivity include patient age <40 and larger tumour size. IMN positivity has been shown to have the same prognostic significance as ALN positivity. The concomitant positivity of ALN and IMN is associated with the worst prognosis.[17]

# Prognostic significance of axillary lymph node involvement

Node-positive breast cancers have a worse prognosis than node-negative cases.[1] An increasing impact on survival is seen as the number of nodes involved increases. For tumours smaller than 2 cm (T1), 5-year survival rates for tumours with no nodal involvement, with one to three involved nodes or more than four involved nodes are 96.3%, 87.4% and 66% respectively. For tumours over 2 cm in diameter, the same three subgroups on the basis of nodal involvement have 5-year survival rates of 89.4%, 79.9% and 58.7% respectively.[18] Surgery and/or radiotherapy to the axilla may affect survival, provide information regarding staging and prognosis, and have implications for locoregional control of breast cancer.

# Staging of axillary lymph nodes

## Introduction

Axillary lymph node dissection (ALND) was, until recently, the most widely used technique for staging the axilla. In some centres, radiotherapy is used as an alternative to ALND to treat axillary nodal disease. Recently, less invasive techniques such as sentinel lymph node biopsy (SLNB) have evolved that have challenged the role of routine ALND in all patients with breast cancer.

## Omitting management of the axilla

It has been suggested that an axillary staging procedure may be omitted in patients with small (<1 cm) tumours of favourable histological grade or type, as a result of the low probability of lymph-node involvement.[19] Judgement as to what constitutes an acceptably low rate of axillary involvement and the cost of identifying the few node-positive patients in these groups is subjective and remains an area of controversy. Furthermore, whether or not any axillary surgery should be done for microinvasive foci has been a subject of debate. Many clinicians intuitively feel that, with the advent of SLNB, all patients with invasive disease should at least have some nodes checked surgically. Others have tried to identify patient categories that may be spared the minor, but finite, morbidity of SLNB.

### Ductal carcinoma in situ (DCIS)

There is consensus that patients with DCIS that is extensive (on imaging) or presents as a palpable mass (about 20%), should have SLNB, but that the majority of patients with small areas of screen-detected DCIS (80% of cases) treated with breast-conserving therapy should not have any axillary surgery.[20] Many reports of node positivity in DCIS relate to isolated tumour cells or micrometastases only,[21] which are almost certainly not clinically significant. An incidental invasive component is more common in patients with widespread high-grade DCIS that requires mastectomy (20%).

### Good-prognosis tumours

The European Society of Mastology guidelines suggest that axillary staging can be omitted for patients with tubular cancers smaller than 1 cm. In a series of patients with mainly T1c mammographically detected tumours, the rate of axillary relapse was only 3% at 5 years. Patients with special types of breast cancer have a risk of nodal metastases of less than 5% and may not need any form of axillary surgery. Similarly, patients with non-high-grade (I and II) T1a and T1b tumours detected mammographically have similar low rates of nodal involvement and it has been suggested that this group may be spared SLNB.[22]

### Patients unfit for general anaesthesia

For selected elderly patients in whom ALND is unlikely to influence the decision to use adjuvant systemic therapy, this may be omitted.

## Preoperative assessment of axillary lymph nodes

Detection of axillary involvement by physical examination has both a high false-positive (25–31%) and false-negative (27–32%) rate.[23–25]

Sentinel lymph node biopsy is the axillary staging procedure of choice in patients with clinically negative axillae. Approximately 30–35% of patients undergoing SLNB are found to have metastatic involvement of the sentinel lymph node (SLN), which means such patients need completion ALND or axillary radiotherapy. In order to spare a proportion of these patients undergoing an unnecessary SLNB, ultrasound scanning (US) of the axilla has been introduced for the preoperative assessment of lymph node involvement. The combination of ultrasound with fine-needle aspiration (FNA) or core biopsy of suspect lymph nodes allows the identification of up to 50% of node-positive patients who can then proceed to ALND and avoid two surgical procedures. Gilissen et al. compared US/FNA findings of 195 patients with their final histopathological outcomes and concluded that US-guided FNA of non-palpable suspicious nodes is a reliable and cost-effective procedure.[26] Other authors have also suggested using US-guided FNA to assess patients with visible but non-suspicious nodes under consideration for neoadjuvant systemic treatment.[27]

## Axillary lymph node dissection (ALND)

The extent of ALND has been defined on the basis on the number of nodes removed or on the location of the nodes excised. An accurate estimate of the level of nodes involved is only possible if the surgeon marks the specimen for the pathologist.

To determine which nodes should be removed when performing an ALND, some investigators have looked at the incidence of involvement of nodes in the upper axilla in the absence of involvement of level I nodes, so-called skip metastases. Isolated level III metastases exist in only 0.2–2% of cases. However, isolated level II metastases have been reported to be present in 1.5–29% of patients.[28–30] Other authors have investigated the distribution of axillary node metastases by studying the incidence of local recurrence after removal of varying levels of nodes. Two studies have reported axillary recurrences in 0.5–1.5% of patients who underwent complete axillary dissection.[5,31] Local recurrence rates following level II clearance are reported to be around 3%.[32]

The data above indicate that dissection of level III nodes is not necessary for staging. If grossly involved nodes are identified intraoperatively, then a level III dissection should be carried out to maximise local control.[33]

## Impact of ALND on survival

It is still unclear whether ALND confers any survival advantage. In the 1970s local treatment was considered to have little impact on survival due to the concept that breast cancer was conceived as a systemic disease from its clinical inception.[9]

The National Surgical Adjuvant Breast and Bowel Project (NSABP) B-04 trial showed no difference in survival between women who had simple mastectomy and those who underwent mastectomy and ALND. However, 33% of women in the non-dissected group did undergo some form of limited axillary surgery and the power of the study may have been insufficient to demonstrate a small but possibly clinically significant difference between groups. Meta-analyses can partly overcome the problem of underpowering, but cannot readily distinguish between the effects of removing nodal tissue per se and the effect of adjuvant systemic treatments on overall survival. One large meta-analysis of about 3000 patients did claim a survival benefit of 5.4% from ALND.[34]

A study by Cabanes et al. at the Institut Curie evaluated lumpectomy and ALND with breast irradiation versus lumpectomy without ALND plus breast and axillary irradiation. A small but significant improvement in survival at 5 years was demonstrated for women who had axillary surgery (96.6% vs. 92.6%) but with longer follow-up any apparent advantage disappeared.[35]

The view that nodal treatment does not influence survival accords with the view that metastatic cells within lymph nodes can remain confined to regional tissues and do not always have the capacity to establish viable metastatic foci at distant sites. Thus, lymph node metastases might not generate foci of distant metastatic disease but might, rather, be indicators of the ability of cancer cell clones (which may include cancer stem cells) to spread from the primary tumour haematogenously and specifically seed to tissues such as bone, lungs and liver.[36]

In summary, the data suggest that ALND is unlikely to have a major impact on survival.

## Morbidity post-ALND

There is significant morbidity associated with ALND, which includes seroma formation, impairment of shoulder movement, neuropathy and arm lymphoedema. Estimates for seroma formation vary from 4% to 52%.[37,38] Shoulder movement is impaired in the majority of patients in the immediate period after ALND, but usually returns to near-normal values within 12 months of surgery.[39,40] Numbness and paraesthesia have been reported in up to 70–80% of patients following division of the intercostobrachial nerve.[39–41] The incidence of lymphoedema ranges from 6% to 30%.[42]

### Seroma formation

Seroma formation is the most frequently occurring complication following ALND. Siegel et al. reported a 4.2% incidence of seroma formation in patients who underwent level II axillary clearance without closed-suction drainage. However, patients were only considered to have seromas if the fluid accumulation was bothersome.[43]

In another study, patients were randomised to either receive an axillary drain for 24 hours or to be followed expectantly. Any palpable fluid collections were aspirated. Drain use was found to decrease the time to seroma resolution, the mean number of aspirations required and the mean volume of fluid aspirated.[44] Relatively recent studies have indicated that not all patients need a drain and that closing the dead space by tacking down the skin flaps reduces the likelihood of seroma development.[45,46]

## Impairment of shoulder movement

The incidence of impairment of shoulder movement is probably underestimated. Patients may be at risk if the position of the arm during surgery is not carefully monitored. Hladiuk et al.[39] prospectively assessed stiffness and objective measures of strength and mobility in 63 patients undergoing axillary dissection using preoperative arm function as a control. Overall, 42% of patients had subjective or objective impairment of arm function 1 year after surgery. In a study by Lin et al.,[40] 17% of patients had greater than 15% restriction of shoulder motion at 1 year. These decreases in mobility can be of particular concern to patients who already have impaired range of upper limb motion due to other diseases or events.

Lotze et al. investigated the benefits of early (1 day postoperatively) versus late (7 days postoperatively) physical therapy on range of motion in 36 patients. No significant differences were noted between the two groups. An increase in the number of days during which a drain was required and greater incidence of seroma were noted in the early mobilisation group.[47] Other studies have failed to confirm this adverse effect of early mobilisation on lymphatic drainage.[48]

## Damage to motor nerves

Three motor nerves are at risk of injury during axillary dissection: the medial pectoral nerve, the long thoracic nerve of Bell and the thoracodorsal nerve.

Damage to the medial pectoral nerve results in minimal morbidity, but leads to unsightly wasting of the lower and lateral fibres of pectoralis major. Loss of pectoralis minor and the lateral third of pectoralis major can cause problems in patients undergoing breast reconstruction using a tissue expansion technique. Damage to the long thoracic nerve results in winging of the scapula and in an unsatisfactory aesthetic outcome. Damage to the thoracodorsal nerve results in minimal impairment, although some reduction in shoulder strength may be noted.

## Neuropathy

Numbness and paraesthesiae in the upper arm are reported in 70–80% of patients following axillary dissection, mostly due to division of the intercostobrachial nerve or more accurately nerves, as there are a number of sensory nerves encountered during axillary dissection. Occasionally sacrifice of this nerve can result in a syndrome, characterised by severe pain and paraesthesia in the upper arm, shoulder, axilla and anterior chest wall.[39–41]

It is usually possible to preserve one or more of the intercostal sensory nerves during dissection. Some units have demonstrated a better outcome at 12 months with intercostobrachial nerve preservation, and randomised studies have shown less sensory loss when the nerve is preserved.[49]

## Breast cancer-related lymphoedema (BCRL)

BCRL is a chronic swelling of the upper limb following surgery to the axillary lymph nodes (**Fig. 7.2**), and was originally described by Handley in 1908.[50] Surgical clearance of axillary lymph nodes as part of the management of invasive breast cancer is the most important aetiological factor in the development of BCRL and the primary initiating event, but it is one of the key puzzles that the majority of patients who undergo this surgical intervention do not develop this problem. Therefore, whilst BCRL may be initiated by removal of lymph nodes, the development of BCRL must depend on other additional factors.[51]

Published rates of the prevalence of BCRL in patients undergoing ALND for breast cancer range

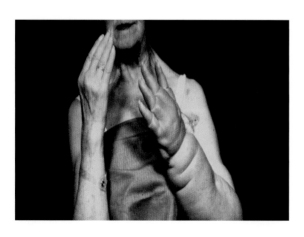

**Figure 7.2** • Breast cancer-related lymphoedema.

from 16% to 28%.[52–54] BCRL develops at a variable rate in individuals. Whilst 75% of women who develop BCRL will have it by 1 year postoperatively, and 90% by 3 years, another puzzling feature of BCRL is that there is often a significant delay in many patients between the initial insult (i.e. surgery) and the development of swelling.[51]

A number of risk factors can be identified for the development of BCRL. The extent of surgery to the breast seems to play a significant role.[52,55]

A correlation between the number of lymph nodes removed at surgery and the development of BCRL has been shown in numerous studies,[56,57] although others have failed to show this relationship.[55] Paradoxically, negative lymph node status has been shown to be related to the development of BCRL.[58] Both four-node axillary sampling[56,57,59] and sentinel lymph node biopsy[60–62] have been shown to reduce the incidence rate of BCRL when compared to ALND.

Using blue dye injected into the arms to visualise and preserve arm lymphatics is one technique being evaluated to reduce the incidence of BCRL.

Management of BCRL

There is a wide range of treatments available for BCRL, reflecting the lack of proven efficacy of any one particular approach. Following ALND, patients are advised to be meticulous with skin care and hygiene, and avoid cuts and injections whenever possible on the operated arm. Although they are also advised to avoid rigorous exercise using this limb, and not to lift heavy weights, there is little evidence base for these precautions and they are primarily based on anecdotal reports by patients about what precipitated their swelling. Once arm swelling has occurred, treatment can be classified into three types: conservative, pharmacological and surgical.[63] Conservative treatment with massage and compression sleeves remains the sheet anchor of treatment.

# Axillary irradiation

## Primary radiotherapy to the axilla

Radiation therapy to the involved axilla, in the absence of axillary surgery, is also effective in preventing recurrence in patients with clinically negative nodes. Retrospective experience has dem-

onstrated an axillary recurrence rate of approximately 1–2% with radiation therapy alone to the axilla. A series from the Joint Centre for Radiation Therapy in Boston described a 0.8% failure rate in 390 node-negative patients, with a median survival of 77 months. N1 patients had a slightly higher recurrence rate at 2.9%.[64]

Spruit et al. compared women treated with breast-conserving surgery combined with radiotherapy to the axilla (plus tamoxifen) to patients treated with breast-conserving surgery and ALND. Local relapse rates were similar in the two groups, 1.1% and 1.5% respectively at 5 years.[65]

Axillary radiotherapy and ALND have been compared in randomised studies. In the NSABP B-04 trial[5] there was no difference in 10-year survival or in axillary failure rate between patients who received radical mastectomy (including ALND) and patients who received total mastectomy (without ALND) plus radiotherapy to the chest wall and regional lymph nodes. A prospective randomised trial was also conducted at the Institut Curie between 1982 and 1987, comparing lumpectomy plus ALND (group A) and lumpectomy plus radiotherapy of regional nodes (group B). The 5-year results of this study were published in 1992.[35] The investigators observed a significant advantage for axillary dissection (ALND) in overall and disease-free survival at 5 years. However, 15-year follow-up results showed no difference in overall survival or disease-free survival. Rates of ipsilateral breast recurrences were the same in the two groups at 60, 120 and 180 months. Rates of isolated axillary recurrences (without concomitant breast recurrence) were 1% in group A versus 3% in group B at 180 months.

## Adjuvant radiotherapy to the axilla

In an overview of randomised trials, the Early Breast Cancer Trialists' Collaborative Group demonstrated that radiotherapy reduced the locoregional relapse rate by about two-thirds, from 19.6% to 6.7%. This was independent of the type of axillary surgery or nodal status, and included breast-conserving surgery and mastectomy.[66] Axillary irradiation may be added to ALND in some cases where women are identified as being at high risk of axillary recurrence, such as where disease is thought to remain after ALND. In these situations, axillary irradiation may confer additional benefits over ALND alone in controlling axillary disease and preventing ensuing symptoms, but there is an increased risk of developing

BCRL (up to 40%). There is no benefit from adding axillary irradiation in women who have ALND with a small number of involved lymph nodes. Most studies have shown at least 50% of recurrences in such women to be on the chest wall, and isolated nodal recurrences are uncommon.[67–71]

 Randomised trials[72,73] have shown an improvement in survival in high-risk disease for patients having the entire lymphatic basin and chest wall irradiated and a reduction in locoregional relapse from 32% to 9% at 10 years.

## Axillary irradiation: complications

Adjuvant radiotherapy to the axilla appears to increase the rate of development of BCRL in many studies.[59,74,75] The pathophysiology of radiation-induced BCRL is related to fibrosis indirectly causing constriction of lymphatic channels[57,76–78] and lymphatic fluid to lymph nodes, which have decreased filter and immune functions as a result.[79] Restriction of shoulder and arm movement is relatively common (approximately 20%), even when the shoulder joint is excluded from the radiation beam.[80] This may be due to the effects of radiation on the pectoral and other muscles associated with shoulder movement. Other complications described for axillary irradiation include rib fractures, pneumonitis, and rarely damage to the brachial plexus and an increased incidence of sarcoma.

## Axillary node sampling

Axillary node sampling refers to the practice of removing a variable amount of the axillary contents without some reference to anatomical structures. Steele et al. reported a randomised trial involving 401 patients who underwent either ALND or axillary node sampling. The incidence of nodal positivity did not differ between the two groups. A subset of patients underwent sampling followed by anatomical dissection, with an increase in the mean number of nodes obtained from 4.1 to 19.7, but none of these patients were upstaged.[81] Similar results had previously been repeated by Forrest et al.[82] A proper axillary node sample as described by Steele et al. removes a minimum of four nodes.[81] The nodes removed are usually from level I, but it differs from a formal level I clearance in that the lateral aspect of the axilla and the subcapsular fossa

are not dissected and individual nodes are 'cherry-picked' from the axilla and only node tissue is removed and sent for pathology. The nerves to latissimus dorsi and serratus anterior are not routinely identified. More elaborate descriptions of this procedure sometimes nominate the intercostobrachial nerve as a landmark of the superior extent of an axillary sample.[83]

In contrast to the results reported by Steele et al., Kissin et al. argued that 24% of patients undergoing axillary node sampling may be erroneously staged.[83] The risk of axillary recurrence seems to be inversely related to the number of nodes removed, with failure rates ranging from 5% to 21% in patients with fewer than five nodes removed.[32,84,85]

An evolution from the 'blind' four-node axillary sampling is the combination of blue dye-directed axillary sampling. Results so far indicate false-negative rates similar to SLNB using dye and radio-activity combined. In a prospective comparison study, Macmillan et al. undertook standard four-node axillary sampling in conjunction with radioisotope localisation and found that the hot node or SLN was present in the excised four-node specimen in more than 75% of cases.[86]

The Edinburgh group recently carried out a study evaluating the combined technique in 434 patients with early breast cancer in a single centre. A blue sentinel node was identified in 394 of 434 cases (91.7%); the false-negative rate was 2.4%. Thirty-six patients had no sentinel node identified. Thirteen of these had positive nodes in the node sample.[87]

## Sentinel lymph node biopsy (SLNB)

SLNB offers the opportunity to identify node-negative breast cancer patients by a surgical procedure that is associated with low morbidity. The concept of the sentinel node being the first node to contain metastatic cancer within a tumour's lymphatic basin was introduced by Cabanas following his work on carcinoma of the penis.[88] Morton et al. subsequently applied this principle to malignant melanoma.[89] The technique was then adapted to the breast by Giuliano et al.[90] An important benefit associated with SLNB is that histopathologists can focus their attention on fewer nodes that are most likely to harbour metastases. SLNB represents a major shift in the surgical management of breast cancer.

Several randomised trials have compared SLNB with ALND and examined the effects on morbidity, recurrence and survival.

A study by Veronesi et al. involving 516 patients with early breast cancer randomised patients to undergo either SLNB and simultaneous completion ALND or SLNB followed by ALND only if the sentinel node contained metastasis. A similar incidence of sentinel node positivity was observed in both groups (32.3% vs. 35.5%). There was less pain and better arm mobility in patients who underwent sentinel node biopsy only than in those who also underwent axillary dissection. Among the 167 patients who did not undergo axillary dissection, there were no cases of overt axillary recurrence during follow-up.[61]

More recently the authors[91] have reported an update on this trial. There was no difference in disease-free or overall survival between the groups. The number of patients with axillary recurrence was very low, and consistent with those of 25-year follow-up of the NSABP B-04 study.[92]

In a further study by Purushotham et al.,[60] 298 patients with early breast cancer (tumours 3 cm or less on ultrasound examination) who were clinically node negative were randomly allocated to undergo ALND (control group) or SLNB followed by ALND if they were subsequently found to be lymph node positive (study group). A detailed assessment of physical and psychological morbidity was performed during a 12-month period postoperatively. A significant reduction in arm swelling, rate of seroma formation, numbness, loss of sensitivity to light touch and pinprick was observed in the study group. Although shoulder mobility was less impaired on average in the study group, this was significant only for abduction at 1 month and flexion at 3 months. Scores reflecting quality of life and psychological morbidity were significantly better in the study group in the immediate postoperative period, with fewer long-term differences demonstrating an overall significant reduction in physical and psychological morbidity.

The ALMANAC trial randomly assigned patients to two groups: (1) standard ALND or (2) SLNB with delayed ALND (or axillary radiation therapy if metastases were found). Researchers evaluated patients in both groups for side-effects and for perceived quality of life. The authors concluded that SLNB is associated with reduced arm morbidity and better quality of life than standard axillary treatment and should be the treatment of choice for patients with early-stage breast cancer and a clinically negative axilla.[62]

The NSABP B-32 trial recruited 5611 women with invasive breast cancer who were randomly assigned to receive either SLN resection followed by immediate conventional ALND (n = 2807; group 1) or SLN resection without ALND if SLNs were negative on intraoperative cytology and histological examination (n = 2804; group 2). Patients within group 2 underwent ALND if no SLNs were identified or if one or more SLNs were positive on intraoperative cytology or subsequent histological examination. Primary end-points included survival, regional control and morbidity. Secondary end-points were accuracy and technical success. SLNs were successfully removed in 97·2% of patients in both groups combined. Identification of a pre-incision hot spot was associated with greater SLN removal (98·9%). Only 1·4% of SLN specimens were outside of axillary levels I and II. In all, 65.1% of SLN specimens were both radioactive and blue; a small percentage was identified by palpation only (3·9%). The overall accuracy of SLN resection in patients within group 1 was 97·1%, with a false-negative rate of 9·8%. Differences in tumour location, type of biopsy and number of SLNs removed significantly affected the false-negative rate.[93] Data relating to survival, regional control and morbidity are not yet available from this trial.

Patients enrolled in the now-closed American College of Surgeons Oncology Group (ACOSOG) Z0010 trial underwent bone marrow aspiration prior to SLNB. Immunocytochemical analysis of the marrow will be compared to the status of SLNBs to determine prognostic accuracy.[94] ACOSOG Z0011 randomised women undergoing breast-conserving therapy with low-volume axillary disease to completion axillary dissection or observation. Overall survival, disease-free survival, local regional control and morbidity were the trial end-points.[95] A total of 891 patients were randomly assigned to SLNB + ALND (n = 445) or SLNB alone (n = 446). Information on wound infection, axillary seroma, paraesthesia, brachial plexus injury (BPI) and lymphoedema was available for 821 patients. Patients who underwent SLNB alone had significantly less surgical morbidity. At 1 year, only 2% of patients who underwent SLNB alone had any evidence of lymphoedema versus 13% of patients following SLNB + ALND. BPIs occurred in less than 1% of patients. The use of SLNB alone resulted in fewer complications.

Ongoing trials, including EORTC 10981 and IBCSG-23-01, are addressing additional issues such as the efficacy of completion ALND versus axillary radiotherapy in sentinel lymph node-positive disease and the impact of ALND in patients with sentinel node micrometastases.[96]

Two issues of importance when considering the applicability of these trials' results to routine clinical practice relate to patient selection and surgical and technical abilities. The 2005 American Society for Clinical Oncology guidelines recommend that patients with clinically node-negative tumours that are 5 cm or smaller are appropriate candidates for lymph node mapping and sentinel node biopsy.[97] Completion ALND remains standard treatment for patients with axillary macrometastases identified on SLNB (**Fig. 7.3**). Appropriately identified patients with a negative SNB, when done under the direction of an experienced surgeon, need not have completion ALND.

The identification of micrometastasis or isolated cancer cells detected by pathological examination of the SLN with use of specialised techniques is currently of unknown clinical significance (**Fig. 7.4**).

Although the data suggest that SLNB is associated with less morbidity than ALND, the comparative effects of these two approaches on tumour recurrence and patient survival requires longer-term follow-up. An important issue regarding widespread utilisation of SLNB relates to surgical quality control, i.e. the demonstration of surgical experience and competence (as determined by the number of cases, the rates of SLN identification and the rate of false negatives).

Data are now available to also support the use of SLNB for multicentric tumours: DCIS, when mastectomy and/or when immediate reconstruction is planned; for older or obese patients; in male breast cancer; and prior excisional or diagnostic biopsy[97] (Table 7.1). SLNB is usually not recommended in T3–4 tumours, inflammatory breast cancer, DCIS not treated by mastectomy, suspicious palpable axillary nodes, pregnancy, previous axillary surgery, previous non-oncological breast surgery and following neoadjuvant treatment. Despite the recommendations following neoadjuvant hormone and chemotherapy and previous axillary sampling, SLNB is being used increasingly and large data sets on these indications are accumulating to show it is safe in these settings.

## Pathological evaluation of sentinel lymph nodes

Pathologists, as part of their standard analysis, must quantify tumour burden in nodes. Consistent reporting, using the American Joint Commission on Cancer (AJCC)/International Union Against Cancer (UICC) staging system, facilitates uniform communication with clinicians and analysis of outcomes.

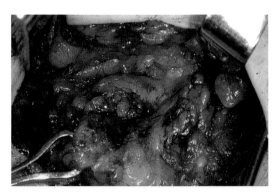

**Figure 7.3** • Sentinel lymph node biopsy – blue-stained lymphatic leading to blue node.

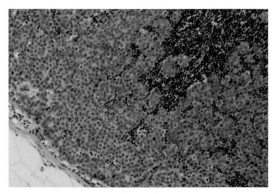

**Figure 7.4** • Axillary lymph node metastasis (haematoxylin/eosin stain).

Table 7.1   Randomised clinical trials involving sentinel lymph node biopsy

| Trial | Phase | Title | ClinicalTrials.gov identifier |
|-------|-------|-------|-------------------------------|
| IBCSG-23-01 | III | Randomised study of surgical resection with or without axillary lymph node dissection in women with clinically node-negative breast cancer with sentinel node micrometastases | NCT00072293 |
| GF-GS-01 | III | Comparing conventional axillary dissection vs. sentinel node resection in clinically node-negative operable breast cancer | NCT00144898 |
| SCCC-2003161 | N/A | Thoracoscopic internal mammary sentinel node biopsy | NCT00450723 |
| MDA-ID-01538 | N/A | Injection methods in finding the sentinel lymph node during lymphatic mapping and sentinel lymph node biopsy in patients with invasive breast cancer | NCT00438477 |
| GUMC-00152 | III | Prognostic study of sentinel lymph node and bone marrow metastases in women with stage I or stage IIA breast cancer | NCT00003854 |
| EU-20006 | II | Sentinel lymph node biopsy to assess axillary lymph nodes in women with stage I or stage II breast cancer | NCT00005821 |
| EU-20214 | N/A | Technetium Tc-99m sulfur colloid and blue dye in detecting sentinel lymph nodes in patients with breast cancer | NCT00052676 |
| NSABP B-32 | III | Surgery to remove sentinel lymph nodes with or without removing lymph nodes in the armpit in treating women with breast cancer | NCT00003830 |
| 07/089 | III | The efficacy of radioguided occult lesion localisation (ROLL) vs. wire-guided localisation (WGL) in breast-conserving surgery for non-palpable breast cancer: a randomised clinical trial | NCT00539474 |
| ACOSOG Z0011 | III | Lymph node removal in treating women who have stage I or stage II breast cancer | NCT00003855 |

Intraoperative assessment of SLNs has been evaluated as part of the development of the modern SLNB technique.[89] It allows immediate completion ALND should the SLNB be positive for tumour. Approximately 75% of patients who undergo SLNB are lymph node negative. In a proportion of the 25% of patients with positive nodes, disease will not be detected intraoperatively because of sampling limitations and the challenge of detecting micrometastases (9% false-negative results).[97] Intra-operative assessment may be by gross inspection, imprint cytology, evaluation of cells scraped from the cut surface of the node, or frozen section.

SLNs that are positive on gross examination are most likely to be associated with positive non-sentinel nodes. It is therefore of real value to identify this category of SLNs early in surgical management. Immediate cytological evaluation or frozen section can confirm suspicious gross appearances. Cut surfaces of SLNs touched to glass slides provide cellular imprints and cell-rich scrapes of the SLN surfaces may be smeared onto a slide. A positive imprint/smear is of immediate practical assistance, but negative imprints/smears are not definitive evidence that a node is tumour free. Intraoperative frozen sections carry the risk of destruction of potentially diagnostic tissue. However, with experienced clinicians, frozen section may be the most desirable intraoperative assessment for some surgeon/pathologist teams, providing slightly higher sensitivity for detection of metastases than immediate cytology alone.[98]

The identification of specific tumour mRNA markers by reverse transcription–polymerase chain reaction has been identified as a potentially valuable diagnostic adjunct for the detection of breast cancer metastases in axillary SLNs in the past.[99] More recently molecular assays for the intraoperative assessment of SLN involvement have become available and have been assessed in a few studies. The assay consists of a reverse transcriptase–polymerase chain reaction that detects the presence of metastasis through the detection of gene-expression markers (mammoglobin and cytokeratin 19) that are present in involved nodal tissue. The assay has been calibrated for the detection of metastasis larger than 0.2 mm.[100] Mansel et al. have found the sensitivity and specificity of the assay to be 100% and 97.6% respectively in interim results from 48 patients, and concluded that the assay allows more thorough node analysis by reducing sampling error and improves intraoperative surgical management of breast cancer patients.[101] Other authors have found similar results[102, 103] and have concluded that the sensitivity of the reverse transcription–polymerase chain reaction assay is comparable to that of the histopathological examination of the entire SLN by serial sectioning at 1.5–2 mm. Hughes et al. have described a similar approach utilising two different markers (TACSTD1 and PIP) that display similar rates of success in the identification of metastatic involvement of SLNs.[104]

Most SLNs with macrometastases or micrometastases are readily identified by examination of haematoxylin/eosin-stained sections.[105] Limited step sections from the block (top level plus one or two sections cut at 200- to 500-µm intervals into the block) enhance detection of micrometastases by allowing evaluation of more of the subcapsular sinus, the location in which micrometastases are most often found. Through this approach, virtually all macrometastases (>2.0 mm) and most micrometastases (>0.2 up to 2.0 mm) will be detected on limited haematoxylin/eosin-stained step sections. In some patients, this technique will allow the detection of isolated tumour cells and clusters of tumour cells (≤0.2 mm), particularly if immunohistochemi-

cal (IHC) analysis is utilised (**Fig. 7.5**). IHC analysis may facilitate screening of SLN sections, but the significance and practical relevance of small clusters of breast cancer cells detected by this method are debated. There is insufficient evidence at present to recommend that IHC for cytokeratins to detect small numbers of cells in a node should be used routinely. Routine IHC is not currently recommended for the evaluation of sentinel nodes from patients with breast cancer.[97]

Results from these assays are available within 30–40 minutes and are being used intraoperatively to decide which patients should proceed to an axillary dissection.

### The impact of nodal micrometastasis and isolated tumour cells

Interest in micrometastasis and isolated tumour cells arises from the fact that women with no evidence of nodal disease have a significant incidence of recurrence (25–30%).[106] The prognostic significance of micrometastases (between 0.2 and 2 mm) and isolated tumour cells is still relatively unclear. Some studies have assigned prognostic significance to nodal micrometastases,[107,108] whereas others have not identified any association between microscopic nodal involvement and prognosis.[106,109] Conflicting opinion exists also on the matter of isolated tumour cells. Whereas some argue that the presence of a few isolated cancer cells in a sentinel lymph node may not be of prognostic significance,[110,111] others believe that the identification of isolated tumour cells requires a completion ALND.[112] The AJCC Cancer Staging Manual recommends more aggressive therapy in these cases. The same guidelines currently classify isolated tumour cells together with node-negative disease.

### Predicting non-sentinel node metastatic disease when the SLN is positive

In patients in whom the SLN is positive for metastatic disease, further options for treatment include completion ALND or radiotherapy. In an overview of 69 reports of SLNB validated by a back-up ALND,[113] residual axillary metastases were found in 53% of SLN-positive cases. Such metastases, if left behind, increase the risk of axillary LR compared with SLN-negative patients, but this may not be true for all patients. Therefore, completion ALND may be unnecessary in a subset of women

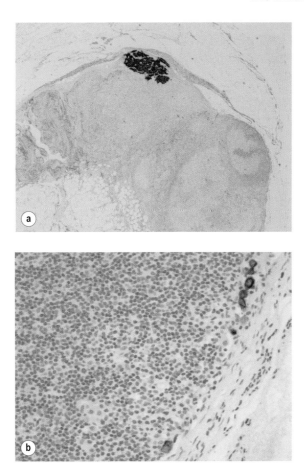

**Figure 7.5** • Axillary lymph node – micrometastasis **(a)** and isolated tumour cells **(b)**.

with SLN metastatic disease in whom the risk of additional non-SLN disease is low.[114]

Several pathological factors have been shown to be associated with a higher risk of non-SLN involvement in the presence of a positive SLN. These include primary tumour-related factors (histological type, invasive carcinoma size, histological grade, presence of lymphovascular invasion and estrogen receptor status) and node-related factors (method of detection of metastasis, size of metastasis, extranodal extension, number of positive SLNs and number of negative SLNs).[115]

The Memorial Sloan-Kettering Cancer Center (MSKCC) has developed a nomogram (www.mskcc.org/nomograms) for predicting the risk of non-SLN involvement in the presence of a positive SLN.[116] The MSKCC nomogram has been tested prospectively and shown to be a valuable method of predicting non-SLN involvement. The predictive power of this nomogram was assessed by calculating the area under the receiver–operator characteristic (ROC) curve.[116] Several studies have attempted to validate this nomogram outside the source institution with mixed results; some of these studies have found the nomogram to be accurate in predicting the likelihood of non-SLN metastases, with an ROC between 0.710 and 0.770,[117–119] others have demonstrated limited predictive accuracy.[115,120] One study described greater predictive ability (ROC 0.840) by using a simplified version of the nomogram incorporating only three features (size of SLN metastasis, grade of primary tumour, proportion of metastatic SLNs) and hypothesised that a potential weakness of the MSKCC nomogram could be the use of the method of initial detection of SLN metastasis as a surrogate for the true size of SLN metastasis, hence limiting interinstitution applicability.[115] The available clinical guidelines on SLNB are listed in Table 7.2.

**Table 7.2** • Clinical guidelines issued on sentinel lymph node biopsy

| Issuing body | Country | Update | Reference |
|---|---|---|---|
| ASCO | USA | 2005 | J Clin Oncol 2005; 23(30):7703–20 |
| NCCN | USA | 2008 | www.nccn.org |
| St Gallen | Switzerland | 2003 | Breast 2003; 12:569–82 |
| NBCC | Australia | 2005 | www.nbcc.org.au/media/Sentinel_node_biopsy.html |
| SCCP | Canada | 2001 | www.cmaj.ca/cgi/content/full/165/2/166 |
| NICE | UK | 2005 | www.nice.org.uk/guidance/IPG147 |
| CAP | USA | 2005 | www.cap.org |

## Controversies in sentinel lymph node biopsy

SLNB in patients with a clinically positive axilla.

> A clinically positive axilla is currently considered an absolute contraindication to SLNB. When axillary metastases are documented by FNA of a clinically palpable node, a routine level II or III ALND is the procedure of choice. However, it would be appropriate to proceed to SLNB plus excision of palpable lymph nodes in patients with non-FNA-documented palpable lymphoadenopathy.

This is justified by the fact that in the absence of FNA-documented metastases, clinical assessment of the presence of axillary metastases is notoriously inaccurate, and the presence of palpable lymphadenopathy is often due to a normal physiological reaction to biopsy of the breast rather than to metastases from cancer. If the SLN and the palpable axillary lymph nodes are negative for metastases, no further axillary surgery would be indicated.

### Multicentric breast cancer

> There is indication that the site of injection of mapping agents is not critical for accurate detection of SLNs. This concept is supported by findings of Kim et al. in a study investigating lymphatic mapping for patients with multicentric tumours. In each patient, blue dye was injected peritumourally around one lesion and isotope injected peritumourally around the second lesion. In all cases at least one SLN demonstrated uptake of both blue dye and isotope.[121] The demonstration that different breast injection sites yield the same clusters of SLNs representing the primary drainage for the entire breast have set the stage for employing lymphatic mapping in patients with multicentric breast cancer. Several investigators have evaluated the

accuracy of lymphatic mapping in this setting.[122–124] Various injection sites and techniques have been employed, including subareolar, peritumoural or intraparenchymal, and dermal. In general, the studies reported thus far support the validity and safety of utilising SLNB to document the nodal status of patients with multiple breast tumours.

The SLN identification rates are 90–100%, the average false-negative rate is less than 10% and, in a substantial proportion of patients, axillary metastases are limited to the SLNs. As was experienced in patients with unifocal disease, results from the procedure are improved with combined use of both an isotope and a blue dye as mapping agents.

### Neoadjuvant systemic therapy

Historically, neoadjuvant systemic therapy was used to treat patients with locally advanced disease with a view to downstaging the tumour. SLNB has been studied in this context in several studies previously and has been shown to yield a slightly higher false-negative rate. However, with better understanding of the technique of lymphatic mapping and SLNB and the increasing use of neoadjuvant systemic therapy in early-stage disease, performing SLNB in this clinical scenario is entirely appropriate.

The appropriate use and optimal timing of SLNB in the setting of neoadjuvant chemotherapy remains controversial. In clinically node-negative patients, an SLNB before neoadjuvant chemotherapy allows accurate nodal staging. Clinically node-positive patients may achieve significant downstaging after neoadjuvant systemic therapy, some of whom may become node negative. The option of SLNB in this group of patients with no further treatment to the node-negative axilla is a possibility.

Studies evaluating SLNB after neoadjuvant chemotherapy have shown wide variability in identification and false-negative rates. The largest series to date consists of patients enrolled in NSABP B-27, in which 428 patients received neoadjuvant chemotherapy followed by SLNB and completion dissection, with an identification rate of 85% and a false-negative rate of 11%.[125] The described false-negative rates are higher than the 5% acceptable rate published by the Consensus Conference on the Role of Sentinel Lymph Node Biopsy in Carcinoma of the Breast in 2002,[126] but similar to those in the large NSABP study of sentinel nodes.

 On the basis of these findings some recommend SLNB for clinically node-negative patients before neoadjuvant treatment. Others prefer to perform SLNB after neoadjuvant systemic therapy, citing a reduced re-operation rate and the avoidance of ALND for node-negative patients as the main motivating factors in their decision.[127]

### SLNB in patients with ductal carcinoma in situ (DCIS)

By definition, DCIS of the breast is a non-invasive lesion that does not have the ability to metastasise. For the most part, this disease is treated to prevent the development of invasive breast cancer. Given this background, ALND or SLNB is inappropriate in patients with DCIS. However, patients with DCIS sometimes have microinvasive or, frankly, invasive carcinoma that can be missed by the pathologist. In a large series from the M.D. Anderson Cancer Center, 399 patients with an initial diagnosis of DCIS underwent determination of which factors were associated with finding invasive carcinoma on final pathological evaluation.[128] On multivariate analysis, significant independent predictors of finding invasive carcinoma were: age younger than or equal to 55 years; diagnosis made with a core biopsy; mammographic size greater than 4 cm; and

high-grade disease. Overall, 20% of the patients with an initial diagnosis of DCIS were found to have invasive carcinoma, and 35% of these patients underwent an SLNB. Patients in this series were more often offered SLNB if they had a mastectomy. Ten percent of patients were found to have a positive SLN and the only independent predictor of finding axillary metastases in patients initially believed to have DCIS only was the presence of a palpable tumour at diagnosis. On the basis of this analysis, the investigators conclude that SLNB should not be performed in all patients with an initial diagnosis of DCIS. Instead, the risks and benefits of SLNB should be discussed with patients scheduled to undergo mastectomy, younger patients, and patients with large or high-grade DCIS. Data from the Moffitt Cancer Center (Tampa, FL) were the first to report the results of SLNB in patients with DCIS, and they identified involved SLNs in 6–9% of consecutive unselected patients.[129] At the Memorial Sloan-Kettering Cancer Center, SLNB was performed in 21% of patients with DCIS who were considered at high risk for the presence of invasion. In this highly selected group of patients, 12% of patients had positive SLNs.[21] At the European Institute of Oncology, approximately 3% of unselected patients with pure DCIS were found to have a positive SLN.[130] Taken together, these studies indicate that lymphatic mapping and SLNB for DCIS should not be routinely done in all patients. However, patients diagnosed with DCIS who are scheduled to undergo mastectomy, and patients considered at high risk of invasive disease, can be offered SLNB as part of their initial surgical management.

In conclusion, there are several options in the management of the axilla in patients undergoing treatment for breast cancer. The treatment should be tailored to the individual patient based on tumour and patient characteristics.

- Approximately 30–40% of symptomatic patients with early breast cancer have axillary nodal involvement. Node-positive breast cancers have a worse prognosis than node-negative cases.
- The likelihood of axillary nodal involvement is directly related to the size of the tumour, date higher histological grade and presence of lymphovascular invasion.
- ALND was, until recently, the most widely used technique for staging the axilla. Recently, less invasive techniques such as SLNB have evolved that have challenged the role of routine ALND in all patients with breast cancer.
- When ALND is indicated, a level II/III anatomical dissection is the preferred operation.
- There is significant morbidity associated with ALND. Both four-node axillary sampling and SLNB have been shown to reduce the incidence rate of complications.
- There is consensus that patients with DCIS that is extensive (on imaging) and treatment is to be by mastectomy or presents as a palpable mass (about 20%) should have SLNB.
- Conservative treatment with massage and compression sleeves remain the main anchor of treatment for BCRL.
- The appropriate staging technique for ALN-negative patients with tumours smaller than 5 cm is SLNB. Completion ALND remains standard treatment for patients with macrometastases identified on SLNB.
- Most SLNs with macrometastases or micrometastases are readily identified by examination of haematoxylin/eosin-stained sections. The presence of isolated tumour cells is currently classified with node-negative disease.
- Studies reported thus far support the validity and safety of utilising SLNB to document the nodal status of patients with multiple breast tumours.
- Several options are available in the management of the axilla in patients undergoing treatment for breast cancer. Treatment should be tailored to the individual patient based on tumour and patient characteristics.

# References

1. Dent DM. Axillary lymphadenectomy for breast cancer. Paradigm shifts and pragmatic surgeons. Arch Surg 1996; 131:1125–7.

2. Halsted WS. A clinical and histological study of certain adenocarcinomata of the breast: and a brief consideration of the supraclavicular operation and of the results of operations for cancer of the breast from 1889 to 1898 at the Johns Hopkins Hospital. Ann Surg 1898; 28:557–76.

3. Eggers C. Cancer surgery: the value of radical operations for cancer after the lymphatic drainage area has become involved. Ann Surg 1937; 106:668–89.

4. Cancer Research Campaign Working Party. Cancer Research Campaign (King's/Cambridge) trial for early breast cancer. A detailed update at the tenth year. Lancet 1980; 2:55–60.

5. Fisher B, Redmond C, Fisher ER et al. Ten-year results of a randomized clinical trial comparing radical mastectomy and total mastectomy with or without radiation. N Engl J Med 1985; 312:674–81.

6. Wood WC, Budman DR, Korzun AH et al. Dose and dose intensity of adjuvant chemotherapy for stage II, node-positive breast carcinoma. N Engl J Med 1994; 330:1253–9.

7. Bonadonna G. Evolving concepts in the systemic adjuvant treatment of breast cancer. Cancer Res 1992; 52:2127–37.

8. Mittra I. Axillary lymph node metastasis in breast cancer: prognostic indicator or lead-time bias? Eur J Cancer 1993; 29A:300–2.

9. Fisher B. The evolution of paradigms for the management of breast cancer: a personal perspective. Cancer Res 1992; 52:2371–83.

10. Hellman S. Karnofsky Memorial Lecture. Natural history of small breast cancers. J Clin Oncol 1994; 12:2229–34.

11. Pickren JW. Significance of occult metastases. A study of breast cancer. Cancer 1961; 14:1266–71.

12. Cruikshank W. The anatomy of the absorbing vessels of the human body. London: G. Nicol, 1786.

13. Mascagni P. Vasorum lymphaticorum corporis humani historia et ichonographiaed. Senis: P. Carli, 1787.

14. Haagensen CD. Diseases of the breast, 3rd edn. London: Saunders, 1986.

15. Ravdin PM. How can prognostic and predictive factors in breast cancer be used in a practical way today? Recent Results Cancer Res 1998; 152:86–93.

16. Carmichael AR, Aparanji K, Nightingale P et al. A clinicopathological scoring system to select breast cancer patients for sentinel node biopsy. Eur J Surg Oncol 2006; 32:1170–4.

17. Cariati M, Purushotham AD. Internal mammary nodes and breast cancer. Br J Surg 2005; 92:131–2.

18. Carter CL, Allen C, Henson DE. Relation of tumor size, lymph node status, and survival in 24,740 breast cancer cases. Cancer 1989; 63:181–7.

19. Della Rovere GQ, Benson JR. A critique of the sentinel node concept. Breast 2006; 15:693–7.

20. Benson JR, della Rovere GQ. Management of the axilla in women with breast cancer. Lancet Oncol 2007; 8:331–48.

21. Klauber-DeMore N, Tan LK, Liberman L et al. Sentinel lymph node biopsy: is it indicated in patients with high-risk ductal carcinoma-in-situ and ductal carcinoma-in-situ with microinvasion? Ann Surg Oncol 2000; 7:636–42.

22. Dabbs DJ, Fung M, Landsittel D et al. Sentinel lymph node micrometastasis as a predictor of axillary tumor burden. Breast J 2004; 10:101–5.

23. Fisher B, Slack NH, Bross ID. Cancer of the breast: size of neoplasm and prognosis. Cancer 1969; 24:1071–80.

24. Butcher HR Jr. Mammary carcinoma. A discussion of therapeutic methods. Cancer 1969; 24:1272–9.

25. Bucalossi P, Veronesi U, Zingo L et al. Enlarged mastectomy for breast cancer. Review of 1,213 cases. Am J Roentgenol Radium Ther Nucl Med 1971; 111:119–22.

26. Gilissen F, Oostenbroek R, Storm R et al. Prevention of futile sentinel node procedures in breast cancer: ultrasonography of the axilla and fine-needle aspiration cytology are obligatory. Eur J Surg Oncol 2007; 34(5):497–500.

27. Jain A, Haisfield-Wolfe ME, Lange J et al. The role of ultrasound-guided fine-needle aspiration of axillary nodes in the staging of breast cancer. Ann Surg Oncol 2008; 15(2):462–71.

28. Rosen PP, Lesser ML, Kinne DW et al. Discontinuous or "skip" metastases in breast carcinoma. Analysis of 1228 axillary dissections. Ann Surg 1983; 197:276–83.

29. Veronesi U, Rilke F, Luini A et al. Distribution of axillary node metastases by level of invasion. An analysis of 539 cases. Cancer 1987; 59:682–7.

30. Smith JA 3rd, Gamez-Araujo JJ, Gallager HS et al. Carcinoma of the breast: analysis of total lymph node involvement versus level of metastasis. Cancer 1977; 39:527–32.

31. Haagensen CD. The physiology of the breast as it concerns the clinician. Am J Obstet Gynecol 1971; 109:206–9.

32. Fowble B, Solin LJ, Schultz DJ et al. Frequency, sites of relapse, and outcome of regional node failures following conservative surgery and radiation for early breast cancer. Int J Radiat Oncol Biol Phys 1989; 17:703–10.

33. NIH Consensus Conference. Treatment of early-stage breast cancer. JAMA 1991; 265:391–5.

34. Orr RK. The impact of prophylactic axillary node dissection on breast cancer survival – a Bayesian meta-analysis. Ann Surg Oncol 1999; 6:109–16.

35. Cabanes PA, Salmon RJ, Vilcoq JR et al. Value of axillary dissection in addition to lumpectomy and radiotherapy in early breast cancer. The Breast Carcinoma Collaborative Group of the Institut Curie. Lancet 1992; 339:1245–8.

36. Cady B, Falkenberry SS, Chung MA. The surgeon's role in outcome in contemporary breast cancer. Surg Oncol Clin North Am 2000; 9:119–32, viii.

37. Say CC, Donegan W. A biostatistical evaluation of complications from mastectomy. Surg Gynecol Obstet 1974; 138:370–6.

38. Tadych K, Donegan WL. Postmastectomy seromas and wound drainage. Surg Gynecol Obstet 1987; 165:483–7.

39. Hladiuk M, Huchcroft S, Temple W et al. Arm function after axillary dissection for breast cancer: a pilot study to provide parameter estimates. J Surg Oncol 1992; 50:47–52.

40. Lin PP, Allison DC, Wainstock J et al. Impact of axillary lymph node dissection on the therapy of breast cancer patients. J Clin Oncol 1993; 11:1536–44.

41. Ivens D, Hoe AL, Podd TJ et al. Assessment of morbidity from complete axillary dissection. Br J Cancer 1992; 66:136–8.

42. Petrek JA, Heelan MC. Incidence of breast carcinoma-related lymphedema. Cancer 1998; 83:2776–81.

43. Siegel BM, Mayzel KA, Love SM. Level I and II axillary dissection in the treatment of early-stage breast cancer. An analysis of 259 consecutive patients. Arch Surg 1990; 125:1144–7.

44. Somers RG, Jablon LK, Kaplan MJ et al. The use of closed suction drainage after lumpectomy and axillary node dissection for breast cancer.

A prospective randomized trial. Ann Surg 1992; 215:146–9.

45. O'Dwyer PJ, O'Higgins NJ, James AG. Effect of closing dead space on incidence of seroma after mastectomy. Surg Gynecol Obstet 1991; 172:55–6.

46. Purushotham AD, McLatchie E, Young D et al. Randomized clinical trial of no wound drains and early discharge in the treatment of women with breast cancer. Br J Surg 2002; 89:286–92.

47. Lotze MT, Duncan MA, Gerber LH et al. Early versus delayed shoulder motion following axillary dissection: a randomized prospective study. Ann Surg 1981; 193:288–95.

48. Petrek JA, Peters MM, Nori S et al. Axillary lymphadenectomy. A prospective, randomized trial of 13 factors influencing drainage, including early or delayed arm mobilization. Arch Surg 1990; 125:378–82.

49. Freeman SR, Washington SJ, Pritchard T et al. Long term results of a randomised prospective study of preservation of the intercostobrachial nerve. Eur J Surg Oncol 2003; 29:213–5.

50. Handley WS. Lymphoangioplasty: a new method for the relief of the brawny arm of breast cancer and for similar conditions of lymphatic oedema. Lancet 1908; 1:783–5.

51. Stanton AW, Levick JR, Mortimer PS. Current puzzles presented by postmastectomy oedema (breast cancer related lymphoedema). Vasc Med 1996; 1:213–25.

52. Schunemann H, Willich N. Lymphoedema of the arm after primary treatment of breast cancer. Anticancer Res 1998; 18:2235–6.

53. Golshan M, Martin WJ, Dowlatshahi K. Sentinel lymph node biopsy lowers the rate of lymphedema when compared with standard axillary lymph node dissection. Am Surg 2003; 69:209–11; discussion 212.

54. MacDonald I. Resection of the axillary vein in radical mastectomy: its relation to the mechanisms of lymphoedema. Cancer 1948; 1:618–24.

55. Clark B, Sitzia J, Harlow W. Incidence and risk of arm oedema following treatment for breast cancer: a three-year follow-up study. Q J Med 2005; 98:343–8.

56. Suneson BL, Lindholm C, Hamrin E. Clinical incidence of lymphoedema in breast cancer patients in Jonkoping County, Sweden. Eur J Cancer Care (Engl) 1996; 5:7–12.

57. Larson D, Weinstein M, Goldberg I et al. Edema of the arm as a function of the extent of axillary surgery in patients with stage I–II carcinoma of the breast treated with primary radiotherapy. Int J Radiat Oncol Biol Phys 1986; 12:1575–82.

58. Purushotham AD, Bennett Britton TM, Klevesath MB et al. Lymph node status and breast cancer-related lymphedema. Ann Surg 2007; 246:42–5.

59. Kissin MW, della Rovere GQ, Easton D et al. Risk of lymphoedema following the treatment of breast cancer. Br J Surg 1986; 73:580–4.

60. Purushotham AD, Upponi S, Klevesath MB et al. Morbidity after sentinel lymph node biopsy in primary breast cancer: results from a randomized controlled trial. J Clin Oncol 2005; 23:4312–21.

61. Veronesi U, Paganelli G, Viale G et al. A randomized comparison of sentinel-node biopsy with routine axillary dissection in breast cancer. N Engl J Med 2003; 349:546–53.

62. Mansel RE, Fallowfield L, Kissin M et al. Randomized multicenter trial of sentinel node biopsy versus standard axillary treatment in operable breast cancer: the ALMANAC Trial. J Natl Cancer Inst 2006; 98:599–609.

63. Pain SJ, Purushotham AD. Lymphoedema following surgery for breast cancer. Br J Surg 2000; 87:1128–41.

64. Recht A, Pierce SM, Abner A et al. Regional nodal failure after conservative surgery and radiotherapy for early-stage breast carcinoma. J Clin Oncol 1991; 9:988–96.

65. Spruit PH, Siesling S, Elferink MA et al. Regional radiotherapy versus an axillary lymph node dissection after lumpectomy: a safe alternative for an axillary lymph node dissection in a clinically uninvolved axilla in breast cancer. A case control study with 10 years follow up. Radiat Oncol 2007; 2:40.

66. Early Breast Cancer Trialists' Collaborative Group. Effects of radiotherapy and surgery in early breast cancer. An overview of the randomized trials. N Engl J Med 1995; 333:1444–55.

67. Fisher BJ, Perera FE, Cooke AL et al. Extracapsular axillary node extension in patients receiving adjuvant systemic therapy: an indication for radiotherapy? Int J Radiat Oncol Biol Phys 1997; 38:551–9.

68. Fowble B, Gray R, Gilchrist K et al. Identification of a subgroup of patients with breast cancer and histologically positive axillary nodes receiving adjuvant chemotherapy who may benefit from postoperative radiotherapy. J Clin Oncol 1988; 6:1107–17.

69. Veronesi U, Luini A, Galimberti V et al. Extent of metastatic axillary involvement in 1446 cases of breast cancer. Eur J Surg Oncol 1990; 16:127–33.

70. Ung O, Langlands AO, Barraclough B et al. Combined chemotherapy and radiotherapy for patients with breast cancer and extensive nodal involvement. J Clin Oncol 1995; 13:435–43.

71. Diab SG, Hilsenbeck SG, de Moor C et al. Radiation therapy and survival in breast cancer patients with 10 or more positive axillary lymph nodes treated with mastectomy. J Clin Oncol 1998; 16:1655–60.

72. Overgaard M, Hansen PS, Overgaard J et al. Postoperative radiotherapy in high-risk premenopausal women with breast cancer who receive

adjuvant chemotherapy. Danish Breast Cancer Cooperative Group 82b Trial. N Engl J Med 1997; 337:949–55.

73. Ragaz J, Jackson SM, Le N et al. Adjuvant radiotherapy and chemotherapy in node-positive premenopausal women with breast cancer. N Engl J Med 1997; 337:956–62.

74. Herd-Smith A, Russo A, Muraca MG et al. Prognostic factors for lymphedema after primary treatment of breast carcinoma. Cancer 2001; 92:1783–7.

75. Ververs JM, Roumen RM, Vingerhoets AJ et al. Risk, severity and predictors of physical and psychological morbidity after axillary lymph node dissection for breast cancer. Eur J Cancer 2001; 37:991–9.

76. Van den Brenk HAS. The effect of ionising radiations on the regenerations and behaviour of mammalian lymphatics. In vivo studies in Sandison Clark chambers. Am J Roentgenol Radium Ther Nucl Med 1957; 78:837–49.

77. Ariel IM, Resnick MI, Oropeza R. The effects of irradiation (external and internal) on lymphatic dynamics. Am J Roentgenol Radium Ther Nucl Med 1967; 99:404–14.

78. Lenzi M, Bassani G. The effect of radiation on the lymph and on the lymph vessels. Radiology 1963; 80:814–17.

79. Fajardo LF. Effects of ionising radiation on lymph nodes. A review. Front Radiat Ther Oncol 1994; 28:37–45.

80. Chetty U, Jack W, Prescott RJ et al. Management of the axilla in operable breast cancer treated by breast conservation: a randomized clinical trial. Edinburgh Breast Unit. Br J Surg 2000; 87:163–9.

81. Steele RJ, Forrest AP, Gibson T et al. The efficacy of lower axillary sampling in obtaining lymph node status in breast cancer: a controlled randomized trial. Br J Surg 1985; 72:368–9.

82. Forrest AP, Stewart HJ, Roberts MM et al. Simple mastectomy and axillary node sampling (pectoral node biopsy) in the management of primary breast cancer. Ann Surg 1982; 196:371–8.

83. Kissin MW, Thompson EM, Price AB et al. The inadequacy of axillary sampling in breast cancer. Lancet 1982; 1:1210–12.

84. Fisher B, Wolmark N, Bauer M et al. The accuracy of clinical nodal staging and of limited axillary dissection as a determinant of histologic nodal status in carcinoma of the breast. Surg Gynecol Obstet 1981; 152:765–72.

85. Graversen HP, Blichert-Toft M, Andersen JA et al. Breast cancer: risk of axillary recurrence in node-negative patients following partial dissection of the axilla. Eur J Surg Oncol 1988; 14:407–12.

86. Macmillan RD, Barbera D, Hadjiminas DJ et al. Sentinel node biopsy for breast cancer may have little to offer four-node-samplers. Results of a prospective comparison study. Eur J Cancer 2001; 37:1076–80.

87. Chetty U, Chin PK, Soon PH et al. Combination blue dye sentinel lymph node biopsy and axillary node sampling: the Edinburgh experience. Eur J Surg Oncol 2008; 34:13–16.

88. Cabanas RM. An approach for the treatment of penile carcinoma. Cancer 1977; 39:456–66.

89. Morton DL, Wen DR, Wong JH et al. Technical details of intraoperative lymphatic mapping for early stage melanoma. Arch Surg 1992; 127:392–9.

90. Giuliano AE, Kirgan DM, Guenther JM et al. Lymphatic mapping and sentinel lymphadenectomy for breast cancer. Ann Surg 1994; 220:391–8; discussion 398–401.

91. Veronesi U, Paganelli G, Viale G et al. Sentinel-lymph-node biopsy as a staging procedure in breast cancer: update of a randomised controlled study. Lancet Oncol 2006; 7:983–90.

92. Fisher B, Jeong JH, Anderson S et al. Twenty-five-year follow-up of a randomized trial comparing radical mastectomy, total mastectomy, and total mastectomy followed by irradiation. N Engl J Med 2002; 347:567–75.

93. Krag DN, Anderson SJ, Julian TB et al. Technical outcomes of sentinel-lymph-node resection and conventional axillary-lymph-node dissection in patients with clinically node-negative breast cancer: results from the NSABP B-32 randomised phase III trial. Lancet Oncol 2007; 8:881–8.

94. White RL Jr, Wilke LG. Update on the NSABP and ACOSOG breast cancer sentinel node trials. Am Surg 2004; 70:420–4.

95. Lucci A, McCall LM, Beitsch PD et al. Surgical complications associated with sentinel lymph node dissection (SLND) plus axillary lymph node dissection compared with SLND alone in the American College of Surgeons Oncology Group Trial Z0011. J Clin Oncol 2007; 25:3657–63.

96. Pater J, Parulekar W. Sentinel lymph node biopsy in early breast cancer: has its time come? J Natl Cancer Inst 2006; 98:568–9.

97. Lyman GH, Giuliano AE, Somerfield MR et al. American Society of Clinical Oncology guideline recommendations for sentinel lymph node biopsy in early-stage breast cancer. J Clin Oncol 2005; 23:7703–20.

98. Van Diest PJ, Torrenga H, Borgstein PJ et al. Reliability of intraoperative frozen section and imprint cytological investigation of sentinel lymph nodes in breast cancer. Histopathology 1999; 35:14–18.

99. Manzotti M, Dell'Orto P, Maisonneuve P et al. Reverse transcription–polymerase chain reaction assay for multiple mRNA markers in the detection of breast cancer metastases in sentinel lymph nodes. Int J Cancer 2001; 95:307–12.

100. GeneSearch™ BLN Assay. Information for physicians, Vol. 2008. Veridex, LLC, 2007.

101. Mansel RE, Goyal A, Douglas-Jones A et al. Intraoperative assessment of sentinel lymph nodes in breast cancer patients using real time RT–PCR: results of the Cardiff Validation Study. 2007 Breast Cancer Symposium. San Francisco, CA: American Society of Clinical Oncology, 2007.

102. Viale G, Dell'Orto P, Biasi MO et al. Comparative evaluation of an extensive histopathologic examination and a real-time reverse-transcription–polymerase chain reaction assay for mammaglobin and cytokeratin 19 on axillary sentinel lymph nodes of breast carcinoma patients. Ann Surg 2008; 247:136–42.

103. Blumencranz P, Whitworth PW, Deck K et al. Scientific Impact Recognition Award. Sentinel node staging for breast cancer: intraoperative molecular pathology overcomes conventional histologic sampling errors. Am J Surg 2007; 194:426–32.

104. Hughes SJ, Xi L, Raja S et al. A rapid, fully automated, molecular-based assay accurately analyzes sentinel lymph nodes for the presence of metastatic breast cancer. Ann Surg 2006; 243:389–98.

105. Recommendations for processing and reporting of lymph node specimens submitted for evaluation of metastatic disease. Am J Clin Pathol 2001; 115:799–801.

106. Herbert GS, Sohn VY, Brown TA. The impact of nodal isolated tumor cells on survival of breast cancer patients. Am J Surg 2007; 193:571–3; discussion 573–4.

107. Susnik B, Frkovic-Grazio S, Bracko M. Occult micrometastases in axillary lymph nodes predict subsequent distant metastases in stage I breast cancer: a case–control study with 15-year follow-up. Ann Surg Oncol 2004; 11:568–72.

108. Cummings MC, Walsh MD, Hohn BG et al. Occult axillary lymph node metastases in breast cancer do matter: results of 10-year survival analysis. Am J Surg Pathol 2002; 26:1286–95.

109. Millis RR, Springall R, Lee AH et al. Occult axillary lymph node metastases are of no prognostic significance in breast cancer. Br J Cancer 2002; 86:396–401.

110. Dowlatshahi K, Fan M, Bloom KJ et al. Occult metastases in the sentinel lymph nodes of patients with early stage breast carcinoma: a preliminary study. Cancer 1999; 86:990–6.

111. Czerniecki BJ, Scheff AM, Callans LS et al. Immunohistochemistry with pancytokeratins improves the sensitivity of sentinel lymph node biopsy in patients with breast carcinoma. Cancer 1999; 85:1098–103.

112. Krauth JS, Charitansky H, Isaac S et al. Clinical implications of axillary sentinel lymph node 'micrometastases' in breast cancer. Eur J Surg Oncol 2006; 32:400–4.

113. Kim T, Giuliano AE, Lyman GH. Lymphatic mapping and sentinel lymph node biopsy in early-stage breast carcinoma: a meta-analysis. Cancer 2006; 106:4–16.

114. Chu KU, Turner RR, Hansen NM et al. Do all patients with sentinel node metastasis from breast carcinoma need complete axillary node dissection? Ann Surg 1999; 229:536–41.

115. Pal A, Provenzano E, Duffy SW et al. A model for predicting non-sentinel lymph node metastatic disease when the sentinel lymph node is positive. Br J Surg 2008; 95(3):302–9.

116. Van Zee KJ, Manasseh DM, Bevilacqua JL et al. A nomogram for predicting the likelihood of additional nodal metastases in breast cancer patients with a positive sentinel node biopsy. Ann Surg Oncol 2003; 10:1140–51.

117. Lambert LA, Ayers GD, Hwang RF et al. Validation of a breast cancer nomogram for predicting nonsentinel lymph node metastases after a positive sentinel node biopsy. Ann Surg Oncol 2006; 13:310–20.

118. Smidt ML, Kuster DM, van der Wilt GJ et al. Can the Memorial Sloan-Kettering Cancer Center nomogram predict the likelihood of nonsentinel lymph node metastases in breast cancer patients in the Netherlands? Ann Surg Oncol 2005; 12:1066–72.

119. Alran S, De Rycke Y, Fourchotte V et al. Validation and limitations of use of a breast cancer nomogram predicting the likelihood of non-sentinel node involvement after positive sentinel node biopsy. Ann Surg Oncol 2007; 14:2195–201.

120. Klar M, Jochmann A, Foeldi M et al. The MSKCC nomogram for prediction the likelihood of non-sentinel node involvement in a German breast cancer population. Breast Cancer Res Treat 2008 (Epub ahead of print).

121. Kim SR, Matsuoka T, Maekawa Y et al. Development of multicentric hepatocellular carcinoma after completion of interferon therapy. J Gastroenterol 2002; 37:663–8.

122. Jin Kim H, Heerdt AS, Cody HS et al. Sentinel lymph node drainage in multicentric breast cancers. Breast J 2002; 8:356–61.

123. Mertz L, Mathelin C, Marin C et al. Subareolar injection of 99m-Tc sulfur colloid for sentinel nodes identification in multifocal invasive breast cancer. Bull Cancer 1999; 86:939–45.

124. Schrenk P, Wayand W. Sentinel-node biopsy in axillary lymph-node staging for patients with multicentric breast cancer. Lancet 2001; 357:122.

125. Mamounas EP, Brown A, Anderson S et al. Sentinel node biopsy after neoadjuvant chemotherapy in breast cancer: results from National Surgical Adjuvant Breast and Bowel Project Protocol B-27. J Clin Oncol 2005; 23:2694–702.

126. Schwartz GF, Giuliano AE, Veronesi U. Proceedings of the consensus conference on the role of sentinel lymph node biopsy in carcinoma of the breast, 19–22 April 2001, Philadelphia, Pennsylvania. Cancer 2002; 94:2542–51.

127. Cody HS 3rd. Sentinel lymph node biopsy for breast cancer: indications, contraindications, and new directions. J Surg Oncol 2007; 95:440–2.

128. Yen TW, Hunt KK, Mirza NQ et al. Physician recommendations regarding tamoxifen and patient utilization of tamoxifen after surgery for ductal carcinoma in situ. Cancer 2004; 100: 942–9.

129. Pendas S, Dauway E, Giuliano R et al. Sentinel node biopsy in ductal carcinoma in situ patients. Ann Surg Oncol 2000; 7:15–20.

130. Intra M, Veronesi P, Mazzarol G et al. Axillary sentinel lymph node biopsy in patients with pure ductal carcinoma in situ of the breast. Arch Surg 2003; 138:309–13.

# 8

# Prevention of breast cancer: the genetics of breast cancer and risk-reducing surgery

D. Gareth R. Evans
Andrew D. Baildam

## Introduction

The last few years have seen a substantial rise in our knowledge of inherited breast cancer. It is now possible to identify women at very high levels of risk of the disease. Whilst there are promising signs for the reduction in risk from hormonal and other manipulations, the level of risk reduction still falls far short of that provided by surgical removal of breast tissue. Until another reliable risk-reducing measure is developed, risk-reducing surgery will remain a mainstay of management in women at very high risk who want to reduce substantially their chances of developing breast cancer.

## Genetic predisposition

The presence of a significant family history is the strongest risk factor for the development of breast cancer. Even at extremes of age, the presence of a *BRCA1* mutation confers significant risks. A 25-year-old woman who carries a mutation in *BRCA1* has a greater risk of developing breast cancer in the following decade than a woman aged 70 years in the general population. About 4–5% of breast cancer is thought to be due to inheritance of a high-penetrance, autosomal-dominant, cancer-predisposing gene.[1,2]

Inheritance of a germline mutation or deletion in a predisposing gene predisposes to early-onset, and frequently bilateral, breast cancer. Certain mutations also confer an increased susceptibility to other malignancies, such as ovary (*BRCA1/2*) and sarcomas (*TP53*)[3–5] (Table 8.1).

Multiple primary cancers in one individual or related early-onset cancers in a family pedigree are highly suggestive of a predisposing gene. It is thought that over 25% of breast cancers in women under 30 years of age are due to mutation in a dominant gene, compared with less than 1% in women who develop the disease over 70 years.[2] It has recently been found that at least 20% of breast cancers under 30 years of age are due to mutations in the known high-risk genes *BRCA1*, *BRCA2* and *TP53*. Nonetheless, this is still largely indicated by family history and the detection rate for mutations in isolated breast cancer cases even at very young ages is considerably less than 10%.[6]

There are few families where it is possible to be certain of a dominantly inherited susceptibility. However, the Breast Cancer Linkage Consortium (BCLC) data suggest that in families with four or more cases of early-onset or bilateral breast cancer, the risk of an unaffected woman inheriting a mutation in a predisposing gene is close to 50%. These studies have estimated that the majority of such families harbour

Table 8.1 • Breast cancer genes: frequency and proportion of risk

| Gene | Other tumour % of susceptibility | Population frequency | Proportion of breast cancer | Proportion of HPHBC | Proportion of familial breast cancer risk | Lifetime risk in women (RR) |
|---|---|---|---|---|---|---|
| BRCA1 AD | Ovary/prostate Colorectal | 0.1% | 1.5% | 40% | 5–10% | 60–85% |
| BRCA2 AD | Ovary/prostate Pancreas HoZ Fanconi (AR) | 0.1% | 1.5% | 40% | 5–10% | 50–85% |
| TP53 LFS AD | Sarcoma, glioma Adrenal | 0.0025% | 0.02% | 2% | 0.1% | 80–90% |
| PTEN Cowden's AD | Thyroid Colorectal | 0.0005% | 0.004% | 0.3% | 0.02% | 25–50% |
| CHEK2 | Colorectal, prostate | 0.5% | 0.5% | 0% | 2% | 18–20% (2.0) |
| ATM AD and AR | HoZ (AR) Lymphoma, leukaemia | 0.5% | 0.5% | 0% | 2% | 20% |
| STK11 AD | Colorectal | 0.001% | 0.001% | 0.6% | 0.04% | 50% |
| BRIP1 | HoZ Fanconi (AR) | 0.1% | 0.1% | 0% | 0.4% | 20% (2.0) |
| PALB2 | HoZ Fanconi (AR) | 0.1% | 0.1% | 0% | 0.4% | 20% (2.0) |
| Five SNPs from GWA | FGFR2, TRCN9, MAP3K, LSP1, 8q128424800 | 30–46% | 0.5–1% | 0% | 2–4% | 11–13% (1.1–1.3) |
| Totals | | 80% for any | 5% | 83% | 27% | |

AD, autosomal dominant; AR, autosomal recessive; GWA, genome-wide association studies; HeZ, heterozygous; HoZ, homozygous; HPHBC, highly penetrant hereditary breast cancer (e.g. more than three affected relatives); LFS, Li–Fraumeni syndrome; RR, relative risk; SNP.

mutations in *BRCA1* or *BRCA2*, especially when male breast cancer or ovarian cancer are present. In breast-only families, the frequency of *BRCA1/2* involvement falls to below 50% in four-case families.[7,8] Family and epidemiological studies have demonstrated that approximately 70–85% of *BRCA1* and *BRCA2* mutation carriers develop breast cancer in their lifetime, although the risk is a little lower for *BRCA2*.[7–9] The very low figures published on small numbers of families from population studies have now been addressed by a meta-analysis,[9] which gives risks to 70 years of age of around 70% for *BRCA1* and 55% for *BRCA2*.

The chances that a family with a history of breast and/or ovarian cancer harbours mutations in *BRCA1* or *BRCA2* can be assessed from computer models.[10,11] We have recently validated these models using a dataset of 258 patients and their samples tested for *BRCA1/2* mutations. We found

that at the lower levels of likelihood for mutations, the computer models substantially overpredict the presence of mutations, particularly for *BRCA1*.[12] Our own manual model was much better at predicting a mutation in both genes and indeed was better than other manual models (Table 8.2). Further indicators for the presence of a *BRCA1* mutation within a family are grade and estrogen receptor status. *BRCA1* tumours are more frequently grade 3 and estrogen receptor negative and often have a medullary-like histology.[13] Ovarian cancers that occur in *BRCA1/2* families are nearly always non-mucinous epithelial cancers.[14]

The likelihood of identifying a *BRCA1/2* mutation should not be confused with the ability to detect a mutation if one is present in the family. No single technique is able to detect all mutations. Even by sequencing the entire gene (exons and intron/exon

Table 8.2 • Scoring system for identification of a pathogenic *BRCA1/2* mutation

| | BRCA1 | BRCA2 |
|---|---|---|
| Female breast cancer <30 years | 6 | 5 |
| Female breast cancer 30–39 years | 4 | 4 |
| Female breast cancer 40–49 years | 3 | 3 |
| Female breast cancer 50–59 years | 2 | 2 |
| Female breast cancer >59 years | 1 | 1 |
| Male breast cancer <60 years | 5 (if *BRCA2* tested) | 8 |
| Male breast cancer >59 years | 5 (if *BRCA2* tested) | 5 |
| Ovarian cancer <60 years | 8 | 5 (if *BRCA1* tested) |
| Ovarian cancer >59 years | 5 | 5 (if *BRCA1* tested) |
| Pancreatic cancer | 0 | 1 |
| Prostate cancer <60 years | 0 | 2 |
| Prostate cancer >59 years | 0 | 1 |

Scores for each cancer in a direct lineage are summated. A score of 10 is equivalent to a 10% chance of identifying a mutation in each gene.

boundaries), the detection rate only equates to about 85%. If a strategy is added to detect large deletions or duplications in *BRCA1*, this can boost detection to around 95%.[15]

The proportion of breast/ovarian cancers attributable to *BRCA1* or *BRCA2* depends on the ethnic origin of families. Many countries or ethnic groups have particular founder mutations that are not seen in other populations. In countries with a small founder population, very few mutations may account for the vast majority of breast cancer families.

The Ashkenazi Jewish population has three founder mutations: 185delAG and 5382insC in *BRCA1*, and 6174delT in *BRCA2*.[16] The three mutations are found in over 2% of the Ashkenazi Jewish population. One study showed that one of the three mutations were present in 59% of high-risk families.[16]

Populations that are more outbred, such as the UK, have larger numbers of mutations, and founder mutations occur at lower frequencies. Nonetheless, many laboratories in the UK have tried to develop a targeted approach to screening, concentrating on the large exons (exon 11 in both genes and exon 10 in *BRCA2*) and the smaller exons commonly reported to be involved, such as exons 2 and 20 in *BRCA1*. This cuts down the number of polymerase chain reactions using the protein truncation test (PTT) to as little as five for *BRCA1* and four for *BRCA2*. However, this strategy reduces the sensitivity of identifying mutations down to as little as 50%.[15]

# Genetic testing

Once a mutation in a predisposing gene like *BRCA1* or *BRCA2* has been identified in a family, definitive genetic testing is possible. This can then more accurately inform women of their risks and give them an informed choice of different options, including risk-reducing surgery. Undertaking mutation analysis on an unaffected individual (without checking an affected relative), particularly in a breast cancer-only family, is problematic. Whilst identifying a pathogenic mutation will confirm a high risk, the absence of a mutation will not exclude the possibility that other genes or even of a mutation refractory to the mutation screening techniques used are present. Although other genes are now being identified (see Table 8.1), many more remain to be found and screening for mutations is not clinically useful outside of *BRCA1/2* and in certain circumstances *TP53*. Nevertheless, the outcomes of genome-wide association studies are suggesting that all breast cancer cases will carry at least one risk allele.[17] Once all the lower risk alleles have been found a definitive genetic test can then be developed.

# Breast cancer risk estimation

Where there is not a dominant family history or it is not possible to identify a mutation in *BRCA1/2*, risk estimation is based on large epidemiological studies, which give a 1.5- to 3-fold relative risk with a family history of a single affected relative.[1,2] Clinicians must be careful to differentiate between lifetime and age-specific risks. Some studies quote ninefold or greater risk associated either with bilateral disease in a mother or with severe benign proliferative breast disease. However, these risks are time limited and if these at-risk individuals are followed up for many years, their relative risk starts to reduce.[18] Clearly, if one uses these risks and multiplies them on a lifetime incidence of 1 in 10–12, some women will apparently have a greater than 100% chance of having the disease. The risks do not multiply and may not even add. Perhaps the best way to assess risk is to take the strongest risk factor, which in most cases is nearly always the family history. If risk is assessed on this alone, minor adjustments can be made for other factors. It is arguable whether these other factors have a major effect on an 80% penetrant gene other than to speed up or delay the onset of breast cancer. Therefore, we can only really assume an effect on non-hereditary elements of risk. Although studies do point to an increase in risk in family history cases associated with some factors, these may just represent an earlier age expression of the gene. Generally, therefore, mutant gene carriers will have risks between 40% and 8–10%, although lower risks are occasionally given. Higher risks are only applicable when a woman at 40% genetic risk is shown to have a germline mutation, to have inherited a high-risk allele or to have proliferative breast disease.

> Within Europe, risk estimation in the family history setting is based mainly on the Claus dataset.[2,19,20] However, within the USA, the Gail model of risk estimation is widely used.[21] As well as these datasets allowing estimation of risk, there are specific computer programs available, including Tyrer–Cuzick,[22] Cyrillic and BRCAPRO.[10]

These programs take into consideration varying permutations of age of onset of diagnosis, number of affected and unaffected women and hormonal factors; as a consequence, different programs result in different risk estimations. The Gail model does not take into account age of relatives or second-degree relatives. A newer model, the Tyrer–Cuzick,[22] incorporates the majority of the currently known risk factors.

A major deficiency of the current genetic models is the assumption that all inherited breast cancer is due to a single high-risk dominant gene or two genes (*BRCA1* and *BRCA2*). The problem this causes in a program like BRCAPRO is that in order to obtain an accurate assessment for identifying a *BRCA1* or *BRCA2* mutation in a family, all other potential genetic factors are overlooked. Therefore, while BRCAPRO provides reasonably accurate estimates for the presence of *BRCA1/2* mutations in high-risk families,[11] its ability to predict breast cancer incidence is substantially hampered in smaller aggregations of breast cancer. We have recently found that BRCAPRO underestimates the risk of breast cancer in moderate/high-risk families by about 50%.[23] The most accurate computer model was the Tyrer–Cuzick model, although a manual model incorporating the Claus tables and data from the BCLC and adjustment for hormonal and reproductive factors was similarly accurate. A fuller explanation of the manual model is available elsewhere.[20,23]

## Management options

Management options available for women at high lifetime risk of breast cancer due to their family history or for those women known to be carrying a mutation in *BRCA1/2* are limited. Screening with mammography or magnetic resonance imaging is one option, and this can be combined with a trial of chemoprevention. However, many women are now seriously considering or undergoing risk-reducing mastectomy (RRM) if found to be mutation carriers for *BRCA1* or *BRCA2*. The efficacy of surgical procedures for reducing the risk of breast cancer was controversial,[24,25] although it would appear that the residual risk of breast cancer depends on the amount of residual breast tissue following the surgical procedure. Recent work suggests that more women are considering RRM,[26,27] although uptake rates vary enormously, with much lower uptake in Israel and southern Europe. Protocols should be in place to deal with requests for RRM at all cancer genetics and oncoplastic clinics. It has been suggested that surgery will increase life expectancy in *BRCA1* or *BRCA2* mutation carriers.[28]

> The first study to demonstrate that women with a high risk of breast cancer can significantly reduce their subsequent incidence of the disease with RRM was only published in 1999.[29] This was followed by a Dutch study that confirmed risk reduction in those at highest risk (*BRCA1/BRCA2* carriers).[30] Current evidence would suggest that RRM is associated with an approximately 90–95% reduction in risk.[31]

# Genetic counselling and the family history clinic

Breast cancer family history clinics started to be established in the UK in 1987,[31,32] and these clinics are now established across Europe and North America. They are generally administered by consultants in medical oncology, clinical genetics and breast surgery, often with a multidisciplinary approach and close involvement of radiologists and a psychiatrist/psychologist. At these clinics unaffected women at increased risk of breast cancer are assessed for their lifetime and shorter-term risks of breast cancer. After assessing risk, women are presented with a number of choices including regular surveillance, usually with a combination of mammography and clinical examination that commences between 30 and 40 years depending on the age of cancers in the family and the overall risk. Women are generally divided into three risk groups: average, moderate and high risk. It is only really in the high-risk group that RRM should be considered. This usually equates to a lifetime risk of 1 in 4 (25%) or greater. As a rough guide, this equates to having a heterozygote risk of 1 in 4 with two relatives including one first-degree relative with breast cancer diagnosed below 50 years of age or three affected relatives under 60 years. All affected relatives should be first-degree relatives or related through a male.

In a survey of 10 European centres,[33] only three (Manchester, Edinburgh, Heidelberg/Dusseldorf) routinely mention the possibility of RRM to those women with a lifetime risk of 1 in 4 or greater. This information is often only given as a single sentence or a statement of the availability of the procedure as an option for prevention of breast cancer. This then allows women to extend the discussion if they wish to do so, or to state that they are not interested in surgery. Many centres only mention risk-reducing surgery to potential mutation carriers undertaking a genetic test. Indeed, there is a cultural shift across Europe from north to south, with RRM becoming less acceptable to both physician and patient as one moves southward.[34,35] In the USA, in centres where mastectomies for severe benign breast disease were commonplace in the 1970s and 1980s,[29] there appears to be less enthusiasm for mastectomy now even among gene mutation carriers.[36] What is absolutely clear is that adequate preparation of a woman contemplating RRM is essential.

# The RRM protocol

If women wish to discuss the surgical procedure in greater detail, most centres in our European survey offered a further appointment at least 1 month later. This gives women time to consider the procedure more fully and to discuss it with appropriate members of their family. Involvement of partners in the decision-making process is encouraged and they are invited to attend each appointment. At the second appointment, with a geneticist or oncologist, a basic description of the surgery is provided, including the potential residual risk of different procedures. It is emphasised that the residual risk and complication rate may be higher if the surgery preserves the nipple–areola complex (NAC). It is also usually made clear that these procedures, although having proven efficacy in reducing the risk of breast cancer, will still leave some residual risk. The patient is also challenged to consider possible complications, which may result in a potentially poor cosmetic result, as well as considering the impact upon her personal life and family dynamics.

The possibility of genetic testing is also discussed in terms of the availability of a living affected member of the family and the basic underlying structure of the family.[20,37,38] If possible, a time scale for genetic testing is discussed, and the woman is asked to consider the potential impact of proceeding with surgery, particularly if she then undergoes genetic testing which finds that she does not in fact carry the causative mutation. It is also emphasised that the genetic risk of breast cancer decreases with age and that the remaining risk of breast cancer if the woman is older (>40 years) is lower than the lifetime risk.[20] Indeed, a mutation carrier for BRCA1 may have no more than a 50% risk of breast cancer in her remaining lifetime if she has reached 50 years. If a woman wishes to proceed, a psychological assessment is arranged.

 At this stage, confirmation of the breast cancers in the family are sought proactively by most centres if this has not already been done. This ensures that the risk assessment is as accurate as possible. We have previously reported the presence of factitious histories within some families where women have fabricated their family history in order to obtain surgery, or are innocently implicated as being at risk by another family member who has promoted an inaccurate family history.[39]

The whole process, from first consultation to the surgical procedure itself, usually takes between 6 and 12 months. This time delay is deliberate; in most centres the greatest delay is at the beginning of the protocol in order to allow women time for the decision-making process. If the protocol is run concurrently with a decision for predictive genetic testing, then the wait will generally be shorter. The full protocol of two sessions at the family history clinic, a session with a psychiatrist and sessions with the surgeon was established in 1993 in Manchester. While only two other centres had a similar written protocol, most clinics adhere to these basic principles. The major difference is that several centres are mainly reactive – in these clinics risk-reducing surgery is usually only formally discussed in women proven to be *BRCA1/2* mutation carriers. Even with a proven mutation carrier no centre actively recommends surgery, but offers it as part of a range of choices.

There is also no clear pattern in terms of the surgical procedure recommended in women who decide on surgery. While some units are cautious about offering skin/nipple-preserving mastectomies, these options are generally available for every case in some centres.

## The surgical consultations

After a psychological assessment, at least two detailed surgical consultations are needed to discuss the types of mastectomy and breast reconstruction procedures available and their techniques, limitations, outcomes and potential complications. These should take place unhurriedly with the specialist surgeon, sometimes together with a plastic surgeon, with time for careful communication, evaluation and reflection. Many women may have little understanding of the extent and nature of risk-reducing surgery, with or without breast reconstruction. They may initially regard RRM as a relatively minor cosmetic procedure, and this may be reinforced by family or social contacts.

The objective of surgery is to reduce the incidence of breast cancer, relieve anxiety and ultimately diminish breast cancer mortality. Any procedure should do so in a way that balances risk reduction with aesthetic outcome and function, and quality-of-life concerns. Whilst high-risk women carry their genotype in all cells and the bilateral incidence of cancer is proven, such women seldom develop multifocal ipsilateral breast cancers. It is impossible surgically to remove completely all breast tissue at risk, with the most complete resection being achieved

by traditional total mastectomy. Some women will choose this as the simplest option, but for most the idea of simple total bilateral mastectomy without breast reconstruction does achieve a balance between risk reduction and cosmetic outcome. Mastectomy with breast reconstruction can be offered to almost all women, with careful evaluation of the breast and body shape to advise on the most appropriate reconstruction options for each individual. The surgical procedure should aim to reduce as substantially as possible the at-risk glandular breast tissue, including the upper outer quadrants, the area with the highest local incidence of cancer. At all stages of preoperative planning women must be fully involved in the decision-making, and must be aware of the reality that no operation completely removes all risk. Conservation of the natural NAC is controversial, as its preservation confers a small but unknown increase in residual risk. If preserved, loss of NAC sensation or even NAC loss from ischaemia may rarely result; nevertheless, a high proportion of women do opt for NAC preservation.

## Contraindications to surgery

Risk-reducing surgery should not be carried out inappropriately. In particular it should not be undertaken in the following circumstances:

- if individual risk cannot be substantiated;
- the family history is found to be fictitious;
- Munchausen's syndrome;
- a gene test result is imminent;
- surgery is not the woman's own choice but that of her partner or family;
- psychiatric disorder, clinical depression, cancer phobia, dysmorphic syndrome;
- comorbidity outweighs potential clinical benefit;
- there is an immovable unrealistic expectation of outcome;
- reasons for choosing surgery are 'cosmetic' rather than 'oncological'.

## Risk-reducing surgery and breast reconstruction

Innovations in breast surgery over the last few years have resulted in a wide range of mastectomy approaches and incisions, and a full repertoire of reconstruction techniques. These should be presented and discussed in detail at the surgical consultation.

Reconstruction often comprises a series of staged procedures extending over a number of months, and it is crucial that realistic outcomes are advised and appreciated. An album of preoperative and postoperative photographs is essential, together with pictures where things have not gone quite so well or complications have occurred. The specialist breast care nurse has an important role during this time of discussion, providing information and facilitating patient–clinician liaison. The offer of a link-up with another woman in a 'buddy system' can be helpful.

Women who opt for RRM with reconstruction have the choice of skin-sparing mastectomy techniques together with immediate reconstruction using expander/implants or myocutaneous flaps, chiefly the latissimus dorsi (LD) flap or the lower abdominal transverse rectus abdominis (TRAM) flap. LD flaps can be used alone if there is sufficient tissue on the back to transfer into the breast defect, the autologous LD flap, or it is used more commonly, with an implant to increase volume and projection when fatty tissue overlying and adjacent to the LD muscle is inadequate. The TRAM myocutaneous flap may be pedicled or a free microvascular transfer, but this escalates substantially the operating time and recovery, and increases risk of major complications. Nevertheless, for some women bilateral autologous LD or TRAM flaps are an excellent choice and result in breast reconstructions that are living tissue throughout, warm, soft in consistency and highly realistic. Other free tissue transfer techniques are technically possible such as rectus muscle-sparing deep inferior epigastric perforator flaps, buttock inferior gluteal artery perforator and superior gluteal artery perforator flaps, and gracilis-based thigh flaps, but these are not widely available.

For a majority the relative 'simplicity' of an implant-based reconstruction makes these the first choice, and many women opt for an immediate submuscular tissue expander placement. The cosmetic key is the match of the skin envelope surface area to that achievable by the expanded muscle pocket that constitutes the neo-breast mound. The concept of a single operation to include mastectomy and reconstruction with an immediate fixed-volume permanent implant is an attractive ideal but only rarely gives good cosmesis, and the aesthetic result of the two-stage process for most women is a significant improvement over a one-stage operation.

Careful preoperative breast evaluation and assessment with accurate skin measuring and marking are

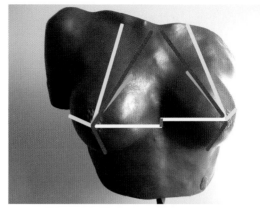

**Figure 8.1** • Detailed assessment of breast size, shape, ptosis and nipple position by surface measurements.

essential to define which skin areas will be resected in association with the breast parenchyma. Skin surface measures of nipple position relative to the midclavicular point and inframammary fold are recorded, together with full breast morphology (**Fig. 8.1**). Photographs are taken preoperatively and there is agreement between the woman and surgeon as to the proposed postoperative breast size.

RRM is a careful time-consuming operation and should not be approached hurriedly. Incisions are planned to optimise glandular access but at the same time placed with appreciation for the need for minimal scarring and long-term aesthetic acceptability. In the Manchester unit there are three main surgical approaches used: horizontal/oblique, Wise pattern incisions and peri/circumareolar approaches, similar to the Benelli mastopexy-type incision. Inframammary incisions are not used for the mastectomy because of two potential failures: firstly, effective access to remove the whole breast parenchyma including the upper outer quadrant and axillary tail; secondly, the danger of ischaemia of the breast lower pole skin between the inframammary incision and the nipple. After early experience in Manchester, when the majority of women having RRM opted to conserve their natural nipples, fewer now do so though some still wish nipple preservation. The main reasons for this are that personal risk reduction is maximised if the nipple is removed and its conservation can result in preservation of some parenchymal and ductal tissue; nipple reconstruction is also usually straightforward and cosmetically very satisfactory.

Women can be advised which of the three surgical approaches for their breast size and shape would be

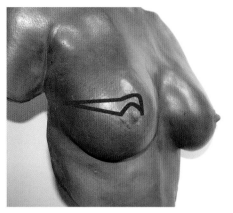

**Figure 8.2** • Horizontal/oblique approach for risk-reducing mastectomy with nipple preservation.

most appropriate. The Wise pattern RRM is based on a classical reduction mammoplasty-type incision. In all operations the nipples can be conserved if desired, utilising de-epithelialised pedicles to perfuse and maintain each NAC. If removed, NACs are subsequently reconstructed using one of a number of small local skin flaps to create the nipple bud, and then tattooed.

Women who choose immediate reconstruction with bilateral LD flaps or bilateral TRAM flaps have a range of skin-sparing mastectomy options open to them, and often choose circumareolar incisions. The circumareolar approach works well with expander/implant breast reconstructions in situations where the NAC is preserved on a superomedial pedicle, but it is more difficult to produce a good cosmetic outcome when the NAC is removed, due to breast coning issues.

## RRM using horizontal/oblique approach

The horizontal/oblique mastopexy incision works best for the breast with little ptosis and a weight of no more than 400–450 g. If the NAC is to be preserved, it can be elevated and maintained on de-epithelialised skin bridges; if not, the NAC can be reconstructed across the scar. If undertaken for the larger breast, the horizontal approach can result in a skin envelope/breast mound disparity, and subcutaneous tissue drop-out in the lower pole can be difficult to correct. If the NAC is preserved in such a breast, it may finish too high relative to the inframammary fold. It is a useful guide to maintain the mid-clavicle to NAC distance in the breast meridian at around 20–23 cm, depending on breast size and chest length.

The patient is positioned on the operating table with partial flexion of elbows and hands tucked into the waistband. The incision follows the carefully marked preoperative skin mark-up, which has been accurately measured, planned and discussed with each patient. The width of skin resected between the incisions tightens the skin and subcutaneous tissue onto the expanded muscle pocket lying beneath (**Fig. 8.2**). If the nipple is preserved, de-epithelialised skin bridges are used to maintain its perfusion. Subcutaneous fat is preserved to keep the deep dermal vasculature, and the breast parenchyma removed from this layer by gentle dissection below the layer of Scarpa's fascia. The skin and subcutaneous tissue should not be buttonholed but removed in parallel and flaps should be of consistent

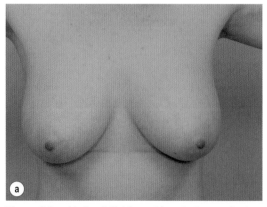

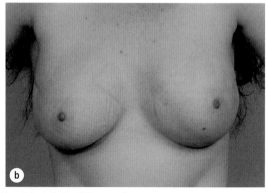

**Figure 8.3** • Horizontal/oblique risk-reducing mastectomy before **(a)** and after **(b)** operation.

thickness extending to the pectoralis fascia. The fascia is preserved and the breast tissue removed and weighed.

The subpectoral space is opened by sharp dissection of the lateral border of pectoralis major, and the submuscular pocket developed by sharp and blunt dissection using an illuminated retractor and direct vision. The submuscular pocket is extended under the upper part of rectus abdominis and the external oblique to recreate the breast lower pole fullness. The tissue expander is placed in the pocket with full aseptic precautions, partially inflated and the subcutaneous space closed over closed vacuum drains. The skin is closed with multiple layers of absorbable sutures and wound dressing strips applied. Cosmetic outcome can be excellent (**Fig. 8.3**).

## Wise pattern RRM

For the breast with greater ptosis and/or greater weight than that amenable to the horizontal/oblique approach, the Wise pattern RRM technique based on a reduction mammoplasty allows unparalleled access to all breast quadrants and the axillary tail, and results in cosmetically concealed scarring away from the upper and medial breast poles, as well as providing an opportunity for accurate matching of the residual skin and subcutaneous tissue to the reconstructed breast cone (**Fig. 8.4**). If required, the NAC can be preserved on a superior or superomedial de-epithelialised pedicle. If the NAC is removed, subsequent bilateral NAC reconstruction can be achieved easily by one

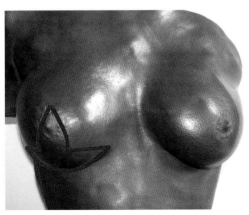

**Figure 8.4** • Wise pattern risk-reducing mastectomy planning.

of the variety of NAC reconstruction techniques available. This and any tattoo procedure effectively covers the upper half of each of the vertical limbs of the mastectomy scar, reducing further the cosmetic disturbance. These procedures have evolved by attention to detail in order to allow risk reduction and correct possible cosmetic inadequacies of conventional approaches.

In common with the horizontal/oblique RRM, resection of the breast gland is achieved by dissecting along the plane of the subtle Scarpa's fascia that separates the fibro-fatty and glandular tissue of the breast from the subcutaneous fat, which should be preserved deep to the dermis. Removal of the subcutaneous fat results in a high incidence of skin damage or frank necrosis, particularly if the subdermal vascular plexus is breached. As always, skin should be closed without undue tension using sutures in layers to create the optimum healing conditions. The mastectomy flaps are retracted gently and handled with great care to minimise trauma from surgical instruments. The plane of dissection is under Scarpa's fascia extending to the pectoralis fascia, and the subpectoral pocket for the tissue expander is created in an identical way to that described earlier. Special care has to be taken with closure so that the T-junctions are not under tension, as this can lead to wound breakdown. The vertical limb of the wound can be drawn together with multiple layers of absorbable subcuticular sutures in order to shorten its length.

Tissue expanders are chosen to match closely the breast base shape as well as diameter. The chosen volume should be determined by the agreed final breast size rather than the size of the natural breast, as there are opportunities for either increasing or decreasing volume if the woman so wishes and it can be safely and realistically achieved. A full layer of muscle cover for protection and smoothing over the expander requires the elevation of both pectoralis major and the upper part of serratus anterior. This can be vascular and needs careful haemostasis and is most easily achieved under direct vision using fibreoptic retractors or headlights and bipolar coagulation. The postoperative result after Wise pattern RRM can be as excellent as that with the horizontal/oblique approach, and has the advantage that there are no scars on the upper or medial breast areas (**Fig. 8.5**). Nipple reconstruction later covers the upper part of each vertical scar, resulting in a highly realistic breast reconstruction (**Fig. 8.6**).

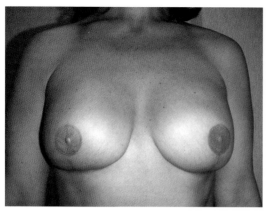

**Figure 8.5** • Wise pattern risk-reducing mastectomies with nipple reconstructions.

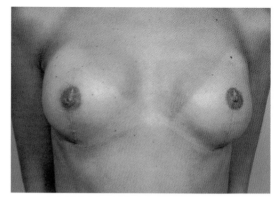

**Figure 8.6** • Wise pattern risk-reducing mastectomy after nipple–areola reconstruction.

After recovery and healing, the tissue expander is inflated cautiously with injectable saline in the outpatient clinic over several weeks or months, and the woman encouraged to use simple skin creams and massage to promote skin softening and elasticity in the neo-breast mound.

## Placement of permanent implants

After full tissue expansion several months later, the tissue expanders are removed and replaced with permanent implants. At full maturation of expansion, permanent implants can be chosen from the extensive ranges now available, with consideration to filler materials, surface textures, size, shape and volume. Permanent implants are specifically ordered for individual women according to breast horizontal width, breast height and projection. For some, round dome-shaped implants are appropriate, for others there is a range of anatomically shaped implants in a wide variety of heights and projections.

This second operation involves accessing the expander pocket either through part of a previous scar or through the inframammary fold, and removing each expander. Shaping of the pocket capsule can be done with bipolar scissors and this helps in forming breast ptosis and filling in and smoothing out areas that may not have expanded fully. Use of implant sizers is helpful prior to permanent implant placement, orientation and closure. Women are sat up on the operating table to judge size, shape and symmetry of the breast reconstructions, and adjustments made accordingly.

For some women the idea of artificially engineered implantable breast prostheses is not acceptable, and they choose instead to undergo breast reconstruction with bilateral LD or TRAM flaps. For this smaller number of women, skin-sparing mastectomy can be achieved through circumareolar incisions in addition to those approaches previously mentioned. Such reconstructions may be very realistic in terms of appearance, shape, movement and warmth (see Fig. 8.6). However, the operation and anaesthesia times associated with bilateral RRM and immediate bilateral myocutaneous flaps are substantial, and there is greater opportunity for perioperative and postoperative complications than with implant-based surgery. The extent and nature of donor-site scarring must be appreciated and understood, as well as the operative, inpatient and subsequent recovery periods and needs. Myocutaneous flap complications do occur and should be discussed, including the uncommon but catastrophic scenario of total flap loss.

## Follow-up

Follow-up of women who have undergone surgery is considered an important part of the protocol. In Manchester, women who have undergone RRM are reviewed annually at a multidisciplinary clinic. As well as discussion of problems/issues with all the relevant clinicians (geneticist, oncologist, psychiatrist, surgeons), each patient is examined. Clinical examination by palpation of the breasts is considered to be adequate, as remaining breast tissue is very superficial in all types of surgical procedure.

The mean expected rate of breast cancer for our cohort of high-risk women is 1% annually, reflecting a lifetime risk that ranges from 25% to 80%. Even though our own cohort has already a follow-up in excess of 1600 woman-years, only 16 cancers would have been expected. If this is to be analysed by type of surgery or confined to known *BRCA1/2* mutation carriers, even longer follow-up will be necessary. Published details of the Manchester protocol are available elsewhere.[40]

## Uptake

Our own data from Manchester show that 6% of women at 1 in 4 (31/906) lifetime risk or above seek further advice about RRM and 3.4% (31/906) have undergone surgery; this rises to 8.5% (65/764) in those at 40% lifetime risk. Of those proven affected mutation carriers aged under 60 years, 74/159 (46%) have now opted for risk-reducing surgery. Results from the Netherlands show a similarly high uptake (52%).[30] Thus far, six mutation carriers in our series and several in the Dutch series that initially opted not to have surgery have developed breast cancer, whereas none of the operated cases have.

## Psychosocial consequences of RRM

 Results from seven studies[41–47] that have evaluated psychosocial outcomes after RRM, two of which had lengthy follow-up periods, show that surgery is associated overall with fairly high levels of satisfaction, reduced anxiety and psychological morbidity among women who undergo this procedure. A number of studies suggest that provision of presurgical multidisciplinary support appears to have had a bearing on outcome. However, a minority of women do express regrets and experience adverse psychosocial events following surgery.

## Surgery for high-risk women with established breast cancer

Women who are under the care of a high-risk breast cancer team and who are considering RRM may have breast cancer diagnosed at some stage during their clinical assessment or on imaging modalities. Surgery then becomes part of the therapeutic management, and such women can no longer be considered to have 'risk-reducing surgery' on the affected breast. The priority is to treat the diagnosed malignancy as effectively as possible, using multimodality treatment within the context of the oncology multidisciplinary team. Therapy will include surgery and any of the adjuvant modalities of radiotherapy, chemotherapy and endocrine manipulation.

Most women will not want breast conservation as primary cancer treatment and will request mastectomy. This is understandable even if the cancer is small and could be effectively managed under other circumstances by breast conservation and radiation therapy.

 These women are often young, and if their family history is attributable to a gene mutation, identified or not, their personal risk of local recurrence or development of a second primary cancer in the same breast is higher than in women with sporadic breast cancer; their risk of contralateral new primary malignancy is also high.[48–50]

Much depends on the stage and grade of the cancer. Nothing is undertaken that might delay or divert necessary adjuvant therapy. Excising the cancer and performing a sentinel lymph node biopsy can provide this information and gives the patient and the clinical team time to discuss and select the most appropriate treatment for the patient and her cancer. Prognosis and life expectancy depend on the recognised prognostic factors of grade, size and lymphovascular invasion. Any reconstructive surgery for the affected breast is considered within the context of total oncology care. It may be that immediate breast reconstruction is not an option, particularly if postoperative radiotherapy is anticipated.

Any request for contralateral RRM, which is entirely understandable, is considered carefully within the context of the overall stage and prognosis. A woman found to have substantial lymph node involvement will be unlikely to benefit from concurrent RRM for the opposite breast; furthermore, any complications arising from contralateral surgery may delay adjuvant treatment. Each request is discussed in detail with the woman and an agreed treatment strategy is formulated, taking into account all factors. One safe approach is to undertake delayed breast reconstruction for the affected breast and to perform RRM with immediate breast reconstruction for the contralateral side at the same operation, after primary adjuvant therapy has been completed. There are many possible permutations and as individual circumstances vary widely, the decision on how to proceed is individual to each patient. Rates of contralateral mastectomy are increasing and the efficacy of contralateral mastectomy is now well established, although proof that this will save lives is still lacking.[51–53]

## Bilateral risk-reducing oophorectomy

Bilateral risk-reducing oophorectomy (including removal of the fallopian tubes) is undertaken in women with *BRCA1/2* mutations in order to reduce the risk of ovarian cancer.

 In addition to reducing the risk of ovarian cancer, prophylactic oophorectomy has also been shown to decrease the risk of breast cancer in women with a *BRCA1/2* mutation.[54]

This amounts to about a 50% reduction with an oophorectomy at 40 years of age and this risk reduction appears to be unaffected by the subsequent use of hormone replacement therapy (HRT).

 However, recent evidence from the Million Women Study would suggest that use of combined estrogen/progesterone HRT doubles the risk of breast cancer after 10 years' use.[55]

Using combined HRT in women who retain their uterus may therefore negate the protective effect of oophorectomy. Bilateral risk-reducing oophorectomy in high-risk women prior to the menopause is therefore likely to decrease the risk of both breast and ovarian cancer.

 Tamoxifen will reduce breast cancer incidence by 40–50%[50,56–58] and this is maintained in long-term follow-up after cessation of treatment.[58] However, this reduction is almost exclusively a reduction in estrogen receptor-positive disease and whether this translates to reduction for *BRCA1* remains unclear.

## Key points

- Gene testing can be useful but may not be possible for many women with a strong family history as no genetic mutation can be identified.
- Between 4% and 5% of breast cancer is due to high-penetrance cancer-susceptibility genes.
- *BRCA1* and *BRCA2* gene mutations result in breast cancer in young women, often bilateral.
- Familial breast cancer can be associated with ovarian and some other malignancies.
- Gail, Claus, Tyrer–Cuzick and BOADICA models predict individual breast cancer risk.
- RRM decreases breast cancer incidence by over 90–95%.
- Common RRM approaches combine breast parenchymal removal with breast reconstruction.
- Breast reconstruction should be appropriate for individual breast morphology.
- RRM can produce profound relief of anxiety, but is major surgery and complications must be avoided wherever possible.
- RRM should be undertaken by multidisciplinary specialised teams working within a protocol.
- Follow-up should ensure that results and outcomes are audited.

# References

1. Newman B, Austin MA, Lee M et al. Inheritance of human breast cancer: evidence for autosomal dominant transmission in high-risk families. Proc Natl Acad Sci USA 1988; 85:3044–8.

2. Claus EB, Risch N, Thompson WD. Autosomal dominant inheritance of early onset breast cancer: implications for risk prediction. Cancer 1994; 73:643–51.

3. Miki Y, Swensen J, Shattuck-Eidens D et al. A strong candidate for the breast and ovarian cancer gene *BRCA1*. Science 1994; 266:66–71.

4. Wooster R, Bignell G, Lancaster J et al. Identification of the breast cancer susceptibility gene *BRCA2*. Nature 1995; 378:789–92.

5. Malkin D, Li FP, Strong LC et al. Germline TP53 mutations in cancer families. Science 1990; 250:1233–8.

6. Lalloo F, Varley J, Ellis D et al. Family history is predictive of pathogenic mutations in BRCA1, BRCA2 and TP53 with high penetrance in a population based study of very early onset breast cancer. Lancet 2003; 361:1011–12.

7. Ford D, Easton DF, Bishop DT et al. Risk of cancer in BRCA-1 mutation carriers. Lancet 1994; 343:692–5.

8. Ford D, Easton DF, Stratton M et al. The Breast Cancer Linkage Consortium: genetic heterogeneity and penetrance analysis of the BRCA1 and BRCA2 genes in breast cancer families. Am J Hum Genet 1998; 62:676–89.

9. Antoniou A, Pharoah PDP, Narod S et al. Average risks of breast and ovarian cancer associated with mutations in BRCA1 or BRCA2 detected in case series unselected for family history: a combined analysis of 22 studies. Am J Hum Genet 2003; 72:1117–30.

10. Parmigiani G, Berry DA, Aquilar O. Determining carrier probabilities for breast cancer susceptibility genes BRCA1 and BRCA2. Am J Hum Genet 1998; 62:145–8.

11. Berry DA, Iversen ES Jr, Gudbjartsson DF et al. BRCAPRO validation, sensitivity of genetic testing of BRCA1/BRCA2, and prevalence of other breast cancer susceptibility genes. J Clin Oncol 2002; 20:2701–12.

12. Evans DGR, Eccles D, Rahman N et al. A scoring system for prioritising breast/ovarian cancer family genetic testing based on detection rates for BRCA1/2 mutations in families from North West and Southern England. J Med Genet 2004; 41:474–80

13. Lakhani SR, Van De Vijver MJ, Jacquemier J et al. The pathology of familial breast cancer: predictive value of immunohistochemical markers, estrogen receptor, progesterone receptor, HER-2, and p53 in patients with mutations in BRCA1 and BRCA2. J Clin Oncol 2002; 20:2310–18.

14. Evans DGR, Young K, Bulman M et al. Mutation testing for BRCA1/2 in ovarian cancer families: use of histology to predict status. Clin Genet 2008; in press.

15. Evans DGR, Bulman M, Gokhale D et al. Sensitivity of BRCA1/2 mutation testing in breast/ovarian cancer families from the North West of England. J Med Genet 2003; 40:107.

16. Struewing J, Hartge P, Wacholder S et al. The risk of breast cancer associated with specific mutations of BRCA1 and BRCA2 among Ashkenazi Jews. N Engl J Med 1997; 336:1401–7.

17. Easton DF, Pharoah PDP, Dunning AM et al. A genome-wide association study identifies multiple novel breast cancer susceptibility loci. Nature 2007; 447(7148):1087–93.

18. Dupont WD, Page DL. Relative risk of breast cancer varies with time since diagnosis of atypical hyperplasia. Hum Pathol 1989; 20:723–5.

19. Vasen HFA, Haites N, Evans DGR et al. Current policies for surveillance and management in women at risk of breast cancer: a survey among 16 European family cancer clinics. Eur J Cancer 1998; 34:1922–6.

20. Evans DGR, Lalloo F. Risk assessment and management of high risk familial breast cancer. J Med Genet 2002; 39:865–71.

21. Gail MH, Brinton LA, Byar DP et al. Projecting individualized probabilities of developing breast cancer for white females who are being examined annually. J Natl Cancer Inst 1989; 81:1879–86.

22. Tyrer JP, Duffy SW, Cuzick J. A breast cancer prediction model incorporating familial and personal risk factors. Stat Med 2004; 23:1111–30.
This model incorporates the majority of currently known breast cancer risk factors.

23. Amir E, Evans DGR, Shenton A et al. Evaluation of breast cancer risk assessment packages in the family history evaluation and screening programme. J Med Genet 2003; 40:807–14.

24. Goodnight JE, Quagliana JM, Morton DL. Failure of subcutaneous mastectomy to prevent the development of breast cancer. J Surg Oncol 1984; 26:198–201.

25. Zeigler LD, Kroll SS. Primary breast cancer after prophylactic mastectomy. Am J Clin Oncol 1991; 14:451–4.

26. Evans DGR, Lalloo F, Shenton A et al. Uptake of screening and prevention trials in women at very high risk of breast cancer. Lancet 2001; 358:889–90.

27. Metcalfe KA, Birenbaum-Carmeli D, Lbiski J et al. International variation in rates of uptake of preventive options in BRCA1 and BRCA2 mutation carriers. Int J Cancer 2008 (Epub ahead of print).

28. Schrag D, Kuntz KM, Garbor JE et al. Decision analysis: effects of prophylactic mastectomy and oophorectomy on life expectancy among women

with BRCA1 or BRCA2 mutations. N Engl J Med 1997; 336:1465–71.

29. Hartmann LC, Schaid DJ, Woods JE et al. Efficacy of bilateral prophylactic mastectomy in women with a family history of breast cancer. N Engl J Med 1999; 340:77–84.

This retrospective US cohort study examined the incidence of, and risk of death from, breast cancer after a median follow-up of 14 years among 639 women who had a family history of breast cancer and who had undergone bilateral subcutaneous or total prophylactic mastectomy. In the mastectomy group, women were divided into high-risk ($n$ = 214) or moderate-risk ($n$ = 425) subgroups, with most women in each subgroup having undergone subcutaneous mastectomy (89% and 90% respectively). The study showed a reduction in the risk of breast cancer of 89.5% ($P$ < 0.001) in moderate-risk women who had undergone prophylactic mastectomy, and a reduction in risk of 90–94% in the high-risk women.

30. Meijers-Heijboer EJ, van Geel B, van Putten WLJ et al. Breast cancer after prophylactic bilateral mastectomy in women with a BRCA1 or BRCA2 mutation. N Engl J Med 2001; 345:159–64.

The incidence of breast cancer after a mean follow-up of 3 years was compared in a Dutch prospective cohort study involving 76 women with BRCA1 or BRCA2 mutations who had undergone bilateral prophylactic mastectomy (total simple, including nipple) and a control group of 63 women with BRCA1 or BRCA2 mutations who underwent surveillance. No cases of invasive breast cancer were observed in the women who had undergone prophylactic bilateral mastectomy, whereas in the surveillance group eight invasive breast cancers were detected. Proportional hazards analysis showed that prophylactic mastectomy significantly ($P$ = 0.003) reduced the incidence of breast cancer.

31. Evans DGR, Fentiman IS, McPherson K et al. Familial breast cancer. Br Med J 1994; 308:183–7.

32. Evans DGR, Cuzick J, Howell A. Cancer genetics clinics. Eur J Cancer 1996; 32:391–2.

33. Evans DGR, Anderson E, Lalloo F et al. Utilisation of preventative mastectomy in 10 European centres. Dis Markers 1999; 15:148–51.

34. Julian-Reynier C, Eisinger F, Moatti J-P et al. Physician's attitudes towards mammography and prophylactic surgery for hereditary breast/ovarian cancer risk and subsequently published guidelines. Eur J Hum Genet 2000; 8:204–8.

35. Julian-Reynier C, Bouchard L, Evans G et al. Women's attitudes toward preventive strategies for hereditary breast/ovarian cancer risk differ from one country to another: differences between Manchester (UK), Marseilles (F) and Montreal (Ca). Cancer 2001; 92:959–68.

36. Evans DGR, Howell A, Baildam A et al. Risk-reduction mastectomy: clinical issues and research needs. J Natl Cancer Inst 2002; 94:307.

37. Eccles DM, Evans DGR, Mackay J. Guidelines for a genetic risk based approach to advising women with a family history of breast cancer. J Med Genet 2000; 37:203–9.

38. Eeles R. Testing for the breast cancer predisposition gene, BRCA1. Br Med J 1996; 313:572–3.

39. Evans DGR, Kerr B, Cade D et al. Fictitious breast cancer family history. Lancet 1996; 348:1034.

40. Lalloo F, Baildam A, Brain A et al. Preventative mastectomy for women at high risk of breast cancer. Eur J Surg Oncol 2000; 26:711–13.

41. Frost MH, Schaid DJ, Sellers TA et al. Long-term satisfaction and psychological and social function following bilateral prophylactic mastectomy. JAMA 2000; 284:319–24.

42. Hatcher MB, Fallowfield L, A'Hern R. The psychosocial impact of bilateral prophylactic mastectomy: prospective study using questionnaires and semi-structured interviews. Br Med J 2001; 322:76–9.

43. Hopwood P, Lee A, Shenton A et al. Clinical follow-up after bilateral risk reducing ('prophylactic') mastectomy: mental health and body image outcomes. Psychooncology 2000; 9:462–72.

44. Stefanek ME, Helzlsouer KJ, Wilcox PM et al. Predictors of and satisfaction with bilateral prophylactic mastectomy. Prev Med 1995; 24:412–19.

45. Borgen PI, Hill ADK, Tran KN et al. Patient regrets after bilateral prophylactic mastectomy. Ann Surg Oncol 1998; 5:603–6.

46. Lloyd SM, Watson M, Oaker G et al. Understanding the experience of prophylactic bilateral mastectomy: a qualitative study of ten women. Psychooncology 2000; 9:473–85.

47. Josephson U, Wickman M, Sandelin K. Initial experiences of women from hereditary breast cancer families after bilateral prophylactic mastectomy: a retrospective study. Eur J Surg Oncol 2000; 26:351–6.

48. Eccles D, Simmonds P, Goddard J et al. Familial breast cancer: an investigation into the outcome of treatment for early stage disease. Fam Cancer 2001; 1:65–72.

49. Metcalfe K, Lynch HT, Ghadirian P et al. Contralateral breast cancer in BRCA1 and BRCA2 mutation carriers. J Clin Oncol 2004; 22(12):2328–35.

50. Narod SA, Brunet JS, Ghadirian P and the Hereditary Breast Cancer Clinical Study Group. Tamoxifen and risk of contralateral breast cancer in BRCA1 and BRCA2 carriers: a case control study. Lancet 2000; 356:1876–81.

51. Heemskerk-Gerritsen BA, Brekelmans CT, Menke-Pluymers MB et al. Prophylactic mastectomy in BRCA1/2 mutation carriers and women at risk of hereditary breast cancer: long-term experiences

at the Rotterdam Family Cancer Clinic. Ann Surg Oncol 2007; 14(12):3335–44.

52. McDonnell SK, Schaid DJ, Myers JL et al. Efficacy of contralateral prophylactic mastectomy in women with a personal and family history of breast cancer. J Clin Oncol 2001; 19(19):3938–43.

53. Herrinton LJ, Barlow WE, Yu O et al. Efficacy of prophylactic mastectomy in women with unilateral breast cancer: a cancer research network project. J Clin Oncol 2005; 23(19):4275–86.

54. Rebbeck TR, Lynch HT, Neuhausen SL et al. Reduction in cancer risk after bilateral prophylactic oophorectomy in BRCA1 and BRCA2 mutation carriers. N Engl J Med 2002; 346:1616–22.

55. Beral V. Breast cancer and hormone-replacement therapy in the Million Women Study. Lancet 2003; 362:419–27.

56. Fisher B, Constantino JP, Wickerham DL et al. Tamoxifen for prevention of breast cancer: report of the National Surgical Adjuvant Breast and Bowel Project P1 study. J Natl Cancer Inst 1998; 90:1371–88.

57. IBIS investigators. First results from the International Breast Cancer Intervention Study (IBIS-I): a randomised prevention trial. Lancet 2002; 360: 817–24.

58. Cuzick J, Forbes JF, Sestak I et al. International Breast Cancer Intervention Study I Investigators. Long-term results of tamoxifen prophylaxis for breast cancer – 96-month follow-up of the randomized IBIS-I trial. J Natl Cancer Inst 2007; 99(4):272–82.

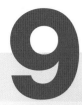

# 9

# Breast reconstruction

Eva M. Weiler-Mithoff

## Introduction

More breast cancers are now detected at an earlier stage and in younger women. Improved survival means that they will live for much longer with the physical defect and the psychological problems of mastectomy. Mastectomy affects body image and feelings of attractiveness, leading to poor self-esteem, low self-confidence and introversion. A woman subsequently has to cope with the indignity and inconvenience of a breast prosthesis, which serves as a constant reminder of the loss of her breast and resulting deformity.

 Breast reconstruction can re-establish body symmetry, eliminate the external prosthesis, diminish anxiety, increase wardrobe flexibility and the feeling of sexual attractiveness, and improve sexual functioning. Breast reconstruction therefore plays a significant role in the woman's physical, emotional and psychological recovery from breast cancer.[1-4]

Even the best reconstruction will not be able to replace the natural breast that has been lost. A totally reconstructed breast will always feel and behave differently and will not have erogenous sensation. Women should be aware of the possibilities of breast reconstruction at the time of planning of the initial surgical treatment, even if it may be their personal preference to have a delayed reconstruc-

tion or no reconstruction at all.[5-7] A final decision regarding the timing and technique of breast reconstruction should be made by the patient and the multidisciplinary oncology team, consisting of ablative surgeon, reconstructive surgeon and oncologist.

 Historically, the goals of breast reconstruction were to improve the appearance when clothed and to avoid an external prosthesis. Surgical advances and increased patient expectations have modified these goals. The current aim is to produce symmetry that satisfies the patient's wishes within the limits of technical feasibility, while matching the remaining breast in terms of its contour, dimension and position. This may involve the use of the patient's own tissues, breast implants and the use of corrective surgery to the opposite breast.[4,8]

## Timing

The fundamental aim of breast cancer surgery must be to provide safe and successful oncological treatment. Breast reconstruction can be performed immediately at the time of mastectomy or delayed.[8]

### Immediate breast reconstruction

Advantages of immediate breast reconstruction include the potential for a single operation and period of hospitalisation. It allows maximum preservation of breast skin and preservation of the inframammary fold. The reconstructive surgeon can then work with good-quality skin flaps that are unscarred and which do not suffer from the effects of radiotherapy. Skin-sparing mastectomy in particular facilitates better cosmetic results, with a reduced need for contralateral symmetrisation surgery.[8–10]

The disadvantages of immediate reconstruction are the limited time for decision-making by the patient, increased operating time and the difficulties of coordinating two surgical teams in those units where there are no 'oncoplastic' surgeons who can perform both the mastectomy and reconstruction.

 Concerns that the more complex nature of surgery may have an increased risk of postoperative complications and may therefore compromise adjuvant treatment are not evidence based, although there is a potential in individual patients for complications to result in a delay in starting adjuvant treatment.[8,11,12]

 Chemotherapy and radiotherapy can have detrimental effects on some types of breast reconstruction, but these can be reduced by judicious choice of type and timing of reconstructive techniques.[13,14]
   Published evidence indicates that immediate breast reconstruction does not adversely affect breast cancer outcome. The reconstruction does not interfere with the delivery of adjuvant treatment and there is no significant difference in the survival rates between patients having immediate or delayed reconstruction.[15–19]

Breast reconstruction may be indicated even in disease with poor prognosis in order to improve the overall psychological rehabilitation and quality of remaining life. It is no longer necessary to make a woman mourn the loss of a breast by experiencing its absence.[4,8,20,21]

## Delayed breast reconstruction

Delayed breast reconstruction, on the other hand, allows the patient unlimited time for decision-making, avoids any potential delay of adjuvant treatment and removes the detrimental affects of radiotherapy or chemotherapy on the reconstruction, but requires replacement of a larger amount of breast skin. The initial mastectomy flaps may be thin, scarred, contracted or irradiated and the end result of the breast reconstruction is thus often not as aesthetically pleasing as that obtained by immediate reconstruction. A second episode of hospitalisation is required and treatment costs are increased compared with immediate reconstruction (Box 9.1).

# Contraindications

Contraindications for breast reconstruction include uncontrolled and non-resectable local chest wall disease, rapidly progressive systemic disease, patients who have serious comorbidity and patients who are psychologically unsuitable.[4]

Box 9.1 • Advantages and disadvantages of immediate and delayed breast reconstruction

### Advantages of immediate breast reconstruction

- Potential for a single operation and one period of hospitalisation
- Maximum preservation of breast skin
- Preservation of the inframammary fold
- Good-quality skin flaps
- Better cosmetic results for skin-sparing mastectomy
- Reduced need for balancing surgery to the contralateral breast
- Lower cost than delayed reconstruction

### Disadvantages of immediate reconstruction

- Limited time for decision-making by patient
- Increased operating time
- Difficulties of coordinating two surgical teams when required
- Potential in individual patients for complications to result in delay of adjuvant treatment

### Advantages of delayed breast reconstruction

- Allows unlimited time for decision-making by patient
- Avoids any potential delay of adjuvant treatment
- Avoids detrimental effects of radiotherapy or chemotherapy on the reconstruction

### Disadvantages of delayed breast reconstruction

- Requires replacement of a larger amount of breast skin
- Mastectomy flaps may be thin, scarred, contracted or irradiated
- Mastectomy scar may be poorly positioned
- May result in a less aesthetically pleasing outcome
- Requires separate episode of hospitalisation
- Increased treatment cost compared with immediate breast reconstruction

# Techniques

Breast reconstruction involves replacement of breast skin and breast volume. Surgical options for reconstruction include the use of tissue expanders and breast implants and the use of autologous tissue. The most commonly used surgical techniques are tissue expansion, latissimus dorsi (LD) myocutaneous flap with or without implant, the use of lower abdominal tissue and other free tissue transfers.

Implant-based techniques require limited surgery initially but have limitations and are not always quick and trouble free. These procedures allow some patient control over breast size, but the quality of the long-term result is directly related to the tolerance of breast implants and often disappointing. Further procedures may be required for complications and maintenance. The aesthetic results from autologous reconstruction are superior to those of implant-based reconstruction due to their versatility, their more natural appearance, consistency and durability. The best results with implants are in patients requiring or requesting bilateral mastectomy and reconstruction. Autologous tissue can also better withstand radiotherapy. The autologous LD flap is highly versatile and has acceptable donor-site morbidity. The skin and fat of the lower abdomen are ideal for autologous breast reconstruction but donor-site morbidity is increasingly being appreciated. Muscle-sparing techniques preserve the abdominal wall function at the cost of a more complex procedure. The effects of adjuvant radiotherapy on breast reconstruction using lower abdominal tissue are still under investigation.[22–26]

 The ultimate choice of technique depends on patient fitness, breast size, body habitus, laxity and thickness of remaining breast skin, the condition of the underlying muscles, availability of flap donor sites, stage of disease and the need for adjuvant radiotherapy. The final decision depends on the personal preference of the patient if more than one reconstructive option is feasible. Because of the variable needs of individual patients, the reconstructive surgical team must be able to provide the full range of reconstructive options.[4,8,27]

## Tissue expansion reconstruction

Tissue expansion is the simplest method of immediate breast reconstruction. An inflatable silicone balloon is placed into a submuscular pocket on the anterior chest wall and subsequently expanded by a series of postoperative saline injections. This ingenious method of breast reconstruction is based on the gradual stretching of the skin with a single- or double-lumen tissue expander to replace the skin loss after mastectomy. The tissue expander or a breast implant will simultaneously replace the breast volume[28] (**Fig. 9.1**). Patient selection and implant selection are crucial. Several techniques are possible:

- fixed volume implant (single stage);
- variable volume expander implant (single stage);

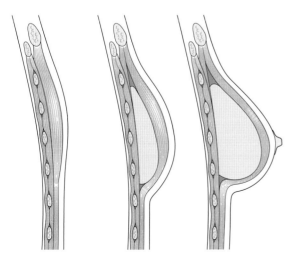

**Figure 9.1** • Breast reconstruction with submuscular tissue expander.

• issue expansion followed by permanent implant (two stage).

Tissue expansion is a simple and flexible technique that does not involve any additional scarring. The breast is reconstructed with local tissues with similar colour and texture. This short procedure requires 1 hour operating time, a short period of hospitalisation and 2–4 weeks recovery time.

## Indications

This technique is suitable for patients with small non-ptotic breasts, when performing bilateral reconstruction or for women who are happy to accept a mastopexy procedure on the opposite breast. This procedure is ideal for patients who want minimal scarring, are not worried about a silicone implant and are unwilling or unfit to undergo autologous tissue reconstruction.[8,27]

## Contraindications

Patients are unsuitable for implant reconstruction if the chest wall tissues are thin, damaged, inelastic or irradiated, if a radical mastectomy has been performed, if there is an extensive infraclavicular tissue deformity after resection or atrophy of the pectoralis major muscle, if there is a vertical mastectomy scar or if they suffer from an autoimmune disease.[8,27]

## Surgical techniques

Tissue expanders are placed under the muscles of the chest wall including pectoralis major, serratus anterior and the external oblique and rectus muscles. A common problem is not getting the expander low enough – the pectoralis major attachment varies between patients and needs to be detached, but the tissue below this is thin, fibrous and does not always expand satisfactorily. One option is to detach the pectoralis major and insert a piece of acellular matrix derived from donated human skin (AlloDerm™). By eliminating the need to elevate the serratus anterior and the external oblique muscles and the rectus abdominus fascia for implant/expander coverage, AlloDerm™ not only reduces morbidity, but it also simplifies expander insertion. The big disadvantage is the cost of the AlloDerm™. There are other options now available including pigskin and these are being evaluated and have the advantage of being cheaper.

Tissue expansion can be used in immediate or delayed breast reconstruction. The expander is only partially inflated at insertion to allow safe closure of overlying muscle and skin. The actual expansion starts 2–4 weeks postoperatively and is usually performed at weekly intervals. Numerous visits to the outpatient department may be required and inflation can sometimes be painful. Overexpansion by 50–200% of the breast volume for several months has been advocated to create a more natural ptosis.[29] Nowadays this is rarely practised. With shaped expanders and matching prostheses expansion is performed as quickly as possible in as few visits as possible and overexpansion is modest, if at all. One concern is that if a shaped prosthesis is placed in a pocket of larger volume it has a greater risk of rotation, so some even advocate replacing an expander with a slightly larger prosthesis. When selecting an expander and prosthesis care must be taken to select devices of the correct width, the correct height and the most appropriate projection. A detailed knowledge of the full range of devices available is essential if the optimum result is to be obtained. Reconstruction of the breast mound can take up to 6 months using tissue expansion. Secondary procedures may be necessary to achieve a more natural appearance of the reconstructed breast. Over one-third of patients require further surgery within the first 5 years after implant-based breast reconstruction.[30] Implant-only breast reconstructions lack ptosis and significant alterations of the contralateral breast to improve symmetry are usually necessary (**Fig. 9.2**).

The long-term results of implant-based reconstruction can be disappointing and are characterised by periods of asymmetry due to continuous changes of the contralateral breast as a consequence of the effects of gravity and fluctuations in weight.[31]

## Complications

The complications of tissue expansion can be grouped into those related to wound failure such as haematoma, wound infection, breast skin necrosis and wound dehiscence, those due to implant failure, and those of breast implants such as capsular contracture, asymmetry, and displacement and thinning of overlying skin. The incidence of skin-flap necrosis and implant exposure can be as high as 10% and

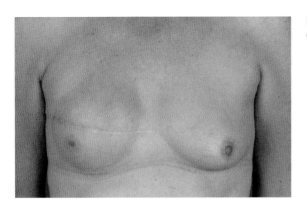

**Figure 9.2** • Delayed breast reconstruction by tissue expansion.

30–50% respectively.[17,32] The commonest and least predictable complication of implant reconstruction is capsular contracture. Hardening of the scar tissue around the implant leads to firmness on palpation and distortion of the breast as well as discomfort and pain. Further surgical revision is necessary in severe cases. The risk of capsular contracture is significantly increased in the presence of preoperative or postoperative radiotherapy.[33,34] Textured implants reduce capsular contracture rates and their use is now routine.

## Latissimus dorsi flap reconstruction

The LD myocutaneous flap, originally described for chest wall reconstruction by Tansini at the turn of the century, was rediscovered and became the standard method of breast reconstruction in the 1970s, allowing the immediate reconstruction of larger, more pendulous breasts[27,35] (**Fig. 9.3**).

The LD muscle is a large triangular back muscle of variable thickness. The cutaneous territory of this flap consists of the skin superficial to the entire muscle and approximately 3 cm beyond. Numerous myocutaneous perforators allow the design of skin islands in various patterns. Orientation of the skin paddle in the skin crease allows maximum skin harvest with a good scar, which can be hidden under the bra strap.

LD flap breast reconstruction is a very versatile, safe and reliable technique with a success rate of over 99%, and is even suitable for high-risk patients. Disadvantages include a donor scar on the back, unless endoscopic techniques are used. The colour match of back and breast skin may not be

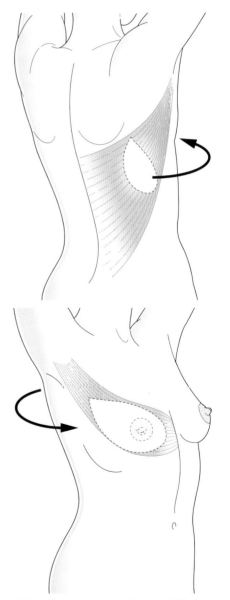

**Figure 9.3** • Breast reconstruction using latissimus dorsi myocutaneous flap.

ideal and there is a potential for further impairment of shoulder movement, which may have already been compromised by previous surgery. The functional deficit after transfer of an LD muscle affects only very specific activities like rowing, cross-country skiing or mountain climbing, but has little effect on most other activities. Additional physiotherapy may be required to restore full shoulder mobility.[8,27,36] LD breast reconstruction is a major operation but a lesser procedure than free tissue transfer. Approximately 3–4 hours operating time, a hospital stay of 5–7 days and a recovery time of 4–8 weeks are required.

## Indications

Indications for this technique include the reconstruction of large breasts where an implant alone would not be sufficient for size, if the chest wall tissues are unsuitable for tissue expansion and if there are additional tissue requirements after mastectomy. Additional indications are congenital breast hypoplasia such as Poland's syndrome, chest wall reconstruction, and partial breast reconstruction after conservation surgery or partial loss of an abdominal tissue flap.[27]

## Contraindications

Contraindications for LD breast reconstruction are previous surgery that may have compromised the vascular supply to the flap such as thoracotomies or extensive and radical axillary surgery, absence of the LD muscle and serious patient comorbidity.[4]

## Surgical techniques

Several variations of this flap are possible. The LD muscle can be transferred as muscle-only flap without a skin island, avoiding a donor-site scar on the back. A myocutaneous flap can be used with or without a breast implant or tissue expander if mus-

cle cover and skin are required. It is also possible to reconstruct a small to moderate-sized breast with an extended or autologous LD flap. This type of reconstruction includes taking the maximum amount of both skin and subcutaneous fat overlying the muscle and avoids the use of implants or tissue expanders (**Fig. 9.4**). A muscle-sparing or perforator-based technique, the so-called thoracodorsal artery perforator (T-DAP) flap, can be employed if preservation of muscle function is desirable.[37–40] The sections that follow describe the technique of autologous LD flap reconstruction.

### Preoperative planning

Preoperative planning takes into account the size and shape of the opposite breast or the planned breast size and, in the case of an immediate breast reconstruction, the area of breast skin excision. In delayed breast reconstruction additional factors such as the thickness and quality of the skin flaps, the condition and function of the pectoralis major muscle, the extent of radiotherapy damage, and the position and quality of the mastectomy scar are assessed and additional soft-tissue requirements noted.

The function of the LD muscle must be tested prior to surgery. If necessary, colour Doppler or magnetic resonance imaging can be used to establish the continuity of the thoracodorsal vessels. The amount and distribution of excess skin and soft tissue are assessed. A lean back can yield 300–400 cm$^3$, an average back 600–800 cm$^3$ and a plump back 1200–1500 cm$^3$.

Prior to surgery, breast base, inframammary fold, anterior axillary fold and the take-off point of the breast from the chest wall are marked with the patient in a sitting or standing position. On the back, the limits of the LD muscle and the skin ellipse are marked. This should be centred over the fat roll on

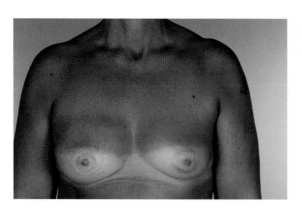

**Figure 9.4** • Immediate right breast reconstruction by autologous latissimus dorsi flap after skin-sparing mastectomy.

the back and positioned in the relaxed skin tension lines. A maximum width of 6–9 cm allows closure without tension. The resulting scar should lie in the middle to lower bra-strap area. The additional areas of soft-tissue harvest such as the parascapular area, fat anterior to the anterior border of the muscle and any supra-iliac fat deposits are marked.

## Positioning in the operating theatre

The patient is positioned in a lateral decubitus position and secured with well-padded table attachments. The arm is suspended or supported with attachments at 90° to allow easy access to the axilla. The mastectomy and any axillary surgery can be performed in this position as well. Such a combined approach in immediate reconstruction can save up to 1.5 hours operating time. A separate incision may be required for axillary clearance in skin-sparing mastectomy and the different spatial orientation has to be taken into account by the surgeon undertaking the axillary surgery.

## Flap harvest

Infiltration of the area of incision and the subcutaneous space overlying the area of soft-tissue harvest with a weak solution of local anaesthetic with or without adrenaline (epinephrine) and normal saline helps to plump up this space and facilitates dissection at the level of Scarpa's fascia. The skin island is incised and Scarpa's fascia is identified. Raising the skin flaps at this level protects the blood supply to the overlying skin flaps and ensures maximum soft-tissue harvest with the flap. At the border of the previously marked soft-tissue harvest the dissection is carried down to the LD muscle, the muscles overlying the scapula and the rhomboid muscles. The superomedial extent of the soft-tissue harvest is the anterior border of the trapezius muscle. The adipofascial parascapular flap extension is lifted caudally until the upper edge of the LD flap is exposed at the tip of the scapula. The proximal portion of the muscle is dissected up to the tendinous junction at the level of the muscle fascia to avoid excess bulk in the axilla after flap transfer. The borders of flap harvest are now marked and the muscle can then be raised from cranial, posterior and inferior. All intercostal perforators are divided and haemostasis is secured. A strip of thoracolumbar fascia can be harvested and protects the posterior and inferior flap borders. The anterior border with the additional soft tissue anterior to the muscle is elevated last, taking care

to identify the posterior border of serratus anterior and avoid harvest of slips of external oblique or serratus posterior muscle. As the LD is lifted off the serratus anterior, the neurovascular pedicle to LD and the serratus branch are identified and carefully preserved. The posterior border of the LD muscle is detached from the teres muscles up to the tendinous insertion. The posterior half of the tendon may be divided if it is very broad in order to provide maximum mobility of the flap. The anterior border of the muscle is freed, carefully avoiding damage to the thoracodorsal neurovascular bundle. A high tunnel to the mastectomy defect is fashioned to position the upper part of the muscle parallel to the anterior axillary fold. The muscle is transferred and the tension on the pedicle is assessed. It is generally not necessary to divide the LD tendon (although some do this routinely) or the serratus branch, which can provide additional vascularity, particularly in delayed reconstruction when the main thoracodorsal vein may be encased by scar tissue. The thoracodorsal nerve is usually preserved to maintain muscular bulk if performing a purely autologous reconstruction. If an implant is being used the nerve can be divided, although muscle twitching tends to decrease with time in those where the nerve is preserved and is rarely a problem. The donor site may be quilted and then closed in three layers with absorbable sutures after insertion of two drains. The flap is secured temporarily on the anterior chest wall to allow repositioning of the patient for the final flap inset.

## Flap inset

The patient is repositioned supine and both breasts are prepared and redraped. The flap is then sutured into position after securing the upper part of the LD muscle to the lateral border of the pectoralis major muscle. The flap is rotated 180° and the scapular adipofascial flap is folded under for extra projection in the lower pole. The edges of the flap are sutured into the medial and superior borders of the mastectomy defect, suturing to the flap or the junction with the chest wall rather than to the chest wall itself. The anterior axillary fold and the inframammary fold are recreated by folding the muscle and attaching it laterally. An upper abdominal advancement flap can provide extra skin for the breast envelope in delayed breast reconstruction or chest wall resurfacing. Any excess skin island is de-epithelialised for additional volume. The projection of the neo-breast can be adjusted with plication sutures. The size of the reconstructed breast should be approximately 25% larger than the opposite breast to allow for some postoperative atrophy. Two drains are inserted and the skin is closed.

## Postoperative management

The patient is encouraged to wear a well-supporting brassiere for the final moulding of the reconstructed breast. Physiotherapy is started on the first postoperative day with shoulder shrugging and exercises up to 90°. Rehabilitation of the scapular region follows after 4 weeks.[8]

## Complications

Potential postoperative complications include wound failure, expander failure and complications of breast implants. Flap-related wound complications include haematoma, infection, partial or total flap necrosis, breast skin-flap necrosis and delayed healing. Donor site-related complications include haematoma, seroma, wound infection and wound dehiscence. Seroma formation is common after extended LD harvest and may require repeated aspiration.

 Several strategies have been suggested in order to reduce the incidence of postoperative seroma, including quilting the skin onto the underlying chest wall and the use of triamcinolone injected into the cavity at first aspiration.[41,42]

 Localised fat necrosis in autologous LD flaps has been reported in up to 14% of cases. Partial flap necrosis occurs in less than 5–7% and total flap necrosis in less than 1%. Implant failure and rates of complications of breast implants are similar to those of implant-only reconstructions (Table 9.1).[37,43,44]

Although short- and medium-term results of LD and implant reconstructions appear quite satisfactory, long-term outcomes are disappointing. There is some evidence that the autologous LD flap may withstand adjuvant radiotherapy better than the LD flap with additional implant.[45–49]

## The silicone issue

All available information on the safety of silicone breast implants has been assessed by the Independent Review Group and the findings published in a very thorough report in 1998.[50]

 This report shows clearly that there is no histopathological or immunological evidence of an abnormal immune response to silicone and no epidemiological evidence of any link between silicone and an established connective tissue disease such as rheumatoid arthritis or autoimmune diseases. There is lack of evidence for an atypical connective tissue disease or

Table 9.1 • Complications of breast reconstruction using latissimus dorsi (LD) flap

| | Autologous LD | LD with implant |
|---|---|---|
| **Flap-related complications (%)** | | |
| Total flap loss | 0–1 | 0.6 |
| Partial flap loss | 1–7 | 3 |
| Fat necrosis | 4–14 | 19 |
| Breast skin necrosis | 10 | 19 |
| Wound infection | 2 | 5 |
| **Donor-site complications (%)** | | |
| Seroma | 20–80 | 9–50 |
| Haematoma | 3–6 | 0.6 |
| Wound dehiscence | 10–25 | 16 |
| **Implant-related complications (%)** | | |
| Capsular contracture | NA | 20–56 |
| Displacement | NA | 1 |
| Implant rupture | NA | 2 |

NA, not appropriate or not relevant.

'silicone poisoning' and no toxic reaction could be found. There is no evidence that children of women with breast implants are at risk of connective tissue disease. However, there is currently not enough information about the actual lifespan of implants and any patient receiving an implant- or tissue expander-based breast reconstruction should be aware that the implant may require replacement.[50]

# Breast reconstruction with lower abdominal tissue

The lower abdomen is often an abundant source of tissue for autologous breast reconstruction. A sizeable and natural-feeling breast mound can be created without any implant or tissue expander with tissue that is usually discarded during an aesthetic abdominoplasty procedure. The donor defect is acceptable and often a cosmetic improvement. Although this technique can provide excellent long-term results, donor-site morbidity should not be underestimated.[51,52]

## Indications

Lower abdominal tissue can be used for immediate and delayed breast reconstruction. Good candidates are young and healthy with sufficient lower abdominal tissue available. It is also indicated if the contralateral breast is large, in bilateral breast reconstruction, if there have been previous complications with breast implants and if the LD muscle has been divided or is atrophic. Reconstructions using lower abdominal tissue can be associated with significant complications and morbidity.[4]

## Contraindications

Contraindications are obesity, smoking, diabetes, autoimmune disease, vasospastic or cardiorespiratory disorders, psychosocial problems, abdominal scars disrupting the vascular anatomy, inadequate

recipient vessels or an inexperienced surgeon. The potentially detrimental effects of adjuvant radiotherapy on the reconstructed breast are currently under investigation.[21,26,53]

## Surgical techniques

Myocutaneous perforators through the rectus abdominis muscle and direct cutaneous vessels provide the blood supply to the lower abdominal apron by three main vascular routes. The deep inferior epigastric artery (DIEA), a branch of the external iliac vessel, is the primary source of circulation to the rectus abdominis muscle. The deep superior epigastric artery (DSEA), the terminal branch of the internal mammary artery and lesser vessel of supply, anastomoses with the DIEA within the substance of the muscle. Additional direct cutaneous supply of the abdominal apron exists through the superficial inferior epigastric artery (SIEA). The triple blood supply to the lower abdominal tissue allows it to be used in a variety of techniques:[54-59]

- pedicled transverse rectus abdominis myocutaneous (TRAM) flap;
- free TRAM flap;
- free deep inferior epigastric perforator (DIEP) flap;
- free SIEA flap.

The reason why surgeons have moved from pedicled TRAM flaps to free perforator flaps is to try to reduce the morbidity of the donor site and preserve abdominal wall integrity and function. The complications encountered with techniques using lower abdominal tissue for breast reconstruction are related to the extent of muscle resection, extent of fascia resection and the use of a mesh to repair the abdominal wall. These factors should be borne in mind when selecting the appropriate procedure for an individual patient (Table 9.2). All these techniques will interfere with abdominal wall sensation (**Fig. 9.5**).

Table 9.2 • Flap survival and donor-site morbidity after breast reconstruction using abdominal tissue

|  | Pedicled TRAM flap | Free TRAM flap | Free DIEP flap |
|---|---|---|---|
| Total flap loss (%) | <1 | 5–7 | 1–5 |
| Partial flap loss (%) | 28–60 | 6–8 | 6 |
| Fat necrosis (%) | 27–40 | 7–13 | 6–10 |
| Abdominal bulge (%) | 8–28 | 5–8 | 0.3–5 |
| Abdominal hernia (%) | >6 | 4–6 | 0–1.4 |

DIEP, deep inferior epigastric perforator; TRAM, transverse rectus abdominis myocutaneous.
Modified from Weiler-Mithoff E, Hodgson ELB, Malata CM. Perforator flap breast reconstruction. Breast Dis 2002; 16:93–106.

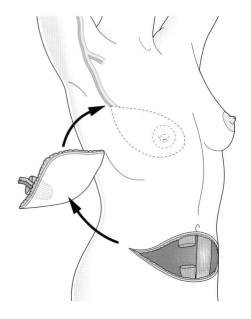

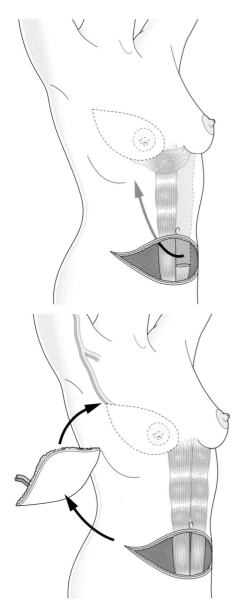

**Figure 9.5** • Techniques of breast reconstruction using abdominal tissue: **(a)** pedicled TRAM flap; **(b)** free TRAM flap; **(c)** free DIEP flap. See text for explanation of abbreviations.

### Pedicled TRAM flap

The pedicled TRAM flap relies on blood flow through the deep superior epigastric vessels within the substance of the rectus abdominis muscle to supply a horizontal ellipse of lower abdominal skin and fat. The flap is transferred onto the chest wall through a large subcutaneous tunnel.[53–55]

The pedicled TRAM flap does not require microvascular skills. However, the perfusion of the flap through microscopic connections only between the DSEA and DIEA results in reduced vascularity and an incidence of fat necrosis of up to 42%. A very large amount of muscle is sacrificed, causing a dramatic reduction in abdominal wall function,

a long recovery time, costal nerve compression and the subsequent complications of the use of mesh, which is usually required to repair the abdominal wall.[55,60,61] The development of reliable free tissue transfer techniques and the autologous LD flap have provided alternatives to the pedicled TRAM flap. The double pedicled flap should be avoided if possible.[62]

### Free TRAM flap

The deep inferior epigastric vessels are the dominant blood supply for a free TRAM flap. The lower abdominal skin is transferred with a segment of rectus abdominis muscle and the deep inferior epigastric vessels, which are anastomosed to the recipient vessels of the subscapular axis or the internal mammary system.[56] The donor site is closed most commonly by insertion of synthetic mesh. This technique provides better tissue perfusion than the pedicled TRAM flap and a larger portion of the abdominal apron can be transferred safely with reduced risks of partial flap necrosis or fat necrosis. This is more appropriate for the reconstruction of a larger breast. A smaller amount of rectus muscle is harvested, causing less interference with abdominal wall function. The free TRAM flap requires a high level of surgical expertise and microsurgical skills.

Free tissue transfer, although routine in many centres, is a major surgical procedure and requires 6–8 hours operating time, hospital stay of 7–10 days and postoperative recovery of 2–3 months. There is an increased risk of general complications, such as deep vein thrombosis, pneumonia or acute respiratory distress syndrome. Specific complications of free TRAM flaps are related to the flap or donor site. Flap-related problems include microsurgical problems with the anastomosis, haematoma, fat necrosis, partial or total flap loss and delayed wound healing. Success rates in many centres are around 98%. Donor-site complications include haematoma, wound infection, problems with mesh closure, asymmetry, bulging, hernia formation and reduced abdominal strength. Although the free flap is preferred to the pedicled variant due to its more reliable blood supply, it still causes some functional impairment of the abdominal wall.[61,63-66]

### Free DIEP flap

The free DIEP flap spares the whole of the rectus abdominis muscle. The flap relies on meticulous dissection of perforating vessels within the rectus abdominis muscle. This technique is particularly indicated for young athletic patients and when performing bilateral breast reconstruction.[57,58] The DIEP flap still has all the potential flap complications of any free tissue transfer but donor-site complications and morbidity are reduced.[61,67,68]

No muscle or fascia is harvested and no mesh is required for donor-site closure.

 Preservation of the rectus muscle preserves abdominal and back extensor muscle strength and reduces donor-site morbidity, postoperative pain and hospital stay. Preliminary studies have shown that this technique is as safe and reliable as the free TRAM flap. The vascularity of the transferred tissue is not compromised and the incidence of fat necrosis is no different from that of the standard free TRAM flap.[4,61,67-69] Disadvantages are increased operating time and an even higher level of surgical expertise requiring specialised training in dissection techniques (**Fig. 9.6**).

### Free SIEA flap

The free SIEA flap does not disturb the rectus abdominis or the abdominal fascia. It relies on a branch of the femoral artery, the SIEA and its vein, which supply the fat and skin of the lower abdomen.[70]

The advantages of this technique are that there is no damage to the muscular or aponeurotic part of the abdominal wall without any risk of postoperative weakness. This operation is also quicker, with an easier dissection of the vascular pedicle, and the postoperative morbidity is comparable to an abdominoplasty procedure. Unfortunately, this vessel is absent in one-third of patients or may have been damaged by previous surgery. The vascular pedicle is short, with a small diameter of 1.5–2 mm. This may result in decreased flap perfusion, with a higher risk of partial or total flap necrosis.[70-72]

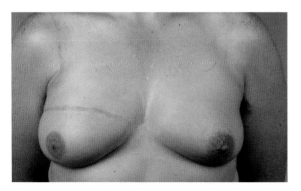

**Figure 9.6** • Delayed breast reconstruction with free DIEP flap.

## Alternative free flap donor sites for breast reconstruction

There are further types of free flap transfer for breast reconstruction. However, the expertise required for these is extremely demanding and the failure rates are potentially higher. They should be reserved for women in whom conventional techniques are deemed inappropriate.

Alternative options of autologous tissue breast reconstruction include the free superior and inferior gluteal flaps, which can be raised as perforator flaps as well. The transverse upper gracilis (TUG) flap uses a transverse skin ellipse from the upper thigh, which is usually discarded in a traditional thigh lift based on myocutaneous perforators through the gracilis flap; the lateral transverse thigh flap, using the so-called saddlebag area of the upper outer thigh; the Rubens peri-iliac fat pad flap; the anterolateral thigh flap; and the free LD flap from the contralateral side. These may be indicated if the lower abdomen or back have insufficient tissue, have already been used, cannot be used due to disruption of the vascular pedicles, or if the patient wants to avoid scars in more obvious parts of the body.[73–78]

# Finishing touches

Further surgery may be necessary to the reconstructed breast, the opposite breast or the donor site of the breast reconstruction. Complete breast reconstruction including nipple–areola reconstruction requires on average 3.3 separate procedures.[79]

## Surgery to the reconstructed breast

The reconstructed breast may require adjustment in size or shape by liposuction, excision of fat necrosis, mastopexy or augmentation. Lipomodelling transfers fat cells which have been harvested by liposuction into autologous breast reconstructions such as the autologous LD flap or the DIEP. This new technique is particularly useful for contour irregularities or generalised volume loss after adjuvant radiotherapy.[80] Further adjustments of the position of the breast on the chest wall, improvement of projection, adjustment of the inframammary fold, or revisional surgery for capsular contracture may be necessary.

## Surgery to the contralateral breast

There are two situations in which contralateral surgery needs to be considered. One is where it is necessary to operate in order to achieve symmetry. The other is where a woman, deemed at high risk of contralateral breast cancer after a formal assessment of genetic risk, wishes a risk-reducing mastectomy with reconstruction.[81]

## Surgery to the flap donor site

Scar revision, liposuction, treatment of persistent seroma, correction of dog ears or repair of an abdominal bulge or hernia may be necessary. Donor-site morbidity is becoming more and more appreciated. Permanent loss of function at the donor site is considered by many almost as serious as failure of the reconstruction itself.[4]

## Nipple–areola reconstruction

The final part of breast reconstruction is restoration of the nipple–areola complex.

 Some patients are happy with a prosthetic nipple but patients should have the opportunity to proceed to nipple–areola reconstruction. This leads to increased satisfaction with the breast reconstruction, a sense of completeness and an enhanced sense of attractiveness, especially unclothed.[82]

The two main options for nipple reconstruction are (i) composite grafts from the opposite breast, toe pulp, ear lobe or dog ears following previous surgery and (ii) local flaps, which have been described in a multitude of variations. Areola reconstruction can be performed by full-thickness skin grafting or by tattooing. Donor sites of skin grafts for areolar reconstruction are selected on the basis of pigmentation. Grafts can be obtained from the contralateral areola, the postauricular area, the upper inner thigh, the labia majora and scarred skin from the mastectomy or old abdominal scars. However, the colour match of these grafts with the contralateral areola may not be acceptable and further tattooing may be necessary. Nowadays skin grafting has been largely abandoned in favour of tattooing, which is a quick and simple technique with minimal morbidity and very few complications apart from colour mismatch. Improved colour match can be achieved by the use of a three-dimensional colour chart.[83,84]

# Salvage surgery

Salvage surgery may be required for complications of the reconstruction or for oncological reasons.

## Complications of breast reconstruction

Where there has been breast skin-flap loss, the situation can be redeemed by advancement of breast skin or flap and direct closure, split-thickness skin graft or LD flap salvage. Implant extrusion due to wound dehiscence may require either implant removal and later reinsertion or conversion to an LD flap. Partial flap loss can be treated with debridement and direct closure, split-thickness skin grafting, or a further flap procedure such as an LD flap or a thoraco-epigastric flap. Unexpected loss of volume in the reconstructed breast after radiotherapy or following atrophy of the muscle components in myocutaneous flaps can be corrected by augmentation or lipo-modelling of the reconstructed breast or additional surgery to the opposite breast in order to achieve symmetry. Complete flap loss can be dealt with by debridement of all necrotic tissues and direct closure or split-thickness skin graft without reconstruction. A further flap procedure or the insertion of tissue expander or implant as a space filler are indicated if the patient wishes a further attempt at breast reconstruction.[8,80]

## Local recurrence

Salvage surgery for chest wall recurrence often creates a surgical dilemma. Although the patient has recurrence, they may have significant life expectancy. These procedures can be difficult because they rely on poor-quality tissues and are often best dealt with in a multidisciplinary setting. The aims of surgery in this situation include local control of disease, palliation of symptoms and enhancement of the quality of remaining life. Resurfacing the chest wall with non-irradiated flap tissues may facilitate further radiotherapy or adjunctive treatment such as brachytherapy. Reconstruction of the resultant defect requires often extensive surgery in the form of local flaps or abdominal advancement, regional flaps such as LD, pectoralis major and parascapular flaps, omental transposition, pedicled or free abdominal flaps or even a combination of these techniques.[8,85–90]

# Summary

Immediate breast reconstruction after mastectomy for breast cancer has been accepted as safe and has no known oncological disadvantages. The ideal breast reconstruction is a soft natural-feeling breast that maintains its characteristics over time as a natural ptosis or droop and a permanent and natural inframammary fold.

It is important for any woman undergoing mastectomy to make an informed decision about reconstruction and to be provided with information about the techniques, advantages and disadvantages. There is a high degree of patient satisfaction with breast reconstruction but high levels of pre-operative information and psychological support are necessary.

Close collaboration between oncological and reconstructive surgeons or management by an oncoplastic surgeon, careful patient selection and counselling, and refinements in surgical techniques can provide a range of safe and predictable techniques for breast reconstruction.

## Key points

- Breast reconstruction plays a significant role in the woman's physical, emotional and psychological recovery from breast cancer.
- Even the best reconstruction will not be able to replace the natural breast that has been lost.
- Surgical options for reconstruction include the use of tissue expanders or breast implants and the use of autologous tissue.
- The most commonly used surgical techniques are tissue expansion, LD myocutaneous flap with or without implant, lower abdominal tissue and other free tissue transfers.

- Implant-based techniques require limited surgery initially but have limitations and are not always quick and trouble free. The quality of the long-term result is directly related to the tolerance of breast implants but is often disappointing unless performed after bilateral mastectomy.
- Further procedures are often required for complications and maintenance. Asymmetry may reoccur due to the effects of gravity on the contralateral breast and fluctuations in body weight.
- The aesthetic results from autologous reconstruction are superior to those of implant-based reconstruction due to their versatility, their more natural appearance, consistency and durability.
- Autologous tissue can better withstand radiotherapy.
- The autologous LD flap is highly versatile and has acceptable donor-site morbidity.
- The skin and fat of the lower abdomen are ideal for autologous breast reconstruction but donor-site morbidity is being increasingly appreciated. Muscle-sparing techniques preserve abdominal wall function at the cost of a more complex procedure.
- Further surgery may be necessary to the reconstructed breast, the opposite breast or the donor site of the breast reconstruction.
- Nipple–areola reconstruction leads to increased satisfaction with breast reconstruction.
- Salvage surgery may be required for complications of the reconstruction or for oncological reasons.
- It is important for any woman undergoing mastectomy to be able to make an informed decision about reconstruction, and information about different techniques, advantages and disadvantages should be freely available.
- Due to the variable needs of individual patients, the reconstructive surgeon must be able to provide the full range of reconstructive options.

# References

1. Schain WS. Breast reconstruction. Update of psychosocial and pragmatic concerns. Cancer 1991; 68(Suppl 5):1170–5.

2. Stevens LA, McGrath MH, Druss RG et al. The psychological impact of immediate breast reconstruction for women with early breast cancer. Plast Reconstr Surg 1984; 73:619–28.

3. Goin MK, Goin JM. Psychological reactions to prophylactic mastectomy synchronous with contralateral breast reconstruction. Plast Reconstr Surg 1982; 70:355–9.

4. Weiler-Mithoff EM. Breast reconstruction: techniques, timing and patient selection. CML Breast Cancer 2001; 13:1–11.

5. Handel N, Silverstein MJ, Waisman E et al. Reasons why mastectomy patients do not have breast reconstruction. Plast Reconstr Surg 1990; 86:1118–22.

6. Scottish Intercollegiate Guidelines Network, Scottish Cancer Therapy Network. Breast cancer in women. Edinburgh: Royal College of Physicians, 1998.

7. Harcourt DM, Rumsey NJ, Ambler NR et al. The psychological effect of mastectomy with or without breast reconstruction: a prospective, multicenter study. Plast Reconstr Surg 2003; 111:1060–8.

8. Baildam A, Bishop H, Boland G et al. Oncoplastic breast surgery – A guide to good practice. EJSO 2007; 33(Suppl):1–23.

9. Kroll SS, Ames F, Singletary SE et al. The oncologic risks of skin preservation at mastectomy when combined with immediate reconstruction of the breast. Surg Gynecol Obstet 1991; 172:17–20.

10. Toth BA, Lappert P. Modified skin incisions for mastectomy: the need for plastic surgical input in preoperative planning. Plast Reconstr Surg 1991; 87:1048–53.

11. Furey PC, Macgillivary DC, Gastiglione CL et al. Wound complications in patients receiving adjuvant chemotherapy after mastectomy and immediate breast reconstruction for breast cancer. J Surg Oncol 1994; 55:194–7.

12. Wilson CR, Brown IM, Weiler-Mithoff EM et al. Immediate breast reconstruction is not associated with a delay in the delivery of adjuvant chemotherapy. Eur J Surg Oncol 2004; 30:324–7.

   No statistically significant difference was found in the time between surgery and first dose of adjuvant chemotherapy in 285 patients undergoing wide local excision, simple mastectomy or mastectomy and immediate breast reconstruction with a variety of techniques.

13. Hussien M, Salah B, Malyon A et al. Impact of adjuvant radiotherapy on the choice of immediate breast reconstruction. Eur J Cancer 2000; 36(Suppl 5):58.

14. Von Smitten K, Sundell B. The impact of adjuvant radiotherapy and cytotoxic chemotherapy on the

outcome of immediate breast reconstruction by tissue expansion after mastectomy for breast cancer. Eur J Surg Oncol 1992; 18:119–23.

15. Malata CM, McIntosh SA, Prurushotham AD. Immediate breast reconstruction after mastectomy for cancer. Br J Surg 2000; 87:1455–72.

16. Rosenquist S, Sandelin K, Wickmann M. Patients' psychological and cosmetic experience after immediate breast reconstruction. Eur J Surg Oncol 1996; 22:262–6.

17. Petit JY, Le MG, Mouriesse H et al. Can breast reconstruction with gel-filled silicone implants increase the risk of death and second primary cancer in patients treated by mastectomy for breast cancer? Plast Reconstr Surg 1994; 94:115–19.

18. Noone RB, Frazier TG, Noone GC et al. Recurrence of breast carcinoma following immediate reconstruction: a 13-year review. Plast Reconstr Surg 1994; 93:90–106.

19. Townsend CM Jr., Abston S, Fish JC. Surgical adjuvant treatment of locally advanced breast cancer. Ann Surg 1985; 201:604–10.

20. Godfrey PM, Godfrey NV, Romita MC. Immediate autogenous breast reconstruction in clinically advanced disease. Plast Reconstr Surg 1995; 95:1039–44.

21. Eberlein TJ, Crespo LD, Smith BL et al. Prospective evaluation of immediate reconstruction after mastectomy. Ann Surg 1993; 218:29–36.

22. Hunt KK, Baldwin BJ, Strom EA et al. Feasibility of postmastectomy radiation therapy after TRAM flap breast reconstruction. Ann Surg Oncol 1997; 4:377–84.

23. Williams JK, Carlson GW, Bostwick J III et al. The effects of radiation treatment after TRAM flap breast reconstruction. Plast Reconstr Surg 1997; 100:1153–60.

24. Tran NV, Evans GRD, Kroll SS et al. Postoperative adjuvant irradiation: effects on transverse rectus abdominis muscle flap breast reconstruction. Plast Reconstr Surg 2000; 106:313–20.

25. Tran NV, Chang DW, Gupta A et al. Comparison of immediate and delayed free TRAM flap breast reconstruction in patients receiving postmastectomy radiation therapy. Plast Reconstr Surg 2001; 108:78–82.

26. Rodgers NE, Allen RJ. Radiation effects on breast reconstruction with the deep inferior epigastric perforator flap. Plast Reconstr Surg 2002; 109:1919–24.

27. Bostwick J III. Plastic and reconstructive breast surgery. St Louis: Quality Medical Publishing, 1990.

28. Radovan C. Breast reconstruction after mastectomy using the temporary expander. Plast Reconstr Surg 1982; 69:195–208.

29. Woods JE, Mangan MA. Breast reconstruction with tissue expanders: obtaining an optimal result. Ann Plast Surg 1992; 28:390–6.

30. Gabriel SE, Woods JE, O'Fallon WM et al. Complications leading to surgery after breast implantation. N Engl J Med 1997; 336:677–82.

31. Clough KB, O'Donoghue JM, Fitoussi AD et al. Prospective evaluation of late cosmetic results following breast reconstruction: implant reconstruction. Plast Reconstr Surg 2001; 107:1702–9.

Prospective evaluation of morbidity and cosmesis of 360 patients with unilateral implant reconstructions for 9 years showed a significant deterioration of long-term results despite a 92.5% rate of symmetry surgery.

32. Slavin SA, Colen SR. Sixty consecutive breast reconstructions with the inflatable expander: a critical appraisal. Plast Reconstr Surg 1990; 86:910–19.

33. Dickson MG, Sharpe DT. The complications of tissue expansion in breast reconstruction: a review of 75 cases. Br J Plast Surg 1987; 40:629–35.

34. Rosato RM, Dowden RV. Radiation therapy as a cause of capsular contracture. Ann Plast Surg 1994; 32:342–5.

35. McCraw JB, Papp CTh. Latissimus dorsi myocutaneous flap. In: Hartrampf CR (ed.) Breast reconstruction with living tissue. Norfolk, VA: Hampton Press, 1991; pp. 211–48.

36. Clough KB, Louis-Sylvestre C, Fitoussi A et al. Donor site sequelae after autologous breast reconstruction with an extended latissimus dorsi flap. Plast Reconstr Surg 2002; 109:1904–11.

37. Delay E, Gounot N, Bouillot A et al. Autologous latissimus breast reconstruction: a 3 year clinical experience with 100 patients. Plast Reconstr Surg 1998; 102:1461–78.

38. McCraw JB, Papp C, Edwards A et al. The autogenous latissimus breast reconstruction. Clin Plast Surg 1994; 21:279–88.

39. Germann G, Steinau HU. Breast reconstruction with the extended latissimus dorsi flap. Plast Reconstr Surg 1996; 97:519–26.

40. Fatah MFT. Extended latissimus dorsi flap in breast reconstruction. Operative Tech Plast Reconstr Surg 1999; 6:38–49.

41. Titley OG, Spyrou GE, Fatah MFT. Preventing seroma in the latissimus dorsi flap donor site. Br J Plast Surg 1997; 50:106–8.

42. Taghizadeh R, Shoaib T, Hart AM et al. Triamcinolone reduces seroma re-accumulation in the extended Latissimus dorsi donor site – a randomised controlled trial. J Plast Reconstr Aesthet Surg; http://www.jprasurg.com/article/PIIS1748681507001994/abstract?source=aemf

43. Kroll SS, Baldwin B. A comparison of outcomes using three different methods of breast reconstruction. Plast Reconstr Surg 1992; 90:455–62.

44. Roy MK, Shrotia S, Holcombe C et al. Complications of latissimus dorsi myocutaneous flap breast reconstruction. Eur J Surg Oncol 1998; 24:162–5.

45. Arnold PG, Lovic SF, Pairolero PC. Muscle flaps in irradiated wounds: an account of 100 consecutive cases. Plast Reconstr Surg 1994; 93:324–7.

46. Scott JR, Malyon A, Hussien M et al. Immediate breast reconstruction: the effect of adjuvant radiotherapy on latissimus dorsi flap reconstructions with and without implants. BAPS Summer Meeting, Stirling, 2001.

47. Brown IM, Hogg FJ, McKeown DJ et al. Long term aesthetic outcome of immediate breast reconstruction with the autologous Latissimus Dorsi flap. BAPS Summer Meeting, Dublin, 2004.

48. Gui GPH, Tan SM, Faliakou EC. Immediate breast reconstruction using biodimensional anatomical permanent expander implants: a prospective analysis of outcome and patient satisfaction. Plast Reconstr Surg 2003; 111:125–38.

49. Tarantino I, Banic A, Fisher T. Evaluation of late results in breast reconstruction by latissimus dorsi flap and prosthesis implantation. Plast Reconstr Surg 2006; 117:1387–94.

50. Report of the Independent Review Group. Silicone gel breast implants. London: HMSO, 1998.

51. Clough BC, O'Donoghue JM, Fitoussi AD et al. Prospective evaluation of late cosmetic results following breast reconstruction. II. TRAM flap reconstruction. Plast Reconstr Surg 2001; 107: 1710–16.

Prospective study of 171 TRAM flap patients for 8 years showed aesthetically pleasing long-term results in 94.2%.

52. Petit JY, Rietjens M, Ferreire MAR et al. Abdominal sequelae after pedicled TRAM flap breast reconstruction. Plast Reconstr Surg 1997; 99:723–9.

53. Hartrampf CR Jr. The transverse abdominal island flap for breast reconstruction. A 7-year experience. Clin Plast Surg 1988; 15:703.

54. Robbins TH. Rectus abdominis myocutaneous flap for breast reconstruction. Aust NZ J Surg 1979; 49:527–30.

55. Hartrampf CR. Breast reconstruction with a transverse abdominal island flap. Plast Reconstr Surg 1982; 69:216–24.

56. Holmstroem H. The free abdominoplasty flap and its use in breast reconstruction. Scand J Plast Reconstr Surg 1979; 13:423–6.

57. Koshima I, Soeda S. Inferior epigastric artery skin flaps without rectus abdominis muscle. Br J Plast Surg 1989; 42:645–8.

58. Allen RJ, Treece P. Deep inferior epigastric perforator flap for breast reconstruction. Ann Plast Surg 1994; 32:32–8.

59. Antia NH, Buch VI. Transfer of an abdominal dermo-fat graft by direct anastomosis of blood vessels. Br J Plast Surg 1971; 24:15–19.

60. Mitzgala CL, Hartrampf CR, Bennett GK. Abdominal wall function after pedicled TRAM flap surgery. Clin Plast Surg 1994; 21:255–72.

61. Futter CM. Abdominal donor site morbidity: impact of the TRAM and DIEP flap on strength and function. Adv Breast Reconstr, Semin Plast Surg 2002; 16:119–30.

62. Jensen JA Is the double pedicle TRAM flap reconstruction of a single breast within the standard of care?. Plast Reconstr Surg 1997; 100:1592–3.

63. Arnez ZM, Bajec J, Bardsley AF et al. Experience with 50 free TRAM flap breast reconstructions. Plast Reconstr Surg 1991; 87:470–8.

64. Schustermann MA, Kroll SS, Weldon ME. Immediate breast reconstruction: why the free TRAM over the conventional TRAM flap? Plast Reconstr Surg 1992; 90:255–61.

65. Grotting JC, Urist MM, Maddox WA et al. Conventional TRAM flap versus free microsurgical TRAM flap for immediate breast reconstruction. Plast Reconstr Surg 1989; 83:828–41.

66. Kroll SS, Schusterman MA, Reece GP et al. Abdominal wall strength, bulging and hernia after TRAM flap breast reconstruction. Plast Reconstr Surg 1995; 96:616–19.

67. Hamdi M, Weiler Mithoff EM, Webster MHC. Deep inferior epigastric perforator flap in breast reconstruction: experience with the first 50 flaps. Plast Reconstr Surg 1999; 103:86–95.

68. Futter CM, Webster MHC, Hagen S et al. A retrospective comparison of abdominal muscle strength following breast reconstruction with a free TRAM or DIEP flap. Br J Plast Surg 2000; 53:578 83.

69. Weiler-Mithoff E, Hodgson ELB, Malata CM. Perforator flap breast reconstruction. Breast Dis 2002; 16:93–106.

70. Stern HS, Nahai F. The versatile superficial inferior epigastric artery free flap. Br J Plast Surg 1992; 95:270–4.

71. Arnez ZM, Khan U, Pogorelec D et al. Breast reconstruction using the free superficial inferior epigastric artery (SIEA) flap. Br J Plast Surg 1999; 52:276–9.

72. Arnez ZM, Khan U, Pogorelec D et al. Rational selection of flaps from the abdomen in breast reconstruction to reduce donor site morbidity. Br J Plast Surg 1999; 52:351–4.

73. Shaw WW. Breast reconstruction by superior gluteal microvascular free flap without silicone implants. Plast Reconstr Surg 1983; 72:490–501.

74. Boustred AM, Nahai F. Inferior gluteal free flap breast reconstruction. Clin Plast Surg 1998; 25: 275–82.

75. Allen RJ, Tucker C Jr. Superior gluteal artery perforator free flap for breast reconstruction. Plast Reconstr Surg 1995; 95:1207–12.

76. Wechselberger G, Schoeller T. The transverse myo-cutaneous gracilis free flap: a valuable tissue source in autologous breast reconstruction. Plast Reconstr Surg 2004; 114:69–73.

77. Elliot LF. The lateral transverse thigh free flap for autogenous tissue breast reconstruction. Perspect Plast Surg 1989; 3:80–4.

78. Hartrampf CR, Elliot LF. Ruben's fat pad for breast reconstruction: a peri-iliac soft-tissue free flap. Plast Reconstr Surg 1994; 93:402–7.

79. Malyon AD, Husein M, Weiler-Mithoff EM. How many procedures to make a breast? Br J Plast Surg 2001; 54:227–31.

80. Delay E. Lipomodelling of the reconstructed breast. In: Spear S (ed.) Surgery of the breast: principles and art. Lippincott, Williams & Wilkins, 2006; pp. 930–46.

81. Sauven P. Guidelines for the management of women at increased familial risk of breast cancer. Eur J Cancer 2004; 40:653–65.

82. Wellisch DK, Schain WS, Noone RB et al. The psychological contribution of nipple addition in breast reconstruction. Plast Reconstr Surg 1987; 80:699–704.

83. Little JW. Nipple–areola reconstruction. In: Spear SL (ed.) Surgery of the breast: principles and art. Philadelphia: Lippincott-Raven, 1998; pp. 661–9.

84. Henseler H, Cheong V, Weiler-Mithoff EM et al. The use of Munsell colour charts in nipple areola tattooing. Br J Plast Surg 2001; 54:338–40.

85. Hathaway CL, Rand RP, Moe R et al. Salvage surgery for locally advanced and locally recurrent breast cancer. Arch Surg 1994; 129:582–7.

86. Burk RW III., Grotting JC. Conceptual considerations in breast reconstruction. Clin Plast Surg 1995; 22:141–52.

87. Sultan MR, Smith ML, Estabrook A et al. Immediate breast reconstruction in patients with locally advanced disease. Ann Plast Surg 1997; 38:345–9; discussion 350–1.

88. Rivas B, Carrillo JF, Escobar G. Reconstructive management of advanced breast cancer. Ann Plast Surg 2001; 47:234–9.

89. Brower ST, Weinberg H, Tartter PI et al. Chest wall resection for locally recurrent breast cancer: indications, technique, and results. J Surg Oncol 1992; 49:189–95.

90. Hasse J. Reconstruction of chest wall defects. Thorac Cardiovasc Surg 1991; 39(Suppl 3): 241–7.

# 10

# Breast cancer treatments of uncommon diseases

Tawakalitu Oseni
Monica Morrow

## Paget's disease

In 1874, Sir James Paget described the clinical entity now known as Paget's disease as 'an eczematous change in the skin of the nipple preceding an underlying mammary cancer'.[1] More than 95% of women with Paget's disease of the nipple have an underlying malignancy, although almost half are clinically and mammographically undetectable.

### Incidence

Paget's disease accounts for 0.7–4.9% of breast malignancies, and has also been reported in males.[2] Since reaching its peak incidence in 1985, the age-adjusted rates of female Paget's disease has decreased from 1.31 to 0.64 per 100 000.[3] The time from first symptoms to treatment is 10–12 months. Misdiagnosis as eczema and treatment with topical steroids is the most common reason for delay in diagnosis.[4,5]

### Pathology

There are two hypotheses regarding the development of Paget's disease of the nipple. The in situ transformation hypothesis suggests that Paget's cells arise from transformed malignant keratinocytes and that it is a type of in situ carcinoma of the skin.[2,4,6]

Consistent with this is that Paget's cells and the underlying cancer are often separated by some distance. The epidermotropic hypothesis of Paget's disease suggests that ductal cells migrate along the basement membrane of ducts into the nipple epidermis. Support for this comes from immunohistochemical studies that show similar staining patterns of Paget's cells and the underlying carcinoma.[7] Proponents of this hypothesis believe that carcinoma is present in 100% of women with pagetoid changes but that it is not always identified during pathological evaluation.

On histological examination, Paget's cells appear as large, round or ovoid intraepidermal cells with abundant clear pale cytoplasm and enlarged pleomorphic and hyperchromatic nuclei with prominent nucleoli. Reactive changes in the dermis, such as plasma cell infiltration, neovascularisation, serous exudate and hyperaemia, result in the characteristic appearance of the nipple in Paget's.[8] One study suggests that Paget's is found in association more often with high-grade ductal carcinoma in situ (DCIS) and high-grade invasive carcinomas than with lower-grade lesions.[1]

## Clinical presentation

Burning, itching and a change in sensation of the nipple and areola are the first symptoms of Paget's disease. This is followed by the development of skin lesions that may be raised and irregular and have a sharp demarcation from the surrounding skin. The nipple may appear erythematous and scaling may be visible. Nipple deformity or retraction may be present if there is tethering from an underlying malignancy, but is not a classic sign. Characteristically, Paget's begins on the nipple and spreads to the areola and subsequently to the surrounding skin. Later stages of Paget's may result in ulceration, bleeding and destruction of the nipple–areola complex (**Fig. 10.1**). Nipple discharge has also been reported in association with Paget's disease but is not common, and bleeding is usually due to ulceration of the nipple epithelium rather than discharge from the underlying ducts.

The differential diagnosis of Paget's disease is chronic eczema, benign papilloma of the nipple, basal cell carcinoma, malignant melanoma and Bowen's disease. Paget's disease can present in association with an underlying mass or calcifications. It can also present as an abnormality of the nipple–areola complex alone or it can be subclinical (reported as a histological finding after a mastectomy for DCIS or invasive cancer). Approximately half of patients with the characteristic nipple changes will have an underlying palpable abnormality at presentation.[9]

## Diagnosis

A full-thickness biopsy of the nipple should be performed to confirm diagnosis. This can be done with a punch biopsy. Exfoliative cytology or incisional biopsy may be done if a punch biopsy is not available. Immunohistochemistry is helpful in differen-

tiating Paget's disease from other nipple pathology. Paget's cells stain positive for CK7, CAM-5.2, AE1/AE3 and S100 but do not express HMB-45 and high-molecular-weight keratins, which helps differentiate them from melanomas.[10–12] As in all patients with breast cancer, bilateral diagnostic mammography is recommended for revealing multicentric disease, suspicious microcalcifications and non-palpable masses, as well as for assessing the contralateral breast. Ultrasound may be useful if mammography is unable to detect an underlying mass. Magnetic resonance imaging (MRI) is a promising method for evaluating patients with Paget's disease due to its high sensitivity in detecting occult malignancy.[13] Currently, there are multiple case reports in the literature documenting the use of MRI in the diagnosis Paget's disease, most in cases where no abnormality could be detected on mammography.[14,15] Because of its greater sensitivity, MRI has the potential to play a significant role in planning surgical therapy.

## Treatment

Treatment of Paget's disease should always include excision of the nipple–areola complex. If a tumour is evident in the periphery of the breast, either clinically or mammographically, mastectomy is the preferred treatment. Some have advocated mastectomy as the procedure of choice in all cases due to the frequent finding of multicentric disease in association with Paget's disease of the nipple. Kothari et al.[4] reported 67 patients with Paget's disease treated by mastectomy. In addition to disease in the central part of the breast, 75% had a malignancy in another quadrant.

However, multiple small studies of breast-conserving therapy in Paget's disease indicate low rates of local recurrence after treatment with excision and irradiation. These are summarised in Table 10.1.[5,16–21] A prospective study of 61 patients with Paget's with no clinically identifiable disease and centrally located DCIS treated with excision of the nipple–areola complex to negative margins, removal of a cone of underlying breast tissue and 50 Gy of irradiation reported a local recurrence rate of 5.2% after a median follow-up of 6.4 years.[17]

Attempts to treat Paget's disease with excision without irradiation have been less successful. Dixon et al.[5] and Polgar et al.[22] reported

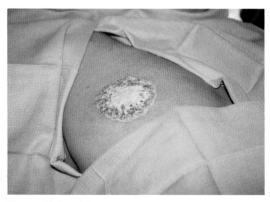

**Figure 10.1** • Advanced changes of Paget's disease with destruction of the nipple and areola and involvement of periareolar skin.

**Table 10.1** • Conservative management of Paget's disease of the nipple

| Reference | Year | n | Median follow-up (months) | Radiation | Recurrence (%) | No. of local recurrences | No. of distant recurrences | No. of deaths |
|---|---|---|---|---|---|---|---|---|
| Kawase et al.[21] | 2005 | 12 | 84 | Yes | 8 | 1 | 0 | 0 |
| Marshall et al.[16] | 2003 | 36 | 113 | Yes | 11 | 4 | 0 | 0 |
| Bijker et al.[17] | 2001 | 61 | 77 | Yes | 5.2 | 4 | 2 | 1 |
| Fu et al.[18] | 2001 | 12 | 42 | No | 25 | 3 | 0 | 0 |
| Kollmorgen et al.[19] | 1998 | 10 | 71 | No | 20 | 0 | 2 | 2 |
| Dixon et al.[5] | 1991 | 10 | 56 | No | 40 | 4 | 0 | 0 |
| Fourquet et al.[20] | 1987 | 20 | 90 | Yes | 6.7 | 3 | 0 | 0 |

recurrence rates of 40% and 33% after excision alone in patients with or without clinical evidence of malignancy in the underlying breast tissue. Similarly, attempts to preserve clinically uninvolved areas of the nipple–areola complex have also resulted in high rates of local recurrence.[18] Overall, at present in the USA breast conservation therapy for the treatment of Paget's disease may be underutilised.[3]

Sentinel lymph node biopsy (SLNB) has become the standard of care in staging the axilla in patients with invasive cancer. In patients with coexisting invasive cancer, axillary staging by SLNB should be undertaken. The prognosis of Paget's disease is determined by the stage of the coexisting carcinoma. Recent studies have shown an 11% incidence of positive lymph nodes when an SLNB is performed in patients identified as having Paget's disease with coexisting invasive carcinoma.[23,24] Sentinel lymph node biopsy should also be undertaken in patients who are undergoing a mastectomy whether or not a preoperative diagnosis of invasive cancer has been made. Guidelines for systemic therapy are the same as those used in women without Paget's disease of the nipple.

# Pregnancy-associated breast cancer

The term 'pregnancy-associated breast cancer' (PABC) includes breast cancer diagnosed during pregnancy, up to 1 year after delivery or at any time while the patient is lactating. Breast cancer is the second most common malignancy in pregnant women after cervical cancer.[25] There is often a delay in diagnosis due to anatomical and physiological changes in the breast and a low index of suspicion of malignancy.

## Epidemiology

The average age of patients with PABC is 32–38 years.[26] The estimated incidence of PABC is 0.2–3.8% of all breast cancers and PABC is reported to occur in 1 in 10 000 to 1 in 3000 pregnancies.[27] The incidence of PABC is expected to increase with the increasing delayed child bearing among women today. PABC is diagnosed at later stages than breast cancer in non-pregnant women of the same age. It is unknown if this is due to a more aggressive biology of PABC or because of a delay in diagnosis.[28]

## Aetiology/risk factors

A case–control study in Japan of 383 patients found that those with PABC were three times more likely than age-matched, non-pregnant, non-lactating women with breast cancer to have a family history of breast cancer.[29] In general, young age of first full-term pregnancy and multiparity are associated with a decrease in the risk of breast cancer. The opposite appears to be true for women who carry the BRCA1/BRCA2 germ-line mutation. Carriers of the BRCA1 or BRCA2 mutation who had a full-term pregnancy were significantly more likely than nulliparous women with the BRCA1 or BRCA2 mutation to develop breast cancer before the age of 40.[30] This may be due to an increased sensitivity of the breast epithelium to estrogen and progesterone in gene carriers.[30]

In general, the infrequent occurrence of PABC has prevented a detailed assessment of the risk factors that differentiate it from breast cancer in general.

## Clinical presentation

The most common presentation of PABC is a painless mass. During pregnancy, levels of estrogen, progesterone, prolactin and chorionic gonadotrophin rise. The breasts undergo marked ductal and lobular proliferation. Mammary blood flow increases by 180% and the weight of the breast can double.[31] Clinical breast examination can be difficult because of the increased nodularity of the breast. Because of these physiological changes and a reluctance to investigate masses discovered during pregnancy, PABC tends to be diagnosed at a more advanced stage and consequently is associated with a worse prognosis. A study of 63 women with PABC indicated that fewer than 20% were diagnosed prior to delivery and the median size of the cancer at diagnosis was 3.5 cm. In the same study, 62% of patients with PABC had lymph node metastasis compared with 39% of matched non-pregnant controls.[27] Additionally, patients with PABC are more likely to have larger tumours, vascular invasion and distant metastasis.[32] It is not known whether these findings are due to a different biology of PABC or because of delay in diagnosis.

## Differential diagnoses

Of breast biopsies performed during pregnancy, 70–80% are benign.[28] The differential diagnosis of a breast mass in pregnancy includes lactating adenoma, fibroadenoma, cystic disease, lobular hyperplasia, galactocele, abscess, lipoma and hamartoma. Rarely, other malignancies present in the breast during pregnancy. A mass in a pregnant woman should be investigated by imaging and biopsy if it has the characteristics of a dominant breast mass. If, clinically, a mass cannot be distinguished from the nodularity of pregnancy, ultrasound is useful in excluding the presence of a suspicious lesion. In women felt to have prominent areas of nodularity, a short-interval follow-up examination in 3–4 weeks is appropriate.

## Diagnostic techniques

Mammography is not routinely used to screen the pregnant woman. In contrast, diagnostic mammography is useful for evaluating masses during pregnancy and can be performed safely with the use of abdominal shielding. Mammography was able to detect 78–88% of palpable breast cancers in reports of 21 and 22 cases respectively.[33,34] A recent retrospective review by Yang and colleagues reiterates the efficacy of mammography in evaluating breast masses in pregnancy. This study showed a 90% sensitivity in detecting suspicious features on a mammogram on preoperative evaluation.[35] Ultrasound is also a safe imaging tool in pregnancy and can reliably identify cystic lesions and help to characterise solid masses. However, dominant solid masses require histological confirmation that they are benign before the decision is made to observe them.[31] As in the non-pregnant patient, core needle biopsy is the preferred method of diagnosis. A study of 331 pregnant women showed that fine-needle aspiration (FNA) is accurate in pregnancy. The increased proliferation of the breast epithelium in pregnancy may result in false-positive cytological diagnosis of carcinoma or atypia unless the cytopathologist is specifically informed of the patient's pregnancy. In addition, benign lesions such as fibroadenomas can increase in size during pregnancy. A specific histological diagnosis by core biopsy will allow continued observation of these lesions, while an increase in size of a lesion diagnosed as 'benign' by FNA is usually an indication for surgical excision. For these reasons, core biopsy is the diagnostic technique of choice in pregnancy. However, there have been case reports of milk fistula formation after core biopsy and this technique should be used with caution for centrally located lesions in lactating women.[36] If FNA and core biopsy are not diagnostic, excisional biopsy should be performed. Breast-feeding should be stopped before biopsy in order to reduce the risk of milk fistula formation. In general, guidelines for the diagnosis of a dominant breast mass in the pregnant woman are the same as those in the non-pregnant woman.

The need for a metastatic work-up should be guided by symptoms and the clinical stage of the cancer, as in non-pregnant patients. Chest radiography can be done safely with abdominal shielding. Bone scans have been performed in pregnant women using lower doses of radioisotope, but their use is generally not recommended during pregnancy.[37] This recommendation was reiterated recently in the international recommendations from an expert meeting regarding breast carcinoma in pregnancy.[38] MRI is promising for use in pregnancy to evaluate liver and bony metastasis, since it does not involve ionising radiation. MRI has also been used for fetal imaging in utero with no untoward effects reported.[39] Gadolinium has been documented to cross the placenta with adverse effects on fetal development in rats. As such, contrast MRI is not recommended in the staging work-up.[38,40] Computed tomography (CT) scans are generally discouraged due to the high radiation exposure. No studies have examined the use of positron emission tomography (PET) during pregnancy.

## Pathology

PABC is histologically similar to carcinoma in non-pregnant patients. PABC tends to be negative for both estrogen receptor and progesterone receptor.[32,40] Conflicting data exist on overexpression of erbB-2 or HER-2/neu in PABC. Tumours associated with PABC are reported to have a high positivity for Ki67 and p53, although the significance of these findings is uncertain.[41]

## Prognosis

Early studies reported a dismal prognosis for PABC. Recent studies indicate a similar prognosis for patients with stage I and II PABC compared with non-pregnant matched controls; however, there appears to be trend towards a worse prognosis in stage III and IV PABC.[27,42] In a study by Petrek et al.,[27] patients with PABC who had negative lymph node involvement had the same 5-year survival as non-pregnant controls. However, the survival of those patients with PABC with positive lymph nodes was 47% vs. 59% in the non-pregnant controls. This may reflect differences in tumour biology or delays in therapy due to concerns about fetal safety. However, some studies suggest that pregnancy is an independent poor prognostic factor.[42,43] Additionally, there appears to be an increased relative risk of dying from breast cancer if it develops within 4 years after giving birth compared with women, matched for age and stage, who have never been pregnant and who develop breast cancer.[32]

## Treatment of the primary tumour

### Local therapy of clinical stage I and II PABC

Treatment should not be delayed because of pregnancy. The risk of spontaneous abortion is highest in the first trimester of the pregnancy and the patient and surgeon may choose to defer surgery until after the 12th week.[44] The approach should involve a multidisciplinary team that includes the surgeon, medical oncologist and high-risk obstetrician. Surgery can be safely performed during all trimesters of pregnancy. Duncan et al.[45] found no increase in congenital anomalies in 2565 pregnant women who underwent surgery compared with pregnant controls who did not have surgery. When planning surgery, the surgical team must be aware of the physiological changes associated with pregnancy, including increased cardiac output, increased blood volume, decreased systemic vascular resistance, hypercoagulable state, delayed gastric emptying and a physiological dilutional anaemia that decreases oxygen-carrying capacity.[45] Additionally, a pillow should be placed on the right side of the patient to relieve pressure on the inferior vena cava. The fetus should be monitored closely during and after surgery.

The type of surgery should be tailored to the gestational age of the fetus and breast cancer stage of the mother. Breast-conserving therapy is generally not recommended in the first trimester of pregnancy because of the need to delay radiotherapy until after delivery, with the potential for increased risk of local recurrence. However, for the patient who receives adjuvant chemotherapy this delay is no longer than that seen in the non-pregnant patient. The effects of increased vascularity of the breast and hormonal changes of pregnancy on local recurrence rates are unknown. The decision to undertake breast-conserving therapy in the pregnant woman is much more complex than in the non-pregnant woman and requires a detailed assessment of the individual tumour characteristics and a frank discussion of the uncertainties associated with this approach. Mastectomy can be performed safely during any trimester of pregnancy, although immediate breast reconstruction is not usually recommended due to the increased operating time and the difficulty in achieving symmetry with the contralateral breast as it continues to change as pregnancy advances.

In the past SLNB has not been recommended in the pregnant or lactating woman. Lymphazurin blue or patent blue V, the dyes most commonly used to localise the sentinel node, have not been studied in pregnant women and therefore their safety has not been established. Technetium-99m, the radioactive tracer commonly used to localise sentinel nodes, results in low doses of radiation (1.85–3.7 MBq) to the breast. Some have advocated its use for SLNB during pregnancy but it is not standard practice and no studies have been conducted to examine the long-term adverse effects on the fetus.[46] Recent studies have shown the exposure to radiation sustained by the fetus to be very small.[47] Keleher and colleagues[48] have estimated the maximum dose absorbed by the fetus in two non-pregnant patients undergoing breast lymphoscintigraphy to be 4.3 mGy. These recent studies have led some to recommend offering SLNB to pregnant patients after extensive counselling on the risks and benefits.[38] However, axillary dissection remains the standard approach in pregnant women with invasive breast cancer.

### Systemic therapy

Chemotherapy is contraindicated in the first trimester of pregnancy. First-trimester exposure to chemotherapy results in a 14–19% risk of fetal malformation,[49] which falls to 1.3% with exposure in the second trimester. Spontaneous abortion has also been reported after first-trimester exposure.[49]

Berry et al.[50] conducted a prospective cohort study of 24 women who received 5-fluorouracil, doxorubicin and cyclophosphamide during the second and third trimesters of pregnancy and found no congenital malformations or postpartum complications in the infants. Hahn et al. recently expanded this study and longer-term follow-up still shows no stillbirths, miscarriages or deaths relating to therapy.[51] Long-term follow-up is still needed to monitor the occurrence of late adverse effects in these children, including the risk of cancer development. In general, methotrexate should be avoided during pregnancy due to a high reported risk of associated abnormalities. Because of limited experience with taxanes during pregnancy their use is not recommended, although cases of normal neonates after taxane exposure during pregnancy have been reported.[52,53] A recent review examined the use of taxanes, vinorelbine and anti-HER-2 agents in PABC.[54] There were no grade 3 or 4 toxicities reported; however, the use of trastuzumab was associated with anhydramnios in 3 of 6 cases.

Chemotherapy should be stopped 3 weeks before delivery to avoid myelosuppression and septic complications in the mother and the newborn infant.[41]

Endocrine therapy is not recommended during pregnancy. Tamoxifen is known to cause spontaneous abortions, birth defects and fetal demise.[55]

The risk–benefit ratio for chemotherapy is shifted during pregnancy because of the potential for fetal injury. While each woman must make an individual decision about the level of risk that is acceptable to her, some general guidelines can be employed. Women with positive lymph nodes should receive chemotherapy after the first trimester of pregnancy. Since adjuvant studies have suggested that chemotherapy is effective if administered within 6 weeks of surgery, short delays to allow treatment to start after delivery are appropriate. For the low-risk node-negative woman, where the survival benefit of chemotherapy is 5% or less, treatment during pregnancy is usually avoided. For the node-negative woman with larger high-grade cancer with unfavourable prognostic features, treatment decisions must be made on an individual basis.

### Locally advanced breast cancer and inflammatory cancer

In women who present with advanced breast cancer during early pregnancy, the need for prompt treatment must be balanced against the risk to the fetus. Termination of pregnancy should be discussed in this circumstance, although it is not an option all women will choose. It is essential that there is a frank discussion with the patient of not only the potential toxicity of chemotherapy to the fetus, but also the risk of death both with and without prompt therapy. After the first trimester, chemotherapy can be administered as discussed above. Surgery as an initial approach to inflammatory cancer should be avoided. **Figure 10.2** is a summary of the management strategy for PABC.

## Termination of pregnancy

In the past, the prognosis of PABC was considered so dismal that therapeutic abortion was advocated in all women. Comparisons of survival in women opting to continue pregnancy and those undergoing abortion do not suggest a survival advantage for abortion.[27,40] Currently, there are no formal recommendations for therapeutic abortion in women with PABC. However, therapeutic abortion can simplify treatment in patients

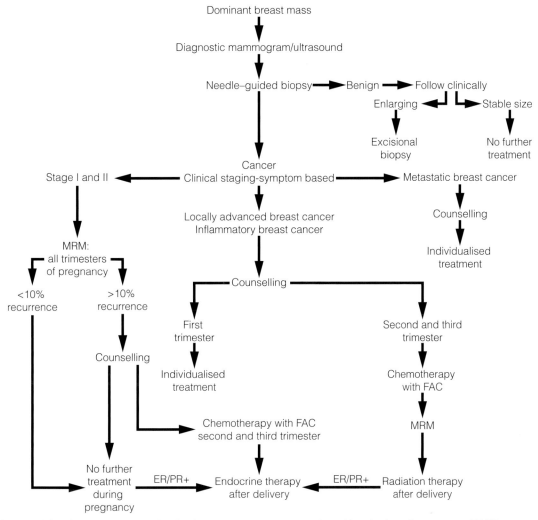

**Figure 10.2** • Management algorithm for the pregnant woman presenting with a dominant breast mass. ER/PR+, estrogen and progesterone receptor positive; FAC, fluorouracil, doxorubicin and cyclophosphamide; MRM, magnetic resonance mammography.

with advanced disease. A detailed discussion about treatment options and the potential risks to the fetus should be undertaken with the patient. Additionally, the patient and family should be informed of the risk of recurrence, overall survival and risk of infertility due to therapy when making a decision regarding termination of pregnancy.

## Pregnancy after breast cancer

Pregnancy after breast cancer appears to be safe. Retrospective studies indicate an equivalent or better survival in patients treated for breast cancer who subsequently become pregnant, although this may be due to selection bias.[27] There is no absolute time interval that is known to be safe for becoming pregnant after a diagnosis of breast cancer. Some advocate waiting 2 years after treatment of PABC for women with low-risk tumours, with a longer waiting period for those with high-risk tumours.[41] However, since the rate of relapse is fairly constant for the first 10 years after breast cancer diagnosis, the rationale for these recommendations is unclear. Ives and colleagues, in their retrospective review of PABC in women in Western Australia, found that for women with localised disease and good prognosis conception 6 months after treatment was unlikely to reduce survival.[56] The ability of the breast cancer survivor to delay pregnancy is often limited by older age and concerns about decreased fertility related to treatment.

# Other breast malignancies

## Primary breast lymphomas

Primary breast lymphoma (PBL) arises from lymphoid tissue in the breast and is defined as lymphoma localised to the breast and its draining lymph node basins.[57] The incidence of PBL is 0.14% of all breast malignancies and 0.65–2% of all non-Hodgkin's lymphomas.[57,58] The most common subtype is diffuse large B-cell lymphoma.[57] The mean age of onset is 65 years. PBL most often presents as a painless, enlarging, rubbery mass. Mammographic and ultrasound findings tend to be non-specific (**Fig. 10.3**). PBLs are categorised using the Working Classification and the Ann Arbor Classification of lymphomas. The international prognostic index is also helpful in predicting aggressiveness of disease.

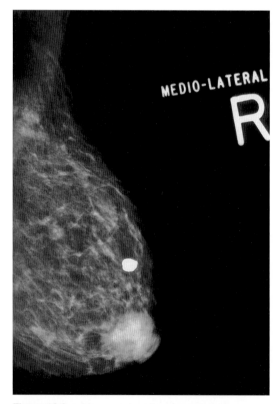

**Figure 10.3** • Mammogram of a primary breast lymphoma in the subareolar space. The appearance is indistinguishable from that of a primary adenocarcinoma.

PBL is usually not suspected in the absence of constitutional symptoms until a core biopsy is obtained. Once the diagnosis is known, a complete history and physical examination should be done, focusing on the presence of constitutional symptoms and evaluation of the lymph node basins. Additionally, CT of the chest, abdomen and pelvis and a bone marrow biopsy are needed to adequately stage the patient. Immunohistochemical studies of PBL have shown that lymphomas co-expressing bcl-6 and CD-10 have a better prognosis.[59] Single-institution reports have indicated that surgery alone or surgery with radiation results in a high incidence of local and disseminated recurrence, and surgery is no longer recommended as a treatment for PBL.[57] The only role of surgery is in obtaining tissue for diagnosis if core biopsy is inadequate. Treatment of PBL consists of chemotherapy with agents appropriate for the histological type of lymphoma followed by appropriately targeted radiation. The 2-year overall survival is 63%, which is comparable to similar lymphomas elsewhere in the body.[57]

## Angiosarcomas of the breast

Although rare, angiosarcoma of the breast is an important clinical entity. Secondary angiosarcoma of the breast is distinguished from primary angiosarcoma by its association with a number of presumed aetiological factors, most commonly radiation and long-standing lymphoedema. The first case of angiosarcoma following radiation to the breast was reported in 1981.[60] The incidence of this problem may be increasing due to the increase in the number of women receiving radiation therapy following breast-conserving surgery. Approximately 100 cases have been reported to date.[61,62] The average time from radiation therapy to diagnosis is 75 months.[61] For an angiosarcoma to be considered radiation induced, it must occur within the radiated field and have a long latency period.

Post-radiation sarcoma usually presents in a multifocal pattern with painless skin nodules. The nodules may be violet, blue, black or red (**Fig. 10.4**). The differential diagnosis includes adenocarcinoma of the breast, radiation-related skin changes and melanoma.[63] The diagnosis is made by full-thickness punch biopsy or incisional or excisional biopsy. FNA is not recommended and mammography and ultrasound are generally not helpful. Molecular markers such as factor VIII-related

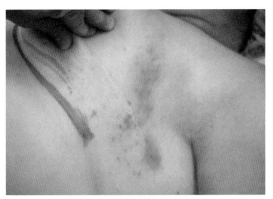

**Figure 10.4** • Appearance of a radiation-induced angiosarcoma on the lateral aspect of a breast treated for adenocarcinoma with lumpectomy and radiotherapy. Multiple reddish-brown cutaneous nodules are visible.

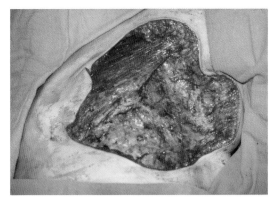

**Figure 10.5** • Extent of resection necessary to obtain negative margins in the patient illustrated in Fig. 10.4.

antigen and CD-34 are positive in most angiosarcomas and can help to distinguish angiosarcomas from other sarcomas.[62] Staging of angiosarcoma follows the guidelines for other sarcomas, where staging is based on size, grade and depth of the tumour. As in other sarcomas, grade is the most important determinant of prognosis. Most radiation-induced angiosarcomas are high grade. Treatment consists of mastectomy with wide resection of the skin of the breast. The microscopic extent of cutaneous angiosarcoma is often greater than clinically evident, so efforts should be made to achieve widely negative skin margins (**Fig. 10.5**). Axillary staging is not recommended since most sarcomas do not metastasise to regional lymph nodes. The recurrence rate is approximately 40% and the prognosis is poor. In a study of 58 patients, almost half had died at an average follow-up period of 15 months.[61] A more recent study of 69 patients revealed an overall 5-year survival of 61%, and a recurrence rate of 55% at a median follow-up of 40 months.[64] Adjuvant treatment follows recommendations for other sarcomas, but individual reports do not indicate a clear benefit. In certain patients adjuvant radiation may be considered given recent case reports of benefit with adjuvant radiotherapy after surgery.[58,64]

## Melanoma of the breast

Primary cutaneous melanoma of the skin of the breast is extremely rare; only 0.28% of all melanomas are reported to occur in this site.[65] Melanoma is more commonly found in the breast as a result of distant metastasis from a primary elsewhere in the body.[66] A history focusing on risk factors for developing melanoma as well as change in the appearance of the lesion should be obtained. Physical examination for the presence of other melanomas and lymphadenopathy should also be performed.

Mammography and ultrasound are generally not helpful in diagnosis and therapeutic planning. Core biopsy or surgical biopsy of the thickest portion of the melanoma should be performed to determine the depth of invasion of the melanoma. Staging follows the American Joint Committee on Cancer (AJCC) or International Union Against Cancer (UICC) guidelines.[67] Immunohistochemistry for HMB-45 and S100 can help differentiate melanoma from other cutaneous lesions.

All patients should undergo measurement of lactate dehydrogenase, and staging with CT or PET is indicated for patients with thick melanomas. Primary treatment for cutaneous melanoma is surgical excision. In the past, mastectomy was the recommended treatment but this is no longer considered necessary. Wide local excision of the lesion is recommended, with margins depending on the depth of invasion. SLNB for intermediate-thickness melanomas and thin melanomas with poor prognostic characteristics should also be done at the time of excision and completion axillary dissection carried out if the sentinel lymph nodes contain metastases.[68] Lymphoscintigraphy should be performed prior to SLNB. Adjuvant treatment for primary melanoma of the breast follows current guidelines for treatment of melanoma found elsewhere in the body.

## Metastasis to the breast

Metastatic disease to the breast is uncommon, with an incidence of 0.5–6.6% of breast malignancies.[69,70] The contralateral breast is the most common site of metastatic malignancy found in the breast.[70] Other common malignancies that metastasise to the breast are lymphoma, melanoma, rhabdomyosarcoma and small cell lung cancer.[66] Physical examination and imaging studies demonstrate masses that are usually indistinguishable from primary breast carcinoma. In most cases, core biopsy is preferred to FNA for pathological diagnosis since molecular studies and immunohistochemistry may play an important role in differentiating primary and metastatic tumours. Treatment is directed at the primary malignancy. Prognosis is poor, with 80% of patients dying within 1 year.[66]

# Male breast cancer

## Epidemiology

The British physician John of Arderne reported the first case of male breast cancer (MBC) in the 14th century. MBC accounts for 1% or less of all breast cancers in Western countries and only 0.1% of male cancer deaths.[71] The prevalence of MBC increases with age. The average age of diagnosis is about 10 years later than in women, but MBC can occur at any age. The incidence has remained stable over the past 40 years.[72] However, this may change given that a recent evaluation of the Surveillance Epidemiology and End Results (SEER) database between 1973 and 2001 revealed an increased incidence of in situ carcinoma in men.[73] The average delay from onset of symptoms to diagnosis is 22 months.[74]

## Risk factors

Alterations in estrogen and testosterone balance appear to play a role in the aetiology of MBCs. An elevated risk of developing MBC has been documented in men with a history of undescended testes, congenital inguinal hernia, orchiectomy, orchitis, testicular injury or infertility.[75,76] Males with Klinefelter's syndrome, which is characterised by gynaecomastia, small firm testes and a 47XXY karyotype, have a 50-fold increased risk of developing breast cancer.[77] Obesity and cirrhosis, which cause a hyperestrogenic state, are also linked to an

elevated risk of developing MBC.[76] Gynaecomastia, once thought to be a risk factor, is now no longer believed to increase the risk of developing MBC.[74,76] Other risk factors include a history of radiation exposure, as in female breast cancer.[76]

Family history is an important risk factor. Between 15% and 20% of male patients with breast cancer have a family history of the disease. The odds ratio for MBC increases with a positive family history and the risk increases as the number of affected first-degree relatives increases and as the age of diagnosis in affected relatives decreases. These factors probably reflect an increasing risk of both BRCA1 and BRCA2 mutations. Inherited mutations such as BRCA1 and BRCA2 predispose men to developing breast cancer. Male carriers of BRCA2 have a 6.3% cumulative risk of developing breast cancer.[78,79] In families with hereditary breast cancer, the presence of MBC increases the likelihood of having a BRCA2 mutation. The number of MBCs attributable to BRCA2 varies among populations and is 4% in the USA. However, in Iceland, the 'founder effect' BRCA2 mutation is present in 40% of MBCs.[79,80] More recent studies suggest that the risk of MBC is roughly equivalent in those with either BRCA1 or BRCA2 mutations.[81]

## Clinical presentation

Of men with MBC, 85% present with a painless mass.[82] Nipple retraction, nipple ulceration, nipple discharge and pain are other presenting signs and symptoms, and 40–50% of men have nipple involvement due to the central location of most tumours.[83] The time from the onset of symptoms to diagnosis is longer in men and, as a result, men often present at later stages.

## Differential diagnosis

Gynaecomastia, abscess, metastatic disease and sarcomas are the main conditions that should be excluded when diagnosing a breast mass in males. Physical examination and FNA or core biopsy are the most useful methods for differentiating MBC from other causes of breast masses in men.

## Diagnosis

The work-up of a breast mass is similar in men and women, although imaging studies are less important in men. Physical examination characterises the size, shape and location of the mass, as well as the presence of nipple discharge, nipple retraction and skin changes. Examination of the axillary, supraclavicular and infraclavicular nodes should also be performed. A diagnostic mammogram and/or focused ultrasound can be used to characterise the lesion, but rarely obviates the need for a histological diagnosis. Since treatment is usually by mastectomy, imaging studies can often be omitted. As in women, diagnosis by needle biopsy, either core biopsy or FNA, is preferred to excisional biopsy. Symptoms and abnormal laboratory values should guide the need for a metastatic work-up.

## Pathology

Almost all pathological types of breast cancer found in women have been described in men. Most MBCs (90%) are invasive and, of these, 80% are infiltrating ductal carcinoma and 5% are papillary.[84] Invasive lobular carcinoma represents only 1% of MBCs, probably due to the paucity of terminal lobules in the male breast. Paget's disease and inflammatory breast cancer are seen with similar frequency in men and women. Less common subtypes such as medullary, tubular, mucinous and squamous carcinomas have also been reported in men, but are found with lower frequencies than seen in women. Of the 10% of MBCs that are non-invasive, almost all are DCIS.[84] Most are of the papillary subtype and are of low or intermediate grade.[85] Lobular carcinoma in situ is rare; when found, it is usually in conjunction with invasive lobular carcinoma.[83]

MBCs have a higher rate of estrogen receptor positivity than that in women when matched for age, stage and grade. Approximately 80% of MBCs are estrogen receptor positive and 75% are progesterone receptor positive.[74] Retrospective study by these same authors and a review of the SEER database over a 25-year period which included 2357 male breast cancers revealed an even greater incidence of estrogen receptor and progesterone receptor positivity, 90% and 80% respectively when compared to 76% and 67% in women.[86] There is limited information about erbB-2 or HER-2/neu overexpression in MBC, and its impact on prognosis is unclear. The initial study by Giordano and colleagues reported greater expression of HER-2, p53 and bcl-2 in male breast cancers when compared to female breast

cancers.[74] Other studies show conflicting results, with some showing less overexpression of HER-2[87] and others showing more.[88] Data on other molecular markers found in female breast cancers, such as p53, bcl-2, cyclin D1 and epidermal growth factor receptor, are limited and their association with prognosis in MBC is inconclusive at this time.[89]

## Prognosis

MBC is staged according to the AJCC or UICC staging system. As with female breast cancer, axillary lymph node status, tumour size, histological grade and hormone receptor status are significant prognostic factors in MBC.[74,90,91]

As in women, axillary lymph node status is the most important prognostic factor in MBC.[91] In one study of 335 cases, node-negative patients had a 90% 5-year survival rate while node-positive patients had a 65% 5-year survival rate.[90] The number of involved axillary nodes also predicts survival. The 10-year survival for patients with involvement of one to three nodes is 44% and this decreases to 14% in patients with four or more positive nodes.[91]

Histological grade of the tumour also predicts prognosis. Giordano et al.[74] reported 5-year survival for patients with grade 1 tumours of 76% compared with 66% for those with grade 2 tumours and 43% for those with grade 3 tumours. Hormone receptor status also appears to be associated with survival. Estrogen receptor-positive and progesterone receptor-positive tumours have significantly improved survival compared with estrogen receptor-negative and progesterone receptor-negative tumours.[92] Overall, stage for stage, MBC has the same prognosis as female breast cancer and the same factors predict outcome.

## Treatment

Treatment of MBC is modelled on the treatment of female breast cancer. However, a retrospective review by Scott-Conner et al.[93] that compared treatment of matched MBC and female breast cancer patients found some significant differences. Males are less likely to have breast-conserving therapy than women, which would be expected given the anatomical considerations in the male breast. Men are also less likely to receive chemotherapy, and are less likely to receive radiation therapy if a lumpectomy is performed.

## Local therapy

Surgery is the primary therapy in MBC and mastectomy the most common procedure employed. Although breast-conserving surgery has been reported, the minimal amount of breast tissue in most male breasts and the central location of the majority of cancers do not make this a particularly attractive option. For stage I and II tumours, total mastectomy is the procedure of choice. If a small tumour is in proximity to the pectoralis major, it is reasonable to resect a small portion of the muscle with the specimen to ensure a negative margin. There is no longer any role for radical mastectomy. Locally advanced disease should be treated with neoadjuvant therapy followed by surgery. In most cases, this will allow a modified radical mastectomy to be performed. If the patient has clinically positive nodes, an axillary dissection should be done. If the axillary lymph nodes are clinically negative, SLNB can be performed. SLNB has been successfully performed in T1 and T2 tumours using a combination of preoperative lymphoscintigraphy, radioisotope tracer and isosulfan blue or patent blue V dye. The sensitivity and specificity are similar to that found in female breast cancer.[94,95]

## Adjuvant therapy

Endocrine therapy is indicated in hormone receptor-positive MBC. Single-institution trials have shown a survival benefit when tamoxifen is given to stage II and III breast cancers.[96] Small single-institution trials also indicate a survival benefit in men who receive cytotoxic chemotherapy.[97] Two comprehensive reviews both confirm a benefit for adjuvant hormone and chemotherapy in men.[98,99] The same guidelines used to make recommendations for women with breast cancer should be used for men.

No formal trials have been conducted to determine the indications for postmastectomy radiation in MBC, but a reduction in local recurrence with the use of radiation has been reported,[100] and the indications for radiation therapy in MBC should be the same as for female breast cancer.

# Metastatic disease

Endocrine therapy is the mainstay of treatment for metastatic MBC. Orchiectomy and other ablative surgeries have been used to treat metastatic disease in the past. More recently, exogenous androgens, antiandrogens, steroids, estrogens, progestins, aminoglutethimide and tamoxifen have been reported to prolong survival.[96,101] Limited information is available on the effectiveness of the newer selective aromatase inhibitors. However, early reports indicate that aromatase inhibitors may not be as successful in men because they only block peripheral estrogen production, which accounts for 80% of estrogen production in men. The presence of an intact feedback loop to the hypothalamus can also lead to hyperstimulation of the testes during treatment with aromatase inhibitors, with increased circulating androgen levels. The remaining 20% of estrogen produced by the testes remains unopposed.[74] Others have suggested that this may not be a problem, but clinical experience remains limited. A phase II trial in male breast cancer examining the use of an aromatase inhibitor combined with goserelin acetate for androgen suppression is ongoing in the USA. In hormone receptor-negative cancers, cytotoxic agents are the mainstay of therapy.[101]

## Key points

### Paget's disease
- Local therapy for Paget's disease consists of mastectomy or breast-conserving therapy that includes excision of the nipple–areola complex followed by radiation therapy.
- SLNB is performed when invasive cancer is present or if mastectomy is planned.
- Adjuvant therapy is based on the stage of the underlying malignancy.

### Pregnancy-associated breast cancer
- A multidisciplinary approach is necessary in managing the woman with PABC. Patient and family counselling is also important.

- Mammography, sonography and image-guided biopsy can be performed safely during pregnancy.
- Surgery can be performed safely during any trimester of pregnancy, while radiation is contraindicated during pregnancy.
- Chemotherapy can be given if necessary during the second and third trimesters.
- Recognising PABC and understanding the management issues associated with it is of increasing importance as more women delay childbirth.

# References

1. Paget J. On disease of the mammary areola preceding cancer of the mammary gland. St Barts Hospital Rep 1874; 10:87–9.

2. Lagios MD, Westdahl PR, Rose MR et al. Paget's disease of the nipple. Alternative management in cases without or with minimal extent of underlying breast carcinoma. Cancer 1984; 54(3):545–51.

3. Chen CY, Sun LM, Anderson BO. Paget disease of the breast: changing patterns of incidence, clinical presentation, and treatment in the U.S. Cancer 2006; 107(7):1448–58.

4. Kothari AS, Beechey-Newman N, Hamed H et al. Paget disease of the nipple: a multifocal manifestation of higher-risk disease. Cancer 2002; 95(1):1–7.

5. Dixon AR, Galea MH, Ellis IO et al. Paget's disease of the nipple. Br J Surg 1991; 78(6):722–3.

6. Fu W, Lobocki CA, Silberberg BK et al. Molecular markers in Paget disease of the breast. J Surg Oncol 2001; 77(3):171–8.

7. Jahn H, Osther PJ, Nielsen EH et al. An electron microscopic study of clinical Paget's disease of the nipple. APMIS 1995; 103(9):628–34.

8. Sakorafas GH, Blanchard K, Sarr MG et al. Paget's disease of the breast. Cancer Treat Rev 2001; 27(1):9–18.

9. Kaelin C. Paget's disease. In: Harris JR, Lippman MF, Morrow M et al. (eds) Diseases of the breast, 2nd edn. Baltimore: Lippincott Williams & Wilkins, 2000; pp. 277–83.

10. Smith KJ, Tuur S, Corvette D et al. Cytokeratin 7 staining in mammary and extramammary Paget's disease. Mod Pathol 1997; 10(11):1069–74.

11. Hitchcock A, Topham S, Bell J et al. Routine diagnosis of mammary Paget's disease. A modern approach. Am J Surg Pathol 1992; 16(1):58–61.

12. Ramachandra S, Gillett CE, Millis RR A comparative immunohistochemical study of mammary and extramammary Paget's disease and superficial spreading melanoma, with particular emphasis on melanocytic markers. Virchows Arch 1996; 429(6):371–6.

13. Friedman EP, Hall-Craggs MA, Mumtaz H et al. Breast MR and the appearance of the normal and abnormal nipple. Clin Radiol 1997; 52(11):854–61.

14. Echevarria JJ et al. Usefulness of MRI in detecting occult breast cancer associated with Paget's disease of the nipple–areolar complex. Br J Radiol 2004; 77(924):1036–9.

15. Frei KA et al. Paget disease of the breast: findings at magnetic resonance imaging and histopathologic correlation. Invest Radiol 2005; 40(6):363–7.

16. Marshall JK, Griffith KA, Haffty BJ et al. Conservative management of Paget disease of the breast with radiotherapy: 10- and 15-year results. Cancer 2003; 97(9):2142–9.

17. Bijker N, Rutgers EJ, Duchateau L et al. Breast-conserving therapy for Paget disease of the nipple: a prospective European Organization for Research and Treatment of Cancer study of 61 patients. Cancer 2001; 91(3):472–7.

18. Fu W, Mittel VK, Young SC. Paget disease of the breast: analysis of 41 patients. Am J Clin Oncol 2001; 24(4):397–400.

19. Kollmorgen DR, Varanasi JS, Edge SB et al. Paget's disease of the breast: a 33-year experience. J Am Coll Surg 1998; 187(2):171–7.

20. Fourquet A, Campana F, Vielh P et al. Paget's disease of the nipple without detectable breast tumor: conservative management with radiation therapy. Int J Radiat Oncol Biol Phys 1987; 13(10):1463–5.

21. Kawase K et al. Paget's disease of the breast: there is a role for breast-conserving therapy. Ann Surg Oncol 2005; 12(5):391–7.

22. Polgar C, Orosz Z, Kovacs T et al. Breast-conserving therapy for Paget disease of the nipple: a prospective European Organization for Research and Treatment of Cancer study of 61 patients. Cancer 2002; 94(6):1904–5.

23. Sukumvanich P et al. The role of sentinel lymph node biopsy in Paget's disease of the breast. Ann Surg Oncol 2007; 14(3):1020–3.

24. Laronga C et al. Paget's disease in the era of sentinel lymph node biopsy. Am J Surg 2006; 192(4):481–3.

25. Antonelli NM, Dotters DJ, Katz VL et al. Cancer in pregnancy: a review of the literature. Part I. Obstet Gynecol Surv 1996; 51(2):125–34.

26. National Cancer Institute. Breast Cancer in pregnancy. Cancer-net. Available at: http://www.cancer/gov/cancerinfo/pdq/treatment/breast-cancer-and-pregnancy#section_63

27. Gemignani ML, Petrek JA, Borgen PI. Breast cancer and pregnancy. Surg Clin North Am 1999; 79(5):1157–69.

28. Woo JC, Yu T, Hurd TC. Breast cancer in pregnancy: a literature review. Arch Surg 2003; 138(1):91–8; discussion 99.

29. Ishida T, Yokoe T, Kasumi F et al. Clinicopathologic characteristics and prognosis of breast cancer patients associated with pregnancy and lactation: analysis of case–control study in Japan. Jpn J Cancer Res 1992; 83(11):1143–9.

30. Jernstrom H, Lerman C, Ghadirian P et al. Pregnancy and risk of early breast cancer in carriers of BRCA1 and BRCA2. Lancet 1999; 354(9193):1846–50.

31. Scott-Conner CE, Schorr SJ. The diagnosis and management of breast problems during pregnancy and lactation. Am J Surg 1995; 170(4):401–5.

32. Guinee VF, Olsson H, Moller T et al. Effect of pregnancy on prognosis for young women with breast cancer. Lancet 1994; 343(8913):1587–9.

33. Liberman L, Giess CS, Dershaw DD et al. Imaging of pregnancy-associated breast cancer. Radiology 1994; 191(1):245–8.

34. Ahn BY, Kim HH, Moon WK et al. Pregnancy- and lactation-associated breast cancer: mammographic and sonographic findings. J Ultrasound Med 2003; 22(5):491–7; quiz 498–9.

35. Yang WT et al. Imaging of breast cancer diagnosed and treated with chemotherapy during pregnancy. Radiology 2006; 239(1):52–60.

36. Schackmuth EM, Harlow CL, Norton LW. Milk fistula: a complication after core breast biopsy. Am J Roentgenol 1993; 161(5):961–2.

37. Baker J, Ali A, Groch MW et al. Bone scanning in pregnant patients with breast carcinoma. Clin Nucl Med 1987; 12(7):519–24.

38. Loibl S et al. Breast carcinoma during pregnancy. International recommendations from an expert meeting. Cancer 2006; 106(2):237–46.

39. Hubbard AM, Crombleholme TM, Adzick NS et al. Prenatal MRI evaluation of congenital diaphragmatic hernia. Am J Perinatol 1999; 16(8):407–13.

40. Barnes DM, Newman LA. Pregnancy-associated breast cancer: a literature review. Surg Clin North Am 2007; 87(2):417–30, x.

41. Keleher AJ, Theriault RL, Gwyn KM et al. Multidisciplinary management of breast cancer concurrent with pregnancy. J Am Coll Surg 2002; 194(1):54–64.

42. Bonnier P, Romain S, Dilhuydy JM et al. Influence of pregnancy on the outcome of breast cancer: a case–control study. Societe Francaise de Senologie et de Pathologie Mammaire Study Group. Int J Cancer 1997; 72(5):720–7.

43. Tretli S, Kvalheim G, Thoresen S et al. Survival of breast cancer patients diagnosed during pregnancy or lactation. Br J Cancer 1988; 58(3):382–4.

44. Tummers P, De Sutter P, Dhont M. Risk of spontaneous abortion in singleton and twin pregnancies after IVF/ICSI. Hum Reprod 2003; 18(8):1720–3.

45. Duncan PG, Pope WD, Cohen MM et al. Fetal risk of anesthesia and surgery during pregnancy. Anesthesiology 1986; 64(6):790–4.

46. Morita ET, Chang J, Leong SP. Principles and controversies in lymphoscintigraphy with emphasis on breast cancer. Surg Clin North Am 2000; 80(6):1721–39.

47. Gentilini O et al. Safety of sentinel node biopsy in pregnant patients with breast cancer. Ann Oncol 2004; 15(9):1348–51.

48. Keleher A et al. The safety of lymphatic mapping in pregnant breast cancer patients using Tc-99m sulfur colloid. Breast J 2004; 10(6):492–5.

49. Ebert U, Loffler H, Kirch W. Cytotoxic therapy and pregnancy. Pharmacol Ther 1997; 74(2):207–20.

50. Berry DL, Theriault RL, Holmes FA et al. Management of breast cancer during pregnancy using a standardized protocol. J Clin Oncol 1999; 17(3):855–61.

51. Hahn KM et al. Treatment of pregnant breast cancer patients and outcomes of children exposed to chemotherapy in utero. Cancer 2006; 107(6):1219–26.

52. Sood AK, Shahin MS, Sorosky JI. Paclitaxel and platinum chemotherapy for ovarian carcinoma during pregnancy. Gynecol Oncol 2001; 83(3):599–600.

53. De Santis M, Lucchese A, De Carolis S et al. Metastatic breast cancer in pregnancy: first case of chemotherapy with docetaxel. Eur J Cancer Care 2000; 9(4):235–7.

54. Mir O, Berveiller P, Ropert S et al. Emerging therapeutic options for breast cancer chemotherapy during pregnancy. Ann Oncol 2008; 19(4):607–13.

55. Isaacs RJ, Hunter W, Clark K. Tamoxifen as systemic treatment of advanced breast cancer during pregnancy – case report and literature review. Gynecol Oncol 2001; 80(3):405–8.

56. Ives A et al. Pregnancy after breast cancer: population based study. BMJ 2007; 334(7586):194.

57. Kuper-Hommel MJ, Snijder S, Janssen-Heijnen ML et al. Treatment and survival of 38 female breast lymphomas: a population-based study with clinical and pathological reviews. Ann Hematol 2003; 82(7):397–404.

58. Ryan G, Martinelli G, Kuper-Hommel M et al. Primary diffuse large B-cell lymphoma of the breast: prognostic factors and outcomes of a study by the International Extranodal Lymphoma Study Group. Ann Oncol 2008; 19(2):233–41.

59. Fruchart C et al. High grade primary breast lymphoma: is it a different clinical entity? Breast Cancer Res Treat 2005; 93(3):191–8.

60. Maddox JC, Evans HL. Angiosarcoma of skin and soft tissue: a study of forty-four cases. Cancer 1981; 48(8):1907–21.

61. Rao J, Dekoven JG, Beatty JD et al. Cutaneous angiosarcoma as a delayed complication of radiation therapy for carcinoma of the breast. J Am Acad Dermatol 2003; 49(3):532–8.

62. Monroe AT, Feigenberg SJ, Mendenhall NP. Angiosarcoma after breast-conserving therapy. Cancer 2003; 97(8):1832–40.

63. Donnell RM, Rosen PP, Lieberman PH et al. Angiosarcoma and other vascular tumors of the breast. Am J Surg Pathol 1981; 5(7):629–42.

64. Sher T et al. Primary angiosarcomas of the breast. Cancer 2007; 110(1):173–8.

65. Ariel IM, Caron AS. Diagnosis and treatment of malignant melanoma arising from the skin of the female breast. Am J Surg 1972; 124(3):384–90.

66. Bartella L, Kaye J, Perry NM et al. Metastases to the breast revisited: radiological–histopathological correlation. Clin Radiol 2003; 58(7):524–31.

67. Balch CM, Buzaid AC, Soong SJ et al. Final version of the American Joint Committee on Cancer staging system for cutaneous melanoma. J Clin Oncol 2001; 19(16):3635–48.

68. Bedrosian I, Faries MB, Guerry D et al. Incidence of sentinel node metastasis in patients with thin primary melanoma (≤1 mm) with vertical growth phase. Ann Surg Oncol 2000; 7(4):262–7.

69. Amichetti M, Perani B, Boi S. Metastases to the breast from extramammary malignancies. Oncology 1990; 47(3):257–60.

70. Paulus DD, Libshitz HI. Metastasis to the breast. Radiol Clin North Am 1982; 20(3):561–8.

71. Weir HK, Thun MJ, Hankey BF et al. Annual report to the nation on the status of cancer, 1975–2000, featuring the uses of surveillance data for cancer prevention and control. J Natl Cancer Inst 2003; 95(17):1276–99.

72. La Vecchia C, Levi F, Lucchini F. Descriptive epidemiology of male breast cancer in Europe. Int J Cancer 1992; 51(1):62–6.

73. Anderson WF, Devesa SS. In situ male breast carcinoma in the Surveillance, Epidemiology, and End Results database of the National Cancer Institute. Cancer 2005; 104(8):1733–41.

74. Pant K, Dutta U. Understanding and management of male breast cancer: a critical review. Med Oncol 2007 (Epub ahead of print).

75. Mabuchi K, Bross DS, Kessler II. Risk factors for male breast cancer. J Natl Cancer Inst 1985; 74(2):371–5.

76. Thomas DB, Jimenez LM, McTiernan A et al. Breast cancer in men: risk factors with hormonal implications. Am J Epidemiol 1992; 135(7):734–48.

77. Lynch HT, Kaplan AR, Lynch JF. Klinefelter syndrome and cancer. A family study. JAMA 1974; 229(7):809–11.

78. Friedman LS, Gayther SA, Kurosaki T et al. Mutation analysis of BRCA1 and BRCA2 in a male breast cancer population. Am J Hum Genet 1997; 60(2):313–19.

79. Thorlacius S, Olafsdottir G, Tryggvadottir L et al. A single BRCA2 mutation in male and female breast cancer families from Iceland with varied cancer phenotypes. Nat Genet 1996; 13(1):117–9.

80. Thorlacius S, Sigurdsson S, Bjarnadottir H et al. Study of a single BRCA2 mutation with high carrier frequency in a small population. Am J Hum Genet 1997; 60(5):1079–84.

81. Brose MS, Rebbeck TR, Calzone KA et al. Cancer risk estimates for BRCA1 mutation carriers identified in a risk evaluation program. J Natl Cancer Inst 2002; 94(18):1365–72.

82. Ribeiro G. Male breast carcinoma – a review of 301 cases from the Christie Hospital and Holt Radium Institute, Manchester. Br J Cancer 1985; 51(1):115–19.

83. Goss PE, Reid C, Pintilie M et al. Male breast carcinoma: a review of 229 patients who presented to the Princess Margaret Hospital during 40 years: 1955–1996. Cancer 1999; 85(3):629–39.

84. Stalsberg H, Thomas SB, Rosenblatt KA et al. Histologic types and hormone receptors in breast cancer in men: a population-based study in 282 United States men. Cancer Causes Control 1993; 4(2):143–51.

85. Hittmair AP, Lininger RA, Tavassoli FA. Ductal carcinoma in situ (DCIS) in the male breast: a morphologic study of 84 cases of pure DCIS and 30 cases of DCIS associated with invasive carcinoma – a preliminary report. Cancer 1998; 83(10):2139–49.

86. Giordano SH et al. Breast carcinoma in men: a population-based study. Cancer 2004; 101(1):51–7.

87. Bloom KJ et al. Status of HER-2 in male and female breast carcinoma. Am J Surg 2001; 182(4):389–92.

88. Rudlowski C et al. Her-2/neu gene amplification and protein expression in primary male breast cancer. Breast Cancer Res Treat 2004; 84(3):215–23.

89. Idelevich E, Mozes M, Ben Baruch N et al. Oncogenes in male breast cancer. Am J Clin Oncol 2003; 26(3):259–61.

90. Guinee VF, Olsson H, Moller T et al. The prognosis of breast cancer in males. A report of 335 cases. Cancer 1993; 71(1):154–61.

91. Cutuli B, Lacroze M, Dilhuydy JM et al. Male breast cancer: results of the treatments and prognostic factors in 397 cases. Eur J Cancer 1995; 31A(12):1960–4.

92. Donegan WL, Redlich PN, Lang PJ et al. Carcinoma of the breast in males: a multiinstitutional survey. Cancer 1998; 83(3):498–509.

93. Scott-Conner CE, Jochimsen PR, Menck HR et al. An analysis of male and female breast cancer treatment and survival among demographically identical pairs of patients. Surgery 1999; 126(4):775–80; discussion 780–1.

94. Port ER, Fey JV, Cody HS III et al. Sentinel lymph node biopsy in patients with male breast carcinoma. Cancer 2001; 91(2):319–23.

95. Goyal A et al. Sentinel lymph node biopsy in male breast cancer patients. Eur J Surg Oncol 2004; 30(5):480–3.

96. Ribeiro G, Swindell R. Adjuvant tamoxifen for male breast cancer (MBC). Br J Cancer 1992; 65(2):252–4.

97. Patel HZ 2nd, Buzdar AU, Hortobagyi GN. Role of adjuvant chemotherapy in male breast cancer. Cancer 1989; 64(8):1583–5.

98. Agrawal A et al. Male breast cancer: a review of clinical management. Breast Cancer Res Treat 2007; 103(1):11–21.

99. Fentiman IS, Fourquet A, Hortobagyi GN. Male breast cancer. Lancet 2006; 367(9510):595–604.

100. Schuchardt U, Seegenschmiedt MH, Kirschner MJ et al. Adjuvant radiotherapy for breast carcinoma in men: a 20-year clinical experience. Am J Clin Oncol 1996; 19(4):330–6.

101. Jaiyesimi IA, Buzdar AU, Sahin AA et al. Carcinoma of the male breast. Ann Intern Med 1992; 117(9):771–7.

# 11

# Treatment of ductal carcinoma in situ

Nicola L.P. Barnes
Nigel J. Bundred

## Background

The introduction of screening mammography has resulted in a marked increase in the detection of ductal carcinoma in situ (DCIS) from 2% of newly diagnosed breast cancers before national screening, to 25–30% of all screen-detected tumours.[1] DCIS is a preinvasive breast cancer; the proliferation of malignant ductal epithelial cells remain confined by an intact basement membrane, with no invasion into the surrounding stroma.[2] Over 90% of DCIS currently diagnosed is impalpable, asymptomatic and detected by screening. These screening-detected cases are frequently small (<4 cm) and localised, and breast-conserving surgery is often possible. The remaining 10% present symptomatically, with a palpable breast lump, nipple discharge or Paget's disease of the nipple. If these symptoms are present, the underlying disease is often extensive and frequently requires mastectomy.

## Risk factors, natural history, pathology and receptors

### Risk factors

Risk factors for the development of DCIS include a family history of breast cancer, older age at first childbirth and nulliparity.[3] Although breast epithelial proliferation is increased by the use of the oral contraceptive pill[4] and hormone replacement therapy (HRT), particularly combined estrogen/progestogen HRT for over 5 years,[5] there is little evidence to date that either the oral contraceptive pill or HRT increases the risk of DCIS.[4] Two studies[6,7] have reported a relative risk of 1.4 for the development of DCIS following estrogen-only HRT preparations and a relative risk of 1.7–2.3 with estrogen- and progestogen-containing preparations. Other studies have shown no increased risk following HRT use.[8,9]

### Natural history

Although factors that pertain to an increased risk of developing DCIS have been identified, the natural history of this heterogeneous disease remains poorly understood.

 A review of DCIS recurrences and their primary lesions from the EORTC 10853 trial[10,11] found concordant histology (similar grade) in 62% of cases, and identical marker expression (estrogen receptor, progesterone receptor, p53 and c-erbB-2/HER-2/*neu*) in 63% of both invasive and non-invasive recurrences.[11] This high percentage of tumours with identical receptor profiles indicates that it is likely that residual disease after initial treatment progresses to either further mammographically detectable DCIS or invasive cancer.

Retrospective studies of cases of low-grade DCIS misdiagnosed as benign found that, 20 years after local excision, approximately 33% of cases had developed an invasive cancer.[12] As not all cases of DCIS progress to invasive disease, detection by mammographic screening could lead to overdiagnosis and treatment of 'non-progressive DCIS', i.e. DCIS that would not have progressed to invasive disease if left untreated. A recent study used statistical modelling (Markov process model) to assess the extent of the overdiagnosis of non-progressive DCIS. This model estimates that a woman attending an incidence screen has a 166 times higher probability of having progressive DCIS or invasive cancer diagnosed than non-progressive DCIS;[13] in addition, although there is an element of overdiagnosis of non-progressive DCIS, this is small compared with the potential benefit of detecting more aggressive disease.

There is increasing evidence that the developmental pathways for low- and intermediate-grade DCIS are distinct from the development of high-grade DCIS. The initial development of low- and intermediate-grade DCIS compared with high-grade DCIS can be partly explained by reference to biological markers. In the sequence of progression from normal breast to DCIS, there is variable loss of chromosomal heterozygosity dependent on nuclear grade. Low- and intermediate-grade tumours show 16q loss, whereas there is 17p loss in high-grade lesions. It is likely that low-grade lesions arise from estrogen receptor-positive atypical ductal hyperplasia or lobular carcinoma in situ (LCIS) and progress to low-grade estrogen receptor-positive DCIS. High-grade lesions have no obvious precursor, unless they arise from usual ductal hyperplasia or atypical ductal hyperplasia that expresses 17p loss. The progression of well-differentiated/low-grade DCIS to poorly differentiated/high-grade DCIS or high-grade invasive cancer is an uncommon event.[11]

## Stem cells

Recent evidence suggests the breast has stem cells that can reconstitute the various cell types within the breast after trauma. Cancers (including DCIS) arise from accumulations of mutations within stem cells which disrupt their tightly controlled self-renewal and proliferation processes. Stem cells (mammospheres) have recently been isolated from human DCIS. In this process, samples of human DCIS tissue are separated into single cells and a subset of these cells (which are putative stem/progenitor cells) grow, in non-adherent culture conditions, to form 3-D branching structures (known as mammospheres). Mammosphere growth is dependent on growth simulation via the epidermal growth factor (EGF) and Notch receptor pathways.[14] The DCIS stem cell paradigm would certainly explain multifocal DCIS and potentially local recurrence. Stem cells survive in non-adherent culture and after wide local excision with clear margins would survive and regrow, which would also explain the 'identical' receptor expression seen in recurrent DCIS as well as early recurrence in high-grade DCIS, as there are more stem cells found in high-grade lesions. Potentially, therefore, targeted inhibition of stem cells may prevent DCIS recurrence.

## Pathology

### Classification and features

DCIS can be often classified into two major subtypes according to the presence or absence of comedo necrosis.[15] A tumour can be designated as comedo if atypical cells with abundant luminal necrosis fill at least one duct. The involved cells are large with pleomorphic nuclei and abnormal mitoses. The necrotic material often calcifies and is subsequently visible on mammography.

Non-comedo tumours encompass all other subtypes of DCIS:

- Solid – where tumour fills extended duct spaces.
- Micropapillary – where tufts of cells project into the duct lumen perpendicular to the basement membrane.
- Papillary – where the projecting tufts are larger than in the micropapillary type and contain a fibrovascular core.
- Cribriform – where the tumour takes on a fenestrated/sieve-like appearance.
- Clinging (flat) – where there are variable columnar cell alterations along the duct margins. (There remains controversy as to whether clinging DCIS is truly an in situ cancer or whether it should be considered as atypical hyperplasia rather than neoplastic.)

Rarer subtypes also exist, including neuroendocrine, encysted papillary, apocrine and signet cell.

The UK- and EU-funded breast-screening programmes use the system of low, intermediate and high nuclear grade to classify DCIS. This definition is based on the characteristics of the lesion as seen with a high-power microscope lens (×40) and uses a comparison of tumour cell size with normal epithelial and red blood cell size:[16]

- Low nuclear grade DCIS has evenly spaced cells with centrally placed small nuclei and few mitoses and nucleoli that are not easily seen.
- High nuclear grade DCIS has pleomorphic irregularly spaced cells with large irregular nuclei (often three times the size of erythrocytes), prominent nucleoli and frequent mitoses. It is often solid with comedo necrosis and calcification.
- Intermediate grade DCIS has features between those seen in low- and high-grade DCIS.

If a lesion contains areas of varying grade, it is awarded the highest grade present. A universally agreed classification system is yet to be established and will need to be observer independent and clinically relevant.

Most cases of DCIS are unicentric.[17] Following extensive pathological sectioning of DCIS mastectomy specimens, only 1% show multicentric disease.[17] A **multicentric** tumour is defined as separate foci of tumour found in more than one breast quadrant, or more than 5 cm away from the initial primary. A tumour is considered **multifocal** if there are separate tumour foci in the same quadrant and close to the original tumour.[18] The local spread of DCIS is along the branching ducts that form the glandular breast. The ducts, which are ill defined, often extend beyond the borders of a quadrant. Most DCIS is continuous along a given ductal segment, but poorly differentiated high-grade lesions can be multifocal.[19] These findings explain why most DCIS recurrences are at or near the site of the initial tumour,[20] but also why recurrences apparently remote from the initial lesion can exhibit similar genotypical and phenotypical characteristics to the primary lesion.[11]

As well as documenting pathological type and grade on the histology report, the pathologist details the presence or absence of microinvasion. If microinvasion is detected histologically, a thorough examination of the entire specimen should be undertaken to exclude other previously unnoticed areas of invasive cancer. Lesions that can be mistaken for microinvasion include DCIS involving lobules, branching of ducts, distortion of ducts by acini or fibrosis, crush or cautery artefacts, and DCIS involving a benign sclerosing process (e.g. radial scar).[21–25]

## Lobular carcinoma in situ

LCIS is a high-risk marker of invasive cancer but is not itself a premalignant lesion. The current classification combines LCIS and atypical lobular hyperplasia into a single group known as lobular intraepithelial neoplasia (LIN). It is often an incidental finding during breast biopsy and accounts for approximately 0.5% of symptomatic and 1% of screen-detected tumours. Ductal and lobular cells are anatomically contiguous in the ducto-lobular unit, but in situ ductal and lobular tumours show different pathological and clinical features. Patients developing LCIS tend to be younger and premenopausal, with bilateral and multicentric disease of lower grade and close to 100% estrogen receptor expression (Table 11.1).[25] Sometimes it is difficult to distinguish histologically between LCIS and DCIS and the pathology report should state this. The clinical interpretation of the report should take into account the increased risks from both tumour subtypes.

If lobular neoplasia is detected at core biopsy, the area of suspicion should be subjected to excision biopsy to confirm the diagnosis and exclude an adjacent invasive focus. If lobular neoplasia is diagnosed coincidentally following excision of a coexisting lesion, no further treatment is necessary (even if the area of lobular neoplasia is not fully excised) and the patient should undergo regular outpatient review

**Table 11.1** • Comparative clinico-pathological features of ductal carcinoma in situ (DCIS) and tabular carcinoma in situ (LCIS)

| Clinico-pathological feature | DCIS | LCIS |
|---|---|---|
| Age at diagnosis (years) | 54–58 | 44–47 |
| Premenopausal | 30% | 70% |
| Absence of clinical signs | 90% | 99% |
| Mammographic findings | Microcalcifications | None |
| Multicentric disease | 30% | 90% |
| Bilateral disease | 12–20% | 90% |
| Histological grade | 65% high grade | 90% low grade |
| Estrogen receptor status | 65% positive | 95% positive |
| Subsequent invasive disease | 30–40% | 25–30% |
| Ipsilateral–contralateral ratio | 9:1 | 1:1 |

on a 'watch and wait' basis. The recent NSABP P-1 prevention trial showed a 56% reduction in risk of developing subsequent invasive cancer with tamoxifen.[26] Further studies are ongoing with aromatase inhibitors in postmenopausal patients with lobular neoplasia. Chemotherapy and radiotherapy have no place in the treatment of lobular neoplasia. A problem area is pleomorphic LCIS, with the current perspective being that this should be treated like DCIS rather than lobular neoplasia.

## Receptors and markers

To advance our understanding of the development and behaviour of DCIS, there has been interest in cell receptor expression and signalling pathways controlling growth. These studies have been mainly based on immunohistochemical assessment but show poorly differentiated high-grade comedo DCIS has low estrogen receptor expression, high rates of cell proliferation[27] (as expressed by Ki67, a nuclear antigen expressed in late $G_1$, S, $G_2$ and M phases of the cell cycle but not in the quiescent $G_0$)[28] and high rates of apoptosis,[29] and over-expresses c-erbB-2 (HER-2/*neu*) and epidermal growth factor receptor (EGFR, a type 1 tyrosine kinase receptor).[27] Low-grade lesions have high estrogen receptor expression, with lower rates of cell proliferation[27] and apoptosis than high-grade lesions,[29] and they rarely express HER-2.[27] Progesterone receptor expression correlates with estrogen receptor expression in both low- and high-grade tumours.[27] In comparison, normal breast epithelium has low expression of estrogen receptor and progesterone receptor,[30] and a very low rate of apoptosis and HER-2 expression.

The increased rate of apoptosis seen in DCIS is lost on progression to invasive cancer, but the high proliferative rate is maintained.[31] Cyclin D1, an oncogene responsible for $G_1$ cell cycle proliferation/progression and induction of apoptosis, is overexpressed in approximately 90% of in situ and invasive ductal cancers.[32] It also appears to be associated with a loss of differentiation (measured by p27[Kip1]).[33] In estrogen receptor-positive tumours, the driving force behind this increase in cell proliferation is the nuclear action of the activated estrogen receptor, which increases growth-promoting gene transcription. In estrogen receptor-negative tumours, the driving pathway is thought to be predominantly via EGFR/HER-2/RAS/MAP kinase activation (**Fig. 11.1**). This leads to a subsequent increase in transcription of both proliferative and, via Akt,

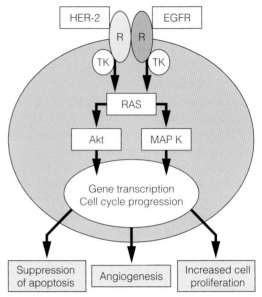

**Figure 11.1** • The basic growth pathway in estrogen receptor-negative breast tumour cells. The estrogen receptor-positive signalling pathway is mediated via estrogen attaching to its receptor, which then moves down its concentration gradient to the cell nucleus. The presence of estrogen receptor in the cell nucleus subsequently increases gene transcription and expression of growth-promoting factors, leading to increased cell proliferation and tumour growth. In cells that do not express estrogen receptors, the main signalling pathway for growth is via the epidermal growth factor (EGF)/c-erbB-2 receptor; this activates the RAS intracellular messenger, which increases cell proliferation and tumour growth via MAP kinase. RAS stimulation also leads to the suppression of the apoptosis cascade via Akt and BAD phosphorylation (an apoptotic protein). MAP K, MAP kinase; R, receptor; TK, tyrosine kinase.

anti-apoptotic genes. Activation of this pathway also induces the expression of cyclo-oxygenase-2 (COX-2), which is an inducible enzyme that converts arachidonic acid to prostaglandins. It has been found to be overexpressed in up to 80% of DCIS.[34] COX-2-positive DCIS shows increased cell proliferation, and is related to increased tumour recurrence and decreased survival in invasive cancer.[35]

In addition to alterations in cell proliferation and apoptosis, the development of neovascularisation is necessary for the growth of solid tumours. It is driven in part by angiogenic factors expressed in hypoxic areas of the tumour. Hypoxic areas of DCIS show a less well differentiated, more malignant phenotype of cells, with increased HIF-1α (a hypoxia-induced transcription factor), decreased estrogen receptor expression and increased expression of cytokeratin-19 (a breast stem cell marker).[23] It is felt that hypoxia-induced dedifferentiation could be a factor promoting tumour progression.[36]

# Presentation, investigation and diagnosis

## Presentation

Over 90% of DCIS is detected at mammographic screening. Approximately 70% of these mammographically detected cases present as microcalcifications with no associated mass lesion. The calcifications may be heterogeneous, fine, linear, branching, malignant or of indeterminate appearance. Microcalcifications with an associated mass lesion are identified in approximately 30% of DCIS mammograms.[37] Atypical mammographic features include circumscribed nodules, ill-defined masses, duct asymmetry and architectural distortion.[38] When diagnosed clinically, DCIS is often extensive or associated with a concurrent invasive tumour. It may present as a palpable mass, Paget's disease of the nipple or nipple discharge.[39]

## Investigation and diagnosis

The importance of thorough clinical examination for detecting the above signs of DCIS or coexisting pathology should not be forgotten. In addition to clinical examination (often normal) and mammographic findings, diagnosis is confirmed by core biopsy, as cytology gives no information on stromal invasion. Image guidance to ensure the accuracy of sampling of these mainly impalpable mammographic lesions is vital. Mammographic magnification views are important in order to delineate accurately the extent of the microcalcifications.

### Stereotactic core biopsy and vacuum-assisted biopsy

In the NHS breast-screening programme, the method of diagnosis is by stereotactic core biopsy with a 14G needle. Simple core biopsy is likely to be superseded by vacuum-assisted biopsy, which takes several contiguous biopsies during a single pass, and a metal clip can be inserted during the procedure to aid future localisation. Vacuum-assisted biopsy has higher sensitivity and specificity than core biopsy,[40,41] but it still underdiagnoses a coexisting invasive tumour in 10–20% of cases due to sampling error.[41] If the area of DCIS is extensive (>4 cm in size), multiple areas of the lesion need to be biopsied preoperatively to ensure that there is unlikely to be an invasive component to the disease and that all the microcalcifications are truly DCIS.

### Localisation-guided biopsy

If a definitive histological diagnosis cannot be made with either core biopsy or vacuum-assisted biopsy, due to failure to sample the calcification adequately, or doubt exists as to whether DCIS is present on histology, then an open biopsy is necessary. Following mammographic magnification views, wires or radioactive tracers are used to localise the lesion and guide the surgeon during open biopsy. For extensive areas of microcalcification, bracketing wires, one at each extent of the area of concern, can aid localisation and enable complete excision of the suspicious area. The excised specimen should be sent for immediate radiography, after careful orientation with Liga-clips or metal markers, to confirm that all the microcalcification of concern has been excised. The guidelines of the British Association of Surgical Oncologists[42] recommend that 90% of diagnostic guided biopsies for screen-detected abnormalities should weigh less than 20 g. Due to improved core biopsy diagnosis, wire-guided localisation procedures are usually therapeutic rather than diagnostic. However, the area of DCIS is often pathologically larger than mammographically suggested; this is especially true if magnification views are not used, and up to 30% of cases need re-excision to clear margins adequately.[43] Accurate orientation of the specimen is essential to direct re-excision of the relevant margins and to minimise the volume of any re-excision.

# Treatment: mastectomy versus breast-conserving surgery

## Mastectomy

The recurrence rate following mastectomy for DCIS is less than 1%.[44] As current evidence (see p. 177) points to DCIS being predominantly unicentric in origin, it is now recognised that mastectomy is overtreatment for the majority of patients.[44] In 1983 mastectomy was performed for 71% of cases of DCIS in the USA but this had dropped to 44% by 1992.[45] The multidisciplinary consensus conference on the treatment of DCIS[1] recommends mastectomy for patients with larger areas of DCIS (arbitrarily considered as >4 cm), for multicentric disease and for patients where radiotherapy is contraindicated. Women should also be offered mastectomy if the excision margins are involved following breast-conserving surgery and cavity re-excision who are not deemed suitable for re-excision. Women with DCIS requiring mastectomy are excellent candidates for skin-sparing mastectomy and immediate breast reconstruction.

## Breast-conserving surgery

Breast-conserving surgery is now the treatment of choice for small localised areas of DCIS (generally those <4 cm in diameter). Larger areas of DCIS can be excised but often require a reshaping or oncoplastic procedure combined with a contralateral breast reduction to achieve symmetry. Areas of DCIS usually need to be radiologically localised preoperatively, as they are predominantly impalpable (see p 175). The lesion should be excised in one piece if possible and orientated with Liga-clips. Before wound closure, the specimen should undergo radiography to ensure that all suspicious microcalcifications have been removed. Many surgeons use a four-quadrant cavity biopsy, with or without India ink staining to assess the surrounding breast. The pathologist should assess the histological margin status and document this in the histology report. If the margins are close (<1 mm), the patient should undergo cavity re-excision, as clear margin status is a key prognostic factor for local recurrence.

The DCIS consensus conference[1] agreed that the following criteria must be met before considering breast-conserving surgery without radiotherapy:
- tumour size must be less than 2 cm (pathological or mammographical);
- excision margins must be greater than 10 mm in each direction;
- the tumour must be of low or intermediate grade (grade I or II).

If these criteria cannot be met, adjuvant treatments, as discussed below, should be considered. The recommended treatment protocol for DCIS is shown in **Fig. 11.2**.

## Axillary staging

The incidence of macroscopic lymph node metastasis in DCIS is less than 1%, and formal axillary staging in women with DCIS should be avoided.[46] Patients found to have positive lymph nodes (perhaps en bloc with the axillary tail at mastectomy) usually have occult invasive disease and should be managed accordingly. A study by Veronesi et al. of 508 patients with pure DCIS found that nine patients (1.8%) had epithelial cells found in the sentinel node (five of these nine cases were micrometastases alone). None of the cases showed further lymph node involvement at formal axillary dissection.[47] A further study which looked retrospectively at the NSABP B-17 and B-24 data, from patients who had undergone local excision of DCIS with clear margins (no axillary surgery at initial treatment), showed that the ipsilateral nodal recurrence rate was 0.83/1000 patient-years in the B-17 trial and 0.36/1000 patient-years in the B-24 trial. The current recommendation is to avoid sentinel node biopsy or any axillary node surgery in DCIS. More effort at preoperative diagnosis of invasive disease rather than sentinel node biopsy is appropriate.[48]

# Recurrence: rates and predictors

No trials have specifically evaluated breast-conserving surgery versus mastectomy in DCIS. The recurrence rate following mastectomy is known to be very low at less than 1%.[44] The overall recurrence for breast-conserving surgery alone is up to 25% at 8 years follow-up, with up to 50% of recurrences (i.e. 12.5% of all cases) being invasive disease.[10,43,49,50] The remaining 50% of recurrences are in situ tumours.[51] Reviews of clinical and pathological variables have demonstrated certain unfavourable tumour characteristics and these are outlined below.

## Assessment of excision margins

A fundamental risk factor for recurrence is inadequate excision following breast-conserving surgery. This is judged as close (<1 mm) or involved margins[43] and/or failure to remove all suspicious microcalcifications.[52] Excision margin width has three times the power of tumour grade in predicting local recurrence.[53] The NSABP-B17, NSABP-B24 and EORTC clinical trials all revealed that the presence of clear margins after local excision significantly decreased tumour recurrence.[10,54–56] On multivariate analysis of the EORTC trial, non-specified, close or involved margins conferred a hazard ratio

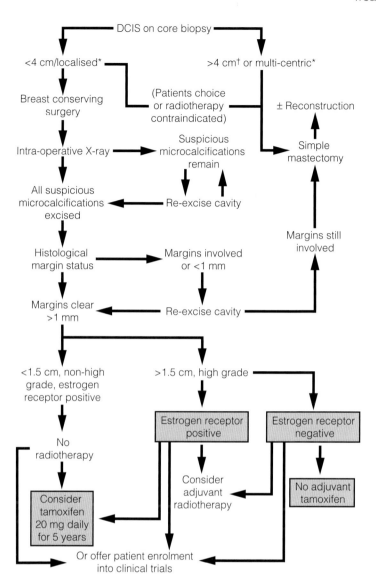

**Figure 11.2** • Recommended treatment algorithm for ductal carcinoma in situ (DCIS). *Determined mammographically. Shaded boxes indicate those treatments suggested by the results of recent trials.[50,58] †Areas of DCIS > 4 cm can be treated by breast conservation if unifocal and patient has large breast, or is suitable for an oncoplastic procedure.

of 2.07 (95% CI 1.35–3.16, $P = 0.0008$) compared with clear margins.[56] The NSABP-B24 trial found a covariate relative risk of 1.68 (95% CI 1.20–2.34) if the margins were involved. No prospective trials have looked at the optimum excision width required for in situ or invasive cancer. When considering the extent of surgical excision there has to be balance between minimising recurrence and producing an acceptable cosmetic outcome. A retrospective study by Chan et al.[43] reported that women with clear margins (judged as greater than 1 mm) had an 8.1% recurrence at a median follow-up of 47 months

compared with 37.9% recurrence where excision margins were close (1 mm). There was no improvement in recurrence rates in more widely excised lesions.

## High-grade/comedo tumours

High-grade tumours and tumours showing comedo necrosis are independent risk factors for recurrence. In a review of the EORTC 10853 trial,[56] high nuclear grade was found to have a hazard ratio of 2.23 (95% CI 1.41–3.51, $P = 0.0011$) for local recurrence, with 22% of high-grade tumours and

11% of intermediate-grade tumours developing either recurrent DCIS or invasive tumour. Comedo necrosis was also shown to be related to local recurrence, 18% of patients with DCIS having comedo necrosis developing recurrence (hazard ratio 1.80, 95% CI 1.08–3.00, P = 0.0183).

## Histological type and tumour architecture

The degree of tumour differentiation is predictive of both local recurrence and metastatic disease. In the EORTC trial,[10,56] poorly differentiated tumours were at significantly higher risk of developing DCIS recurrence (hazard ratio 3.58, 95% CI 1.68–7.62, P = 0.0001) and metastasis (hazard ratio 6.65, 95% CI 1.46–30.22, P = 0.00083) compared with well-differentiated tumours. In this same trial, histological type was also strongly related to DCIS recurrence, though not to invasive recurrence. Both solid/comedo DCIS (hazard ratio 4.40, 95% CI 2.28–8.48, P = 0.0001) and cribriform DCIS (hazard ratio 3.74, 95% CI 1.91–7.30, P = 0.0001) were found to be much more likely to recur than clinging or micropapillary tumours. Within the well-differentiated group, no tumours with clinging DCIS recurred.[56] It has been suggested that this well-differentiated clinging DCIS should be reclassified separately as 'columnar alteration with prominent apical snouts and secretion',[57] with debate as to whether this subtype would be more appropriately managed as atypical ductal hyperplasia or LCIS.

## Age at diagnosis

A further risk factor for recurrence irrespective of tumour grade or type is a young age (<40 years) at diagnosis. The EORTC 10853 trial[10,56] found that women less than 40 years at diagnosis were more likely to recur (hazard ratio 2.54, 95% CI 1.53–4.23, P = 0.010) than older women. The NSABP B-24 trial[54] found that the rate of ipsilateral breast tumours (in the placebo population) in women aged 49 years or less at diagnosis was 33.3 per 1000, compared with 13.0 for those aged 50 and above. In the UK/ANZ DCIS trial,[58] only a small proportion (9.5%) of the women were less than 50 years old at diagnosis. The power of this study is thus limited, but of these younger women, 26% recurred after excision and

tamoxifen compared with only 17% of women older than 50 years. Rodrigues et al.[59] studied women aged 42 years or less (mean age 38.5) or women aged 60 years or more (mean age 67.8) at diagnosis. They found that although there was no difference in tumour grade, comedo necrosis or overall histology (as also found in the EORTC trial) between the groups, compared with older patients c-erbB-2 or HER-2 was overexpressed in the younger patient population. Approximately 65% of the younger age group were c-erbB-2 or HER-2 positive compared with 38% of the older age group (P = 0.06). No significant difference was found between estrogen receptor, progesterone receptor, p53, Ki67, cyclin D1 or bcl-2 expression.

## Tumour size and palpability

None of the major trials have found any statistical significance between recurrence and tumour size. The NSABP-B17 trial[50] found that the size of mammographically detected tumours was not significant in predicting ipsilateral recurrence. However, when the researchers examined the clustering of microcalcifications in women whose mammograms did not show a tumour mass, they found that clustered microcalcifications greater than 10 mm (relative risk 2.06, 95% CI 1.36–3.10) or scattered calcifications (relative risk 2.41, 95% CI 1.40–4.16) had a significantly higher ipsilateral recurrence than clustered calcifications of 10 mm or less. The EORTC 10853 trial[56] found no difference in recurrence rates between tumours less than 10 mm in size and those 10–20 mm or greater than 20 mm in size (P = 0.2127). However, the tumours that were clinically apparent rather than mammographically detected were more likely to recur (covariate relative risk 2.17, 95% CI 1.53–3.08).[56]

## Scoring systems

In order to bring together the most clinically relevant risk factors, Silverstein at al.[15] developed the Van Nuys Prognostic Index, with the aim of predicting which women would be at risk of recurrence following breast-conserving surgery. This numerical algorithm was derived from regression analysis of retrospective data pooled from patients with DCIS treated at two centres in the USA.

The study was not randomised and used historical controls. The formula encompassed tumour size, margin width and pathological classification. The index has since been modified as the University of Southern California/Van Nuys Prognostic Index (USC/VNPI) and now includes patient age.[60] Each criterion is weighted with a score of 1, 2 or 3 and the individual scores combined to give an overall score from 4 to 12. Scores of 4–6, 7–9 and 10–12 are said to be at low, moderate and high risk of 5-year recurrence respectively. The data are skewed by the fact that 80% of large tumours (>4 cm) recurred, whereas in the UK these women would have undergone mastectomy. The value of the scoring system for a UK population, where the majority of cases of DCIS are small (<2 cm) and screen-detected (patients usually over 50 years old), may be limited. Boland et al.[53] were unable to demonstrate that size was a marker of recurrence in screen-detected DCIS in the UK.

## Markers of recurrence

To improve the detection of specific patient groups at increased risk of recurrence, biological markers that could help determine recurrence potential in DCIS are being investigated. Provenzano et al.[61] found that estrogen receptor, progesterone receptor and bcl-2 negativity and HER-2 and p21 positivity were associated with an increased risk of clinical recurrence. This was irrespective of tumour grade. Estrogen receptor, progesterone receptor, bcl-2 and HER-2 were found to be interdependent on each other, whereas p21 was found to be independent of the above associations, which is thought to reflect the differing biological pathways of action between the markers.

There has also been recent interest in another member of the type 1 tyrosine kinase receptor family, c-erbB-4/HER-4. DCIS and invasive tumours that show coexpression of HER-2 and HER-4 have a better prognosis (reduced recurrence) than HER-2-positive, HER-4-negative tumours.[62–64] A summary of the risk factors for DCIS recurrence is shown in Table 11.2.

**Table 11.2** • Risk factors for recurrence of ductal carcinoma in situ

| **Excision margins** | Margins ≤1 mm after breast-conserving surgery |
|---|---|
| **Tumour grade** | High grade (III) |
| **Comedo necrosis** | Present |
| **Histological type** | Poorly differentiated |
| **Patient age** | Younger age at diagnosis (≤40 years) |
| **Biological markers** | |
| Negativity | Estrogen receptor |
| | Progesterone receptor |
| | bcl-2 |
| | HER-4 |
| Positivity | HER-2 |
| | p21 |
| | p53 |
| | Ki67 (high-percentage expression) |
| **Patient presentation** | Symptomatic |
| **Tumour size** | Not significant |

Poor-prognosis tumours often possess multiple bad prognostic features, i.e. they tend to be poorly differentiated, high-grade, comedo tumours that are estrogen receptor negative and overexpress c-erbB-2.

# Adjuvant therapy

## Radiotherapy

Three main trials have examined the value of radiotherapy following breast-conserving surgery for DCIS. The NSABP-B17,[50] EORTC 10853[10] and UK/ANZ DCIS[58] trials each studied a radiation dose of 50 Gy in 25 fractions. All found a significant reduction in ipsilateral recurrence following radiotherapy (Table 11.3, **Fig. 11.3**).

The reduction was similar for both in situ and invasive recurrence. In the EORTC trial, the risk of DCIS recurrence was reduced by 48% ($P = 0.0011$) and invasive local recurrence by 42% ($P = 0.0065$) at a median of 10.5 years follow-up.[65]

Both groups had similar low risks of metastases and death. No actual survival advantage following radiotherapy was found in either the NSABP-B17 or EORTC 10853 trials (the UK/ANZ DCIS trial has had too few deaths to reach any conclusions). The DCIS consensus statement[1] and pathological review

Table 11.3 • Summary of major radiotherapy/tamoxifen clinical trials following breast-conserving therapy for ductal carcinoma in situ

| | NSABP-17* | | NSABP-24* | | EORTC 10853† | | UK/ANZ DCIS‡ | | | |
| --- | --- | --- | --- | --- | --- | --- | --- | --- | --- | --- |
| | BCS alone | BCS and XRT | BCS and XRT | BCS, XRT and tamoxifen | BCS alone | BCS and XRT | BCS alone | BCS and XRT | BCS and tamoxifen | BCS, XRT and tamoxifen |
| Number of patients | 403 | 411 | 899 | 899 | 500 | 502 | 544 | 267 | 567 | 316 |
| Number of local recurrences at median follow-up: | | | | | | | | | | |
| 43 months | 64 | 28 | – | – | – | – | – | – | – | – |
| 48 months | – | – | – | – | 83 | 53 | – | – | – | – |
| 53 months | – | – | – | – | – | – | 119 | 22 | 101 | 21 |
| 74 months | – | – | 130 | 84 | – | – | – | – | – | – |
| 90 months | 140 | 47 | – | – | – | – | – | – | – | – |
| 126 months | – | – | – | – | 132 | 75 | – | – | – | – |
| Local recurrence rates: | | | | | | | | | | |
| 4-year all recurrences | – | – | – | – | 16% | 9% | – | – | – | – |
| 4-year invasive | – | – | – | – | 8% | 4% | – | – | – | – |
| 5-year all recurrences | – | – | 13% | 8.2% | – | – | 15% | 3% | 12% | 3% |
| 5-year invasive | – | – | 7% | 4.1% | – | – | 5% | 1% | 5% | 2% |
| 8-year all recurrence | 27% | 12% | – | – | – | – | – | – | – | – |
| 8-year invasive | 13% | 4% | – | – | – | – | – | – | – | – |
| 10-year all recurrences | – | – | – | – | 26% | 15% | – | – | – | – |
| 10-year invasive | – | – | – | – | 13% | 8% | – | – | – | – |

| | | | | | | | | | | |
|---|---|---|---|---|---|---|---|---|---|---|
| Number of distant metastases | 6 | 9 | 7 | 3 | 20 | 23 | – | – | – | – |
| Total number of contralateral breast events | 19 | 20 | 36 | 18 | 28 | 39 | 17 | 5 | 6 | 5 |
| Number of contralateral invasive breast cancers | 16 | 12 | 23 | 15 | 19 | 28 | 10 | 5 | 5 | 5 |
| Bilateral event-free survival at: | | | | | | | | | | |
| 4 years | – | – | – | – | 82% | 86% | – | – | – | – |
| 5 years | 74% | 84% | 83% | 87% | – | – | 85% | 97% | 88% | 97% |
| 8 years | 60% | 75% | – | – | – | – | – | – | – | – |
| 10 years | – | – | – | – | 74% | 85% | – | – | – | – |

BCS, breast-conserving surgery; XRT, radiotherapy.

*Fisher ER, Dignam J, Tan-Chiu E et al. Pathologic findings from the National Surgical Adjuvant Breast Project (NSABP) eight-year update of Protocol B-17: intraductal carcinoma. Cancer 1999; 86:429–38.

†Julien J, Bijker N, Fentimen I et al. Radiotherapy in breast-conserving treatment for ductal carcinoma in situ: first results of the EORTC randomized phase III trial 10853. EORTC Breast Cancer Cooperative Group and EORTC Radiotherapy group. Lancet 2000; 355:528–33. Bijker N, Meijnen P, Peterse JL et al. Breast-conserving treatment with or without radiotherapy in ductal carcinoma-in-situ: ten-year results of European Organisation for Research and Treatment of Cancer randomized phase III trial 10853 – a study by the EORTC Breast Cancer Cooperative Group and EORTC Radiotherapy Group. J Clin Oncol 2006; 24(21):3381–7.

‡UK Coordinating Committee on Cancer Research (UKCCCR). Ductal carcinoma in situ (DCIS) Working Party on behalf of DCIS trialists in the UK, Australia and New Zealand, Radiotherapy and tamoxifen in women with completely excised ductal carcinoma in situ of the breast in the UK, Australia and New Zealand: randomised controlled trial. Lancet 2003; 362:95–103.

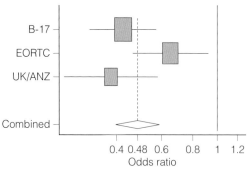

**Figure 11.3** • Radiotherapy trials overview: ipsilateral ductal carcinoma in situ (DCIS) and invasive recurrences. This Forrest plot of the major randomised controlled trials of radiotherapy in DCIS (B17,[50] EORTC[10] and UK/ANZ[58]) shows a significant reduction in ipsilateral recurrence risk following radiotherapy for all trials, with a combined odds ratio for the reduction in recurrence of DCIS and invasive disease of 0.48 for all trials. Reproduced from Cuzick J. Treatment of DCIS – results from clinical trials. Surg Oncol 2003; 12:213–19. With permission from Elsevier.

of the EORTC trial suggested that completely excised low-grade DCIS has a recurrence rate of just 4% at 5 years, making adjuvant radiotherapy difficult to recommend due to the associated morbidity. In the USA, it is recommended that all patients who have undergone breast-conserving surgery for DCIS receive a course of radiotherapy.[50] In Europe, adjuvant radiotherapy is recommended for all high-grade DCIS. Intermediate- and low-grade DCIS is selected for adjuvant radiotherapy on an individual patient basis.

## Endocrine therapy

Although radiotherapy reduces tumour recurrence following breast-conserving surgery, there is still an overall recurrence rate of between 3% and 13%[10,50,58] at 5 years, and research into the use of additional adjuvant therapies for DCIS remains important.

In this trial, 30% of women were younger than 50 years at diagnosis and the effect of tamoxifen

The NSABP-B24 trial compared breast-conserving surgery and radiotherapy with or without adjuvant tamoxifen. The study found that tamoxifen following breast-conserving surgery and radiotherapy was of benefit in reducing recurrence. There were 43% fewer invasive breast cancer events and 31% fewer non-invasive events in the tamoxifen-treated group.[54] The main advantage was in reducing invasive recurrence in the ipsilateral breast, although there was a significantly lower cumulative incidence of all breast cancer-related events in the tamoxifen group.

was largely due to a 40% reduction in this younger age group, with only a 20% reduction in the age group greater than 50 years. Adjuvant tamoxifen after wide local excision for DCIS should therefore be offered in this younger (under 50) age group. A retrospective review of the NSABP-B24 results showed that tamoxifen was only beneficial in estrogen receptor-positive cases. The relative risk of recurrence of any breast cancer in the estrogen receptor-positive cohort was 0.41 (95% CI 0.25–0.65, $P = 0.0002$), whereas there was little benefit in the estrogen receptor-negative cases (relative risk 0.80, $P = 0.51$).[66] The UK/ANZ DCIS trial found that adjuvant tamoxifen reduced overall DCIS recurrence (hazard ratio 0.68, 95% CI 0.49–0.96, $P = 0.03$) but not invasive disease[58] (see Table 11.3).

The UK/ANZ DCIS trial has not yet published a breakdown of tamoxifen response in relation to estrogen receptor status. A further study showing that response to tamoxifen is confined to estrogen receptor-positive DCIS also examined estrogen withdrawal (i.e. stopping HRT) in women with estrogen receptor-positive or -negative DCIS. There was a significant decrease in cell proliferation in the estrogen receptor-positive group but no change in proliferation was observed in estrogen receptor-negative tumours.[67] Results of the Canadian RTOG 98-04 trial comparing tamoxifen with or without radiotherapy following breast-conserving therapy are awaited.

In the randomised controlled trials, the rate of contralateral breast cancer after DCIS is 0.5% per year for 10 years. As tamoxifen can halve the risk of breast cancer in the contralateral breast, it could also be regarded as a chemopreventive agent. This could potentially justify its use in all estrogen receptor-positive women. However, approximately 60% of DCIS express HER-2. Estrogen receptor-positive tumours that also express HER-2 are often resistant to tamoxifen therapy but do respond to therapy with aromatase inhibitors. The ERISAC trial has shown that exemestane (a steroidal aromatase inhibitor), at a dose of 25 mg/day, inhibits epithelial proliferation in DCIS by 39% (hazard ratio 0.61, 95% CI 0.41–0.91, $P = 0.016$) compared with placebo.[68] This suggests that aromatase inhibition of estrogen receptor-positive DCIS could potentially be used to prevent local recurrence. A comparison of tamoxifen with anastrozole (a third-generation aromatase inhibitor), after complete excision of DCIS, is being tested in the IBIS II trial.

# Follow-up and prognosis

Following primary treatment for DCIS and radiological and pathological confirmation that there has been complete excision of all suspicious microcalcifications with clear margins, patients should be given the opportunity to participate in clinical trials. Follow-up in outpatient clinics, after the initial postoperative reviews, should be by annual bilateral two-view mammography to detect recurrence. Although most DCIS recurrence is impalpable, clinical examination may be important for detecting invasive recurrences, especially in the premenopausal breast. Breast cancer-specific mortality following breast-conserving surgery for DCIS is low at less than 2% at 10 years and is not influenced by adjuvant radiotherapy.[69] This figure is similar to that following mastectomy for DCIS.

# Management of recurrence

## In situ recurrence

Patients with an in situ recurrence where the primary was treated with breast-conserving surgery alone can be offered re-excision (ensuring clear margins) followed by postoperative radiotherapy. Patients who have already received radiotherapy following their primary excision should be advised to have completion mastectomy. A skin-sparing mastectomy with a myocutaneous flap breast reconstruction gives excellent results.

## Invasive recurrence

The management of invasive recurrence is again dependent on the initial therapy for DCIS. If the patient did not receive radiotherapy after initial DCIS excision, then wide local excision and radiotherapy may still be an option depending on the size and location of the invasive tumour. If wide local excision is not an option, then mastectomy and axillary staging is the treatment of choice, with adjuvant therapy dictated by the standard protocols for primary invasive cancers. Studies following salvage treatment for both in situ and invasive recurrences of DCIS have shown overall

cause-specific survival rates in excess of 90% at 8 years after recurrence.[51]

# DCIS of the male breast

DCIS accounts for 1.9–15% of breast cancers in men. It usually presents clinically with symptoms of a retro-areola cystic-type mass or bloody nipple discharge. The clinical, rather than mammographic, detection possibly accounts for the different incidence of DCIS between men and women. The predominant histological subtypes in pure DCIS in men are papillary and cribrifrom, the standard treatment being total mastectomy with excision of the nipple–areola complex.[70] Pure DCIS is nearly all of low or intermediate grade; less than 3% of cases are high grade.[69] In a series of 114 patients, 84 with pure DCIS and 30 with DCIS and invasive cancer, there were no cases of high-grade comedo DCIS without an invasive tumour.[71] The percentage of men with DCIS that eventually develop an invasive cancer is not known.

# The future

## Radiotherapy trials

The benefits of radiotherapy following breast-conserving surgery for DCIS are now clear, although clarification is needed as to which subsets of women definitely do or do not require radiotherapy. The role of boost in addition to whole breast radiotherapy, particularly in younger women, needs further study. A UK trial has been proposed with the aim of studying the need for radiotherapy in women with estrogen receptor-positive low/intermediate-grade disease who are receiving adjuvant systemic hormonal therapy following local excision with clear margins.

## Chemoprevention trials

The aim of adjuvant therapy for in situ breast cancer is the prevention of progression to invasive malignancy. The NSABP P-1 chemoprevention trial[72] compared tamoxifen to placebo in patients at high risk of breast cancer. The study reported a 49% reduction in incidence of invasive cancer and a 50% reduction of DCIS in the tamoxifen-treated group. The reduction in contralateral breast cancer was only seen in estrogen receptor-positive cases and no benefit was seen for estrogen receptor-negative patients. There is also interest in the potential use of aromatase inhibitors, which have a better side-effect profile than tamoxifen. The IBIS II trial, currently underway, randomises postmenopausal women with estrogen receptor-positive DCIS treated with breast-conserving surgery to receive tamoxifen (20 mg daily) or the aromatase inhibitor anastrozole (1 mg daily) for 5 years. It also stratifies women between anastrozole and placebo for high-risk postmenopausal chemoprevention.

The results of the NSABP B-35 trial, which compared tamoxifen versus anastrozole in postmenopausal women following breast-conserving surgery and radiotherapy for DCIS, are awaited.[73] The Canadian-based RTOG 98-04 trial is studying women with 'good-risk' DCIS (unicentric, low/intermediate grade, ≤2.5 cm) with clear margins following breast-conserving surgery and randomising them to receive tamoxifen alone or tamoxifen and radiotherapy.

## UK National DCIS audit (Sloane Project)

The Sloane Project aims to audit all screen-detected DCIS in the UK over the course of 5 years. This will potentially collect data on 2000 cases per year. All 98 screening units in the country are expected to take part. For each case the clinical, pathological, radiological and treatment characteristics are being documented following the NHS Breast Screening Programme guidelines. The aim is then to correlate these with clinical outcomes – specifically recurrence and invasive cancer development.

## Novel therapies

A number of new classes of agent are being developed for use in chemoprevention or therapy for DCIS. The compounds targeted are selective blockers of either the estrogen receptor-dependent or the estrogen receptor-independent growth pathways (see Fig. 11.1) and include selective estrogen receptor down-regulators, new aromatase inhibitors (which prevent estrogen biosynthesis by inhibiting the conversion of adrenal androgens to estrogens), signal transduction inhibitors (e.g. EGFR tyrosine kinase inhibitors, RAS farnesylation transferase inhibitors, MAP kinase inhibitors) and COX-2 inhibitors. If disrupted, the RAS/MAP kinase pathway may have a strong chemopreventive/chemotherapeutic effect and is an important target pathway in estrogen-independent (estrogen receptor-negative) tumours. Treatment of human DCIS xenografts with the EGFR/tyrosine kinase inhibitor Iressa has been shown to inhibit cell proliferation and MAP kinase activation.[74] Farnesyltransferase inhibitors (e.g. R115777, which blocks the farnesylation step in the RAS activation pathway[75]) are also being investigated; HER-2 also signals via RAS activation and around 60% of DCIS express HER-2. Due to the possible protective effect of HER4 (c-erbB-4) on recurrence, 'selective c-erb receptor' inhibition, rather than 'pan c-erb receptor' blockade, may be an ultimate goal when precise pathways of action are known. COX-2 inhibitors (e.g. celecoxib) have been shown to prevent tumour formation in *HER2* transgenic mice; they have been found to be pro-apoptotic, anti-angiogeneic and anti-lymphangiogeneic,[76] but in a small preoperative trial celecoxib did not affect proliferation or apoptosis.[14,68]

## Optimising treatment

Controversies regarding the optimum management of this heterogeneous preinvasive lesion still reign. The surgeon should ensure complete pathological and radiological excision of DCIS and discuss appropriate adjuvant therapy (radiotherapy or endocrine) with the patient in a multidisciplinary setting in order to minimise recurrence without overtreatment.

## Key points

- DCIS is a preinvasive breast tumour; the proliferation of malignant epithelial cells is confined within an intact basement membrane. The developmental pathway for low- and intermediate-grade DCIS is different from that for high-grade DCIS.
- DCIS accounts for approximately 25% of new screen-detected cancers.
- Small localised areas of DCIS (<4 cm) should be treated with breast-conserving surgery with or without radiotherapy. Larger lesions need to be treated by mastectomy. Axillary surgery should be avoided.
- Up to 13% of cases recur at 5 years following breast-conserving surgery and radiotherapy, 50% of which (i.e. up to 6.5% of all cases) may be invasive disease.
- The key factor for decreasing tumour recurrence is clear margins at the time of surgery.
- Bad prognostic factors include younger age at diagnosis (<40 years), poorly differentiated high-grade tumours, the presence of comedo necrosis, HER2 positivity and estrogen receptor negativity.
- Tamoxifen is not indicated after mastectomy for DCIS but is valuable in estrogen receptor-positive lesions treated by breast-conserving surgery.

# References

1. Schwartz GF, Solin LJ, Olivotto IA et al. and the consensus conference committee. The consensus conference on the treatment of in situ ductal carcinoma of the breast, 22–25 April 1999. Cancer 2000; 88:946–54.

2. Lagios MD. Heterogeneity of ductal carcinoma in situ of the breast. J Cell Biochem Suppl 1993; 17G:49–52.

3. Rakovitch E. Part 1. Epidemiology of ductal carcinoma in situ. Curr Probl Cancer 2000; 24:100–11.

4. Williams G, Anderson E, Howell A et al. Oral contraceptive (OCP) use increases proliferation and decreases oestrogen receptor content of epithelial cells in the normal human breast. Int J Cancer 1991; 48:206–10.

5. Hofseth LJ, Raafat AM, Osuch JR et al. Hormone replacement therapy with oestrogen or oestrogen plus medroxyprogesterone acetate is associated with increased epithelial proliferation in the normal post-menopausal breast. J Clin Endocrinol Metab 1999; 84:4559–65.

6. Schairer C, Byrne C, Keyl PM et al. Menopausal estrogen and estrogen–progestin replacement therapy and the risk of breast cancer (United States). Cancer Causes Control 1994; 5:491–500.

7. Longnecker MP, Bernstein L, Paganini-Hill A et al. Risk factors for in situ breast cancer. Cancer Epidemiol Biomarkers Prev 1996; 5:961–5.

8. Henrick JB, Kornguth PJ, Viscoli CM et al. Postmenopausal estrogen use and invasive versus in situ breast cancer risk. J Clin Epidemiol 1998; 51:1277–83.

9. Gapstur SM, Morrow M, Sellars TA. Hormone replacement therapy and risk of breast cancer with a favourable histology: results of the Iowa Women's Health Study. JAMA 1999; 281:2091–7.

10. Julien J, Bijker N, Fentimen I et al. Radiotherapy in breast-conserving treatment for ductal carcinoma in situ: first results of the EORTC randomized phase III trial 10853. EORTC Breast Cancer Cooperative Group and EORTC Radiotherapy Group. Lancet 2000; 355:528–33.

    The results of a multicentre, randomised, controlled trial of 1010 patients with DCIS treated with breast-conserving surgery, randomised to receive no further treatment or radiotherapy. The study found that radiotherapy reduced overall invasive (40% reduction, $P = 0.04$) and non-invasive (35% reduction, $P = 0.06$) ipsilateral recurrences (median follow-up 4.25 years).

11. Bijker N, Peterse JL, Duchateau L et al. Histological type and marker expression of the primary tumour compared with its local recurrence after breast-conserving therapy for ductal carcinoma in situ. Br J Cancer 2001; 84:539–44.

12. Page DL, Dupont WD, Rogers LW et al. Continued local recurrence of carcinoma 15–25 years after a diagnosis of low grade ductal carcinoma in situ of the breast treated only by biopsy. Cancer 1995; 76:1197–200.

13. Yen M-F, Tabár L, Vitak B et al. Quantifying the potential problem of over diagnosis of ductal carcinoma in situ in breast cancer screening. Eur J Cancer 2003; 39:1746–54.

14. Farnie G, Clarke RB, Spence K et al. Novel cell culture technique for primary ductal carcinoma in situ: role of Notch and epidermal growth factor receptor signaling pathways. J Natl Cancer Inst 2007; 99:616–27.

15. Silverstein MJ, Lagios MD, Craig PH et al. A prognostic index for ductal carcinoma in situ of the breast. Cancer 1996; 77:2267–74.

16. Pathology reporting in breast cancer, 2nd edn. Sheffield: National Health Service Breast Screening Programme Publications, Report No. 3, 1995; pp. 22–7.

17. Holland R, Hendriks JH, Vebeek AL et al. Extent, distribution, and mammographic/histological correlations of breast ductal carcinoma in situ. Lancet 1990; 335:519–22.

18. Steering Committee on Clinical Practice Guidelines for the Care and Treatment of Breast Cancer. The management of ductal carcinoma in situ (DCIS). Can Med Assoc J 1998; 158(Suppl):S27–34.

19. Faverley DRG, Burgers L, Bult P et al. Three dimensional imaging of mammary ductal carcinoma in situ: clinical implications. Semin Diagn Pathol 1994; 11:193–8.

20. Holland PA, Ghandi A, Knox WF et al. The importance of complete excision in the prevention of local recurrence of ductal carcinoma in situ. Br J Cancer 1998; 77:110–14.

21. Kerner H, Lichtig C. Lobular cancerisation: incidence and differential diagnosis with lobular carcinoma in situ of the breast. Histopathology 1986; 10:621.

22. Fischer ER. Pathobiological considerations relating to the treatment of carcinoma of the breast. CA 1996; 47:52.

23. Eusebi V, Collina G, Bussolati G. Carcinoma in situ in sclerosing adenosis of the breast. An immunocytochemical study. Semin Diagn Pathol 1989; 6:146.

24. Youngston BJ, Cranor M, Powell C et al. Epithelial displacement in surgical breast specimens following needling procedures. Am J Surg Pathol 1994; 18:896.

25. Akashi-Tanaka S, Fukotomi T, Nanasawa T et al. Treatment of non-invasive carcinoma: fifteen-year results at the National Cancer Centre Hospital in Tokyo. Breast Cancer 2000; 7:341–4.

26. Dunn BK, Ford LG. Breast cancer prevention: results of the National Surgical Adjuvant Breast and Bowel Project (NSABP) breast cancer prevention trial (NSABP P-1: BCPT). Eur J Cancer 2000; 36(Suppl 4):49–50.

27. Millis RR, Bobrow LG, Barnes DM. Immuno-histochemical evaluation of biological markers in mammary carcinoma in situ: correlation with morphological features and recently proposed schemes for histological classification. Breast 1996; 5:113–22.

28. Sullivan RP, Mortimer G, Muircheartaigh IO. Cell proliferation in breast tumours: analysis of histological parameters Ki67 and PCNA expression. Ir J Med Sci 1993; 162:343–7.

29. Boland GP Knox WF, Bundred NJ. Molecular markers and therapeutic targets in ductal carcinoma in situ. Microsc Res Tech 2002; 59:3–11.

30. Shoker BS, Jarvis C, Clarke RB et al. Estrogen receptor-positive proliferating cells in the normal and pre-cancerous breast. Am J Pathol 1999; 155:1811–15.

31. Parton M, Dowsett M, Smith I. Studies of apoptosis in breast cancer. Br Med J 2001; 322:1528–32.

32. Weinstat-Saslow D, Merino MJ, Manrow RE et al. Overexpression of cyclin D mRNA distinguishes invasive and in situ breast carcinomas from non-malignant lesions. Nat Med 1995; 1:1257–60.

33. Zhou Q, Hopp T, Fuqua SA et al. Cyclin D1 in breast pre-malignancy and early breast cancer: implications for prevention and treatment. Cancer Lett 2001; 162:3–17.

34. Soslow RA, Dannenberg AJ, Rush D et al. COX-2 is expressed in human pulmonary, colonic and mammary tumours. Cancer 2000; 89:2637–45.

35. Ristimaki A, Sivula A, Lundin J et al. Prognostic significance of elevated COX-2 expression in breast cancer. Cancer Res 2002; 62:632–5.

36. Helcynska K, Kronblad Å, Jögi A et al. Hypoxia induces a dedifferentiated phenotype in ductal carcinoma in situ. Cancer Res 2003; 63:1441–4.

37. Dershaw DD, Abramson MD, Kinne DW. Ductal carcinoma in situ: mammographic findings and clinical implications. Radiology 1989; 170:411–15.

38. Ikeda DM, Andersson I. Ductal carcinoma in situ: atypical mammographic appearances. Radiology 1989; 172:661–6.

39. Schuh ME, Nemoto T, Penetrante RB et al. Intraductal carcinoma. Analysis of presentation, pathologic findings, and outcome of disease. Arch Surg 1986; 121:1303–7.

40. Silverstein MJ, Parker R, Grotting JC et al. Ductal carcinoma in situ (DCIS) of the breast: diagnostic and therapeutic controversies. J Am Coll Surg 2001; 192:196–214.

41. Lee CH, Carter D, Philpotts LE et al. Ductal carcinoma in situ diagnosed with stereotactic core needle biopsy: can invasion be predicted?. Radiology 2000; 217:466–70.

42. Blamey RW. The British Association of Surgical Oncology Guidelines for surgeons in the management of symptomatic breast disease in the UK (1998 revision). BASO Breast Speciality Group. Eur J Surg Oncol 1998; 24:464–76.

43. Chan KC, Knox WF, Sinha G et al. Extent of excision margin width required in breast conserving surgery for ductal carcinoma in situ. Cancer 2001; 91:9–16.

44. Silverstein MJ, Barth A, Poller DN et al. Ten year results comparing mastectomy to excision and radiation therapy for ductal carcinoma in situ of the breast. Eur J Cancer 1995; 31A:1425–7.

45. Fonseca R, Hartmenn L, Petersen I et al. Ductal carcinoma in situ of the breast. Ann Intern Med 1997; 127:1013–22.

46. Kitchen PR, Cawson JN, Krishnan CM et al. Axillary dissection and ductal carcinoma in situ of the breast: a change in practice. Aust NZ J Surg 2000; 70:419–22.

47. Veronesi P, Intra M, Vento AR et al. Sentinel lymph node biopsy for localised ductal carcinoma in situ? Breast 2005; 14(6):520–2.

48. Julian TB, Land SR, Fourchotte V et al. Is sentinel node biopsy necessary in conservatively treated DCIS? Ann Surg Oncol 2007; 14(8):2202–8.

49. Ottesen GL, Graversen HP, Blichert-Toft M et al. Carcinoma in situ of the female breast. 10 year follow-up result of a prospective nationwide study. Breast Cancer Res Treat 2000; 62:197–210.

50. Fisher ER, Dignam J, Tan-Chiu E et al. Pathologic findings from the National Surgical Adjuvant Breast Project (NSABP) eight-year update of Protocol B-17: intraductal carcinoma. Cancer 1999; 86:429–38.

The 8-year update of 623 women in a randomised controlled trial of 814 women with DCIS treated with local excision who were randomised to receive radiotherapy or no additional treatment. The study found that women who received additional radiotherapy following breast-conserving surgery had a significant reduction in ipsilateral breast tumours (31% vs. 13% at 8 years, $P = 0.0001$). The authors also analysed a range of clinico-pathological characteristics of the patients and the tumours to assess predictors of recurrence; findings suggested that the presence of comedo necrosis was an independent risk factor for recurrence.

51. Solin LJ, Fourquet A, Vincini FA et al. Salvage treatment for local recurrence after breast-conserving surgery and radiation as initial treatment for mammographically detected carcinoma in situ of the breast. Cancer 2001; 91:1090–7.

52. Waldman FM, DeVries S, Chew KL et al. Chromosomal alterations in ductal carcinomas in situ and their in situ recurrences. J Natl Cancer Inst 2000; 92:313–20.

53. Boland GP, Chan KC, Knox WF et al. Value of the Van Nuys Prognostic Index in prediction of recurrence of ductal carcinoma in situ after breast-conserving surgery. Br J Surg 2003; 90:426–32.

54. Fisher B, Dignam J, Wolmark N et al. Tamoxifen in the treatment of intraductal breast cancer: National Surgical Adjuvant Breast and Bowel Project B-24 randomised controlled trial. Lancet 1999; 353:1993–2000.

Double-blind, randomised, controlled trial of 1804 women with completely or incompletely excised DCIS at breast-conserving surgery who were randomised to receive radiotherapy plus or minus tamoxifen. The women receiving tamoxifen had fewer breast cancer events at 5 years compared with placebo (8.2 vs. 13.4, $P = 0.0009$), mainly due to a decrease in invasive cancer in the ipsilateral breast. A retrospective review of the results (Ref. 68) showed that this benefit was confined to estrogen receptor-positive cases.

55. Fisher B, Constantino J, Redmond C et al. Lumpectomy compared with lumpectomy and radiation therapy for the treatment of intraductal breast cancer. N Engl J Med 1993; 328:1581–6.

56. Bijker N, Peterse JL, Duchateau L et al. Risk factors for recurrence and metastasis after breast conserving therapy for ductal carcinoma in situ: analysis of EORTC trial. J Clin Oncol 2001; 19:2263–71.

A review of 843 women of the 1010 randomised cases from the EORTC 10853 trial (local excision of DCIS plus or minus radiotherapy) that examined the clinico-pathological characteristics of the women. The authors found that clear margins were the most important factor in reducing local recurrence (hazard ratio 2.07, $P = 0.0008$). Patients with poorly differentiated DCIS were at higher risk of metastatic disease (hazard ratio 6.57, $P = 0.01$) and other poor prognostic factors included young age (<40 years) at diagnosis (hazard ratio 2.14, $P = 0.02$) and symptomatic detection (hazard ratio 1.8, $P = 0.008$).

57. Fraser J, Raza S, Chorny K et al. Columnar alteration with prominent apical snouts and secretions: a spectrum of changes frequently present in breast biopsies with microcalcifications. Am J Surg Pathol 1998; 22:1521–7.

58. UK Coordinating Committee on Cancer Research (UKCCCR). Ductal Carcinoma In Situ (DCIS) Working Party on behalf of DCIS trialists in the UK, Australia and New Zealand. Radiotherapy and tamoxifen in women with completely excised ductal carcinoma in situ of the breast in the UK, Australia and New Zealand: randomised controlled trial. Lancet 2003; 362:95–103.

A 2 × 2 factorial design, randomised controlled trial of 1701 screen-detected patients with completely excised DCIS, randomised to receive tamoxifen, radiotherapy, both treatments or none. The authors found that radiotherapy reduced the incidence of both ipsilateral invasive recurrence (hazard ratio 0.45, $P = 0.01$) and DCIS recurrence (hazard ratio 0.36, $P = 0.0004$). Tamoxifen reduced overall DCIS recurrence (hazard ratio 0.68, $P = 0.03$) but not invasive disease. The trial has not yet published results with regard to estrogen receptor status.

59. Rodrigues N, Dillon D, Parisot N et al. Differences in the pathologic and molecular features of intraductal breast carcinoma between younger and older women. Cancer 2003; 97:1393–403.

60. Silverstein MJ. The University of Southern California/Van Nuys Prognostic Index for ductal carcinoma in situ of the breast. Am J Surg 2003; 186:337–43.

61. Provenzano E, Hopper JL, Giles GG et al. Biological markers that predict clinical recurrence in ductal carcinoma in situ of the breast. Eur J Cancer 2003; 39:622–30.

62. Witton CJ, Reeves JR, Going JJ et al. Expression of the HER1–4 family of receptor tyrosine kinases in breast cancer. J Pathol 2003; 200:290–7.

63. Suo Z, Risberg B, Kalsson M et al. EGFR family expression in breast carcinomas. C-erbB-2 and c-erbB-4 have different effects on survival. J Pathol 2002; 196:17–25.

64. Barnes NLP, Khavari S, Boland GP et al. Absence of HER4 expression predicts recurrence of ductal carcinoma in situ of the breast. Clin Cancer Res 2005; 11:2163–8.

65. Bijker N, Meijnen P, Peterse JL et al. Breast-conserving treatment with or without radiotherapy in ductal carcinoma-in-situ: ten-year results of European Organisation for Research and Treatment of Cancer randomized phase III trial 10853 – a study by the EORTC Breast Cancer Cooperative Group and EORTC Radiotherapy Group. J Clin Oncol 2006; 24(21):3381–7.

66. Allred DC, Bryant J, Land S et al. Estrogen receptor expression as a predictive marker of the effectiveness of tamoxifen in the treatment of intraductal breast cancer: findings from NSABP Protocol B-24 (abstract). Breast Cancer Res Treat 2002; 76(Suppl 1):S36.

67. Boland GP, McKeowan A, Chan KC et al. Biological response to hormonal manipulation in oestrogen receptor positive ductal carcinoma in situ of the breast. Br J Cancer 2003; 89:277–83.

68. Bundred NJ, Cramer A, Cheung KL et al. ERISAC trial: evidence exemestane effects oestrogen receptor (ER) positive ductal carcinoma in situ (DCIS) proliferation. Breast Cancer Res Treat 2007; 106(Suppl 1):S5043.

69. Allred DC, Mohsin SK, Fuqua SA. Histological and biological evolution of human premalignant breast disease. Endocr Relat Cancer 2001; 8:47–61.

70. Simmons RM. Male ductal carcinoma in situ presenting as bloody nipple discharge: a case report and literature review. Breast J 2002; 8:112–14.

71. Hittmair AP, Liniger RA, Tavassoli FA. Ductal carcinoma in situ (DCIS) in the male breast. A morphological study of 84 cases of pure DCIS and 30 cases of DCIS associated with invasive carcinoma: a preliminary report. Cancer 1998; 83:2139–49.

72. Fisher B, Constantino JP, Wickerman DL et al. Tamoxifen for prevention of breast cancer: report of the National Surgical Adjuvant Breast and Bowel Project P-1 Study. J Natl Cancer Inst 1998; 90:1371–88.

73. Vogel VG, Constantino JP, Wickerham DL et al. National Surgical Adjuvant Breast and Bowel Project Update: prevention trials and endocrine therapy of ductal carcinoma in situ. Clin Cancer Res 2003; 9(Suppl):495s–501s.

74. Chan KC, Knox WF, Ghandi A et al. Blockade of growth factor receptors in ductal carcinoma in situ inhibits epithelial proliferation. Br J Surg 2001; 88:412–18.

75. Johnston S. Farensyl transferase inhibitors: a novel targeted therapy for cancer. Lancet Oncol 2001; 2:18–26.

76. Masferrer JL, Leaky KM, Koki AT et al. Antiangiogenic and anti-tumour activities of COX-2 inhibitors. Cancer Res 2000; 60:1306–11.

# 12

# The role of adjuvant systemic therapy in patients with operable breast cancer

Ian E. Smith
Monica Arnedos

## Introduction

The mortality from breast cancer has fallen by over 15% in the UK over the last 15 years, and this has occurred in the face of a rising incidence. This fall coincides with the widespread national uptake of adjuvant systemic therapy and increasing evidence of its survival benefit. The basis for this treatment is that over half of women with operable breast cancer who receive local regional treatment alone will die from metastatic disease, indicating the presence of micrometastases at the time of initial clinical presentation. Traditionally, the major risk factors for recurrence have been the involvement of axillary nodes, poor histological grade, large tumour size and histological evidence of lymphovascular invasion around the tumour site. The absence of estrogen and progesterone receptor and the overexpression of human epidermal growth factor receptor 2 (HER-2) also carry an adverse prognosis. The only way to improve survival for these women is to administer effective systemic medical treatment, using endocrine therapy, chemotherapy and targeted biological therapies, combined with locoregional treatment by surgery and radiotherapy. More recently, gene expression has emerged as a new determinant of recurrence risk and a major current challenge is to assimilate this new technology into treatment planning.

## Adjuvant endocrine therapy

Approximately 75% of invasive breast cancer patients present with hormone receptor-positive disease.[1] As the estrogen receptor (ER) pathway is key to the growth of these cancers, modulation of ER activation is an essential component of treatment for these women. Since the observation by Beatson more than 100 years ago that oophorectomy could induce regression of advanced breast cancer,[2] endocrine treatment has been one of the most valuable therapies in cancer medicine.

### Tamoxifen

Until recently tamoxifen has been the standard adjuvant endocrine therapy.

 The results of an overview of tamoxifen trials involving more than 33 000 women carried out by the Early Breast Cancer Trialists' Collaborative Group (EBCTCG) have shown that tamoxifen for about 5 years reduces the risk of recurrence by 11.8% and the absolute risk of death by 9.2%.[3]

The proportional reduction is not significantly affected by age or nodal status; the absolute benefit of course relates to the absolute risk. Tamoxifen is associated with a small but significantly increased incidence of uterine carcinoma (0.13% per year) and of thromboembolism and stroke.

## Tamoxifen duration

The overview data indicate that 5 years of tamoxifen is more effective than less. Until very recently, there was no convincing evidence that more than 5 years of tamoxifen had a further advantage. Indeed, the largest published trial so far of tamoxifen for more than 5 years (National Surgical Adjuvant Breast and Bowel Project (NSABP) B-14) showed that tamoxifen for more than 5 years had an unexpected adverse influence on disease-free survival (DFS; 78% vs. 82% with placebo, P = 0.03) and this was also associated with higher rates of endometrial cancer, ischaemic heart disease and cerebral vascular disease.[4] Recently, however, a much larger international trial involving 11 500 patients, the Adjuvant Tamoxifen Longer Against Shorter (ATLAS) trial, has also addressed the question of long-term tamoxifen duration. Results, so far presented only in abstract, have shown a small but significant further reduction in recurrence with more than 5 years treatment (hazard ratio (HR) 0.88).[5]

## Aromatase inhibitors

### First line

The aromatase inhibitors anastrozole and letrozole have each been shown to improve DFS compared with tamoxifen when given as first-line adjuvant therapy for a planned 5 years in postmenopausal women with hormone receptor-positive early breast cancer[6,7] (**Fig. 12.1**).

In the ATAC (Arimidex, Tamoxifen, Alone or in Combination) trial involving over 9000 women, anastrozole was compared with tamoxifen and with a combination of the two drugs and was shown to be superior to both in terms of DFS. With a median follow-up of 68 months, a 5-year DFS benefit of 2.8% (HR 0.83) has emerged.[7]

In the BIG1-98 trial involving more than 8000 women, letrozole was compared with tamoxifen in a four-arm trial as follows: letrozole monotherapy; tamoxifen monotherapy; sequential tamoxifen then letrozole; sequential letrozole then tamoxifen; all for a total of 5 years. So far the two monotherapy arms show results very similar to those from ATAC

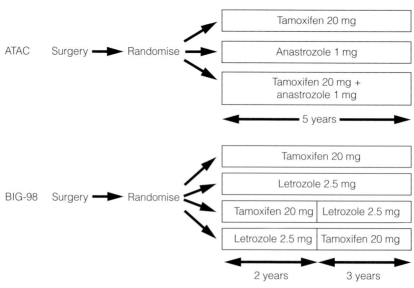

**Figure 12.1** • Schematic of the ATAC and BIG1-98 trials.

and with a median follow-up of 51 months, letrozole resulted in an absolute 5-year DFS improvement of 2.9% over tamoxifen (HR 0.82).[6] Neither trial has so far shown a significant overall survival (OS) improvement (HR 0.97 and 0.91 respectively; Table 12.1).

First-line aromatase inhibitors: bad prognosis subgroups

ER-positive, progesterone receptor (PgR)-negative breast cancers are recognised as having more aggressive features.[8] In the EBCTCG analysis, patients with PgR-poor tumours had a worse prognosis but nevertheless had a similar proportional benefit to adjuvant tamoxifen compared with control.[3]

In an initial analysis of the ATAC trial based on locally defined PgR levels derived from case record forms, the major benefit of anastrozole over tamoxifen was found in patients with a low PgR.[9] A subsequent analysis based on central review confirmed that patients with a low PgR had a worse prognosis, but failed to confirm a relative benefit for anastrozole over tamoxifen.[10] Likewise, in the BIG1-98 trial there was no relative benefit for letrozole over tamoxifen in patients with PgR-negative tumours.[11]

HER-2-positive tumours are recognised as having a worse prognosis and in a neoadjuvant endocrine therapy trial comparing letrozole with tamoxifen, a large and highly significant difference was seen for letrozole over tamoxifen in terms of clinical response in this small subgroup (88% vs. 21%, $P = 0.0004$).[12] In a similar neoadjuvant trial comparing anastrozole with tamoxifen, the IMmediate Preoperative Arimidex Compared with Tamoxifen (IMPACT) trial, a numerically large although non-significant trend was again seen in favour of the aromatase inhibitor for HER-2-positive tumours (58% vs. 22%, $P = 0.09$).[13]

These results were not, however, confirmed in the equivalent adjuvant trials.

 In the ATAC trial there was no evidence of a proportionately greater benefit for anastrozole over tamoxifen in HER-2-positive tumours compared with other subtypes.[10] A similar finding was made for letrozole compared with tamoxifen in the BIG1-98 trial.[11]

Comparative toxicities of front-line anastrozole/letrozole and tamoxifen

The ATAC and BIG1-98 trials have both shown that tamoxifen is associated with a small but significant increase in the incidence of hot flushes compared with anastrozole or letrozole (4.5–5% increase), vaginal bleeding (3.3–3.7% increase), vaginal discharge (8.6% increase), endometrial carcinoma (0.2–0.4% increase) and venous thromboembolism (1.4–2% increase). The ATAC trial has likewise shown a small but significant increase in ischaemic cerebral vascular disease (1.1% increase) with tamoxifen compared with anastrozole, but this has not been confirmed in the BIG1-98 trial with letrozole. In contrast, anastrozole and letrozole have been shown to be associated with a small but statistically significant increase in the incidence of musculoskeletal problems (6.5–8% increase) and fractures (1.7–2.2% increase).

 Of note, tamoxifen is associated with a significant increase in gynaecological surgery compared with either of the aromatase inhibitors. In the ATAC trial 5.1% of women have had hysterectomies compared with 1.3% on anastrozole.[14] In the BIG1-98 trial 288 women (9.1%) have required endometrial biopsies compared with 77 (2.3%) with letrozole.[15]

## Sequential therapy with aromatase inhibitors after tamoxifen

Four trials have so far reported on results following sequential adjuvant aromatase inhibitors 2–3 years after tamoxifen (**Fig. 12.2**). In the first, the Intergroup Exemestane Study (IES), patients who had already been on tamoxifen for around 2 years were randomised double-blind to continuing on tamoxifen or switching to exemestane to complete 5 years treatment.[16] A total of 4274 patients were involved and updated results with a median follow-up of 55.7 months have been published. The event-free survival

Table 12.1 • Results from the ATAC and BIG1-98 trials

|  | ATAC* | BIG1-98† |
|---|---|---|
| No. of patients | 9366 | 8010 |
| Median follow-up (months) | 68 | 51 |
| DFS (hazard ratio) | 0.83 | 0.82 |
| 5-year DFS difference (%) | 2.8 | 2.9 |
| OS (hazard ratio) | 0.97‡ | 0.91‡ |

* Hormone receptor-positive group.
† Only monotherapy groups.
‡ Non-significant.

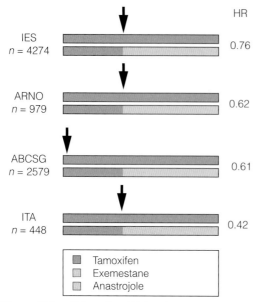

| | | HR |
|---|---|---|
| IES n = 4274 | | 0.76 |
| ARNO n = 979 | | 0.62 |
| ABCSG n = 2579 | | 0.61 |
| ITA n = 448 | | 0.42 |

■ Tamoxifen
□ Exemestane
□ Anastrojole

**Figure 12.2** • Schematic of trials using aromatase inhibitors in sequential therapy.

difference was 3.3% with unadjusted HR 0.76 (95% CI 0.66–0.88, P = 0.0001). In the intention-to-treat (ITT) analysis, there was a 15% relative reduction in risk of death for patients receiving exemestane (HR 0.85, 95% CI 0.71–1.02, P = 0.08). In the subgroup of patients who were ER positive or unknown, the HR was 0.83 (95% CI 0.69–1.00, P = 0.05).

The other three sequential trials involved anastrozole. In the ARNO (Arimidex-Nolvadex 95) and the ITA (Italian Tamoxifen Anastrozole) trials, randomisation was also carried out at the 2- to 3-year point in women remaining in remission on tamoxifen.[17,18] Both of these trials showed a significant reduction in DFS with respective HR of 0.66 (ARNO) and 0.42 (ITA).

The ABCSG (Austrian Breast Cancer Study Group) 8 trial differed from the others in that randomisation was carried out at the start of treatment to 5 years of tamoxifen versus 2 years followed by 3 years of anastrozole. Event-free survival from the point of switching again showed a significant advantage for anastrozole over tamoxifen with an HR of 0.63.[19,20]

These results at first sight suggest superiority to the benefit achieved with first-line aromatase inhibitor therapy in ATAC and BIG1-98. It must, however, be remembered that these trials represent a selective group of patients with some high-risk women already having relapsed. This point is emphasised

in the ABCSG 8 analysis from the start of therapy (at the time of randomisation). The event-free survival difference was only 1.5% at 5 years in this study and was no longer significant (P = 0.07, HR 0.76).[20]

Currently there is therefore no convincing evidence to suggest that a switch policy to aromatase inhibitors after 2 years of tamoxifen is superior to front-line therapy. Two trials are addressing this issue directly. BIG1-98 compares tamoxifen for 2 years followed by letrozole (arm C) with letrozole alone for 5 years (arm B). Likewise, the TEAM (Tamoxifen Exemestane Adjuvant Multinational) trial has an amended design and is comparing tamoxifen for 2–3 years followed by exemestane to complete 5 years with exemestane alone for 5 years.

## Extended adjuvant therapy with aromatase inhibitors

The risk of recurrence of early breast cancer continues for at least 10 years after diagnosis and is greater in patients with hormone receptor-positive cancers.[21] In the EBCTCG overview analysis more than half of breast cancer recurrences occur after the 5-year mark.[3]

Against this background, the results of the MA17 trial evaluating the benefit of extended adjuvant therapy with letrozole in women still in remission after 5 years of tamoxifen were of great importance in that they demonstrated a significant DFS benefit in favour of letrozole.[22] This benefit has continued and indeed increased with duration of therapy with an initial HR of 0.52 (0.40–0.64) 12 months after randomisation, increasing to 0.19 (0.04–0.34) after 48 months.

The optimal duration of adjuvant aromatase inhibitor therapy has not yet been established. It is possible that for some women very lengthy or even lifelong treatment might be the most appropriate, but this has to be balanced against the potential risks of very-long-term usage. Clinical trials are essential in this area. In this context, the MA17 trial is now running a second randomisation for women still in remission after 5 years of letrozole. Other trials are also addressing this key issue, including NSABP B-42 (5 vs. 10 years of letrozole) and ABCG-16 Secondary Adjuvant Long-term Study with Arimidex (SALSA) comparing a further 2 years vs. a further 5 years of adjuvant treatment with anastrozole after an initial 5 years of adjuvant endocrine therapy.

## Other aromatase inhibitor issues

Aromatase inhibitors are contraindicated in pre-menopausal women. The temptation, however, has been to extrapolate these results to younger women following chemotherapy-induced amenorrhoea.

In an audit carried out at The Royal Marsden Hospital, 12 of 45 younger women (27%), median age 47, treated with an aromatase inhibitor following chemotherapy-induced amenorrhoea (27%) developed clinical or biochemical return of ovarian function (including up to the age of 53 years).[23]

Aromatase inhibitors should therefore be used with great caution in this group of women and ideally serum estradiol should be monitored using a high sensitivity assay.

Vaginal dryness, atrophy and dyspareunia are significant issues in women on aromatase inhibitors. In a small study 6 of 7 women given vaginal estradiol while on an aromatase inhibitor developed a significant rise in serum estradiol from less than 5 pmol/L to a mean of 72 pmol/L (maximum 219 pmol/L) at 2 weeks.[24] Vaginal estrogen preparations should not be used with caution in women on aromatase inhibitors unless serum estradiol levels can be monitored with a high sensitivity assay.

# Endocrine therapy in premenopausal women

In premenopausal women, the emphasis has often been more on adjuvant chemotherapy than on endocrine therapy. Recently, however, there has been renewed interest in the value of ovarian ablation in addition to chemotherapy or tamoxifen, or both. A key current question for all women with hormone receptor-positive disease is to determine which groups do not require chemotherapy and can be adequately treated with endocrine therapy alone.

The 2005 EBCTCG overview analysis reports on almost 8000 women under the age of 50 with ER-positive or ER unknown disease randomised into trials of ovarian suppression (surgery, irradiation or luteinising hormone-releasing hormone analogues). These show a reduction in the risk of

recurrence of around 11.5% after 20 years of follow-up (2P < 0.000001) in women who did not also receive chemotherapy, but a reduction of only 0.6% (2P = 0.04) in women treated with chemotherapy as well.[3]

Some trials have suggested that ovarian suppression with goserelin is as effective as adjuvant chemotherapy with CMF (cyclophosphamide, metothrexate and 5-fluorouracil) in young women with ER-positive disease (e.g. ZEBRA, ABCSG 5).[25,26]

CMF is no longer optimal adjuvant chemotherapy, but these trials nevertheless raise the important issue of which women with hormone receptor-positive disease, both premenopausal and postmenopausal, will benefit from endocrine therapy alone, without the addition of chemotherapy. There are several approaches to this problem. The ATAC trial, as reported above, shows a striking correlation between the degree of PgR positivity and long-term outcome. It has been suggested that the degree of proliferation as assessed by Ki67 before treatment or indeed after 2 weeks of endocrine therapy may also correlate well with long-term outcome.[27] Another approach involves gene expression microarray as a predictor of outcome[28,29] and trials are planned to test this hypothesis (e.g. MINDACT, TAILOR X).

The converse question, addressing the need for ovarian suppression in addition to chemotherapy and/or tamoxifen, is also a key current issue in the management of premenopausal breast cancer. In the INT-101 trial, the addition of goserelin and tamoxifen to standard adjuvant therapy with CAF (cyclophosphamide, adriamycin and fluorouracil) significantly improved DFS.[30] The gain was most marked in women under the age of 40 and specifically in those who failed to achieve amenorrhoea after chemotherapy alone (40% 9-year DFS vs. 55% with the addition of goserelin and 64% with the addition of goserelin and tamoxifen).

A prospective trial, SOFT (Suppression of Ovarian Function), is currently addressing this question; 3000 premenopausal women with hormone-receptor positive disease are being randomised to tamoxifen alone for 5 years or tamoxifen with ovarian suppression, or exemestane for 5 years with ovarian suppression, either after chemotherapy in women who are still menstruating or in women who have not received chemotherapy. This trial also addresses the important question of whether an aromatase inhibitor is superior to tamoxifen in premenopausal patients who have undergone ovarian suppression.

# Chapter 12

## Adjuvant chemotherapy

Adjuvant chemotherapy is of major importance in the treatment of early breast cancer.

 The 2005 Oxford Overview analysis[3] has shown that combination chemotherapy reduces the proportional annual risk of recurrence by almost 25% and risk of death by around 17%.

The absolute reduction in risk of recurrence for women under 50 is 12.3% after 15 years (53.5% control vs. 41.5% treated) and 10% for breast cancer mortality (42.4% vs. 32.4%). Women over the age of 50 have a smaller benefit, with a 4% reduction in risk of recurrence and a 3% reduction in breast cancer mortality. Most of the effect of adjuvant chemotherapy on the risk of recurrence is seen within the first 5 years after randomisation.

However, the crucial factor with adjuvant chemotherapy is patient selection. For some subgroups the benefit is very much larger than this and for others smaller. Adjuvant chemotherapy began in women with involved nodes for whom recurrence risk was highest. It is now clear that many women with node-negative disease also benefit; conversely, it is likely that some with node-positive disease do not. Currently a great deal of research is focused on identifying with more precision than in the past which patients are likely to benefit from chemotherapy and, particularly in those with estrogen receptor-positive cancers, for whom adjuvant endocrine therapy is also of benefit.

## Age and chemotherapy

Younger women in general gain more from chemotherapy compared with women who are older. Women under 40 achieve a 40% reduction in the risk of recurrence and a 29% reduction in mortality. The benefit reduces with each decade. In the 60–69 age group the proportional reduction in recurrence is only 13% and in mortality 9%, and so far there is no evidence from the Overview of a significant benefit in those over 70 (although the numbers are small).

## Nodal status

In the early years, adjuvant chemotherapy tended to be reserved for patients with axillary node involvement on the basis of higher risk. It is now clear that the proportional reduction in the risk of recurrence is similar for those with node-negative as for node-positive disease (rate ratio for recurrence in women under 50 is 0.64 if node negative and 0.63 if node positive; respective values for women 50 or over are 0.72 and 0.70) and many patients with node-negative disease also gain significant benefit. Nevertheless, since the absolute risk is greater in women with node-positive disease, so is the absolute benefit. Thus in women aged less than 50 the absolute reduction in the risk of recurrence with node-positive disease is 14.6% compared with 9.9% for node-negative disease.

## ER status

There has been considerable controversy over the years as to whether patients with ER-positive disease gain as much from adjuvant chemotherapy as those whose tumours are ER negative. The most recent Oxford Overview data with 15-year follow-up indicate that the proportional benefits are very similar, at least in younger women. In those less than 50 the proportional reduction in recurrence risk for ER-poor tumours is 39% compared with 44% for ER-positive tumours.

In contrast, in older women aged 50–69 there is the suggestion that those with ER-poor tumours gain more with a proportional reduction in recurrence of 33% compared with only 16% for those with ER-positive tumours, although the errors overlap.

## Chemotherapy in the presence of tamoxifen

 The Overview indicates an additional benefit for combination chemotherapy over tamoxifen alone for ER-positive tumours, but again more so for younger than for older women. In those under the age of 50 the additional proportional reduction in recurrence was 36%, with a 5-year absolute gain of 7.6%. In older women aged 50–69 the additional proportional reduction was 15% with tamoxifen given concurrently and 23% when given sequentially, with an absolute 5-year gain of 4.9%.

## Anthracycline-based chemotherapy

For the last decade or more, anthracyclines have replaced older CMF regimens.

The 2005 Overview data, including trials involving a total of around 40 000 women, indicate an additional proportional risk reduction of recurrence of around 11% and a proportional reduction in mortality of around 16%. This equates to an absolute reduction in the risk of recurrence and mortality of around 3% in 5 years and 4% in 10 years.

Since this overview, other supportive studies have confirmed the benefit of anthracycline-based therapy.[31,32]

For example, in the UK, the National Epirubicin Adjuvant Trial (NEAT) and the BR9601 trial compared either six cycles of classic CMF (cyclophosphamide 100 mg/m$^2$ orally for 14 days or 600 mg/m$^2$ i.v. on days 1 and 8, methotrexate 40 mg/m$^2$ and fluorouracil 600 mg/m$^2$ i.v. on days 1 and 8) (NEAT) or eight cycles of modified CMF (cyclophosphamide 750 mg/m$^2$, methotrexate 50 mg/m$^2$ and fluorouracil 600 mg/m$^2$ i.v. every 3 weeks) with four cycles of epirubicin 100 mg/m$^2$ followed by four cycles of the same CMF.[33] The joint analysis of the 2391 eligible patients after a 2-year follow-up reported a benefit in favour of the anthracycline combination arm compared with the CMF treatment group in terms of median relapse-free survival (RFS) (91% vs. 85%; HR 0.69, 0.95% CI 0.58–0.82, P < 0.001) and OS (95% vs. 92%; HR 0.67, 95% CI 0.55–0.82, P < 0.001).

In a multivariate analysis, prognostic factors associated with RFS and OS were nodal status, tumour grade and size, treatment administered and ER status. In relation to adverse events there was more severe alopecia, more nausea (15% vs. 7%) and more vomiting (12% vs. 4%) in the anthracycline arm. No differences were reported for fatigue, infection, neutropenia or neutropenic sepsis. Deaths attributed to chemotherapy were higher in the CMF-alone arm (14 vs. 6), and all the six deaths in the combined arm occurred while on the CMF treatment.

A randomised trial conducted by the National Cancer Institute of Canada Clinical Trials Group (NCIC-CTG) compared CEF (cyclophosphamide 75 mg/m$^2$ orally on days 1–14, epirubicin 60 mg/m$^2$ i.v. on days 1 and 8 and fluorouracil 500 mg/m$^2$ on days 1 and 8) with classic CMF (cyclophosphamide 100 mg/m$^2$ orally on days 1–14, methotrexate 40 mg/m$^2$ i.v. on days 1 and 8, and fluorouracil 600 mg/m$^2$ i.v. on days 1 and 8).[32] A total of 716 pre- or perimenopausal women with axillary involvement were included. After a median follow-up of 59 months

there was a benefit in RFS and OS for patients receiving the CEF regimen, with a 29% relative risk reduction in recurrence (P = 0.009) and a 19% relative reduction in mortality (P = 0.03). This benefit was associated with more acute toxicity in the CEF arm, with more alopecia, nausea, vomiting and febrile neutropenia than the CMF regimen. There was also an increase in the incidence of acute myelogenous leukaemia for the patients receiving this high-dose anthracycline regimen; this issue is discussed below.

## Dose of anthracyclines

The two main anthracyclines in current use are adriamycin (doxorubicin) and epirubicin.

The Cancer and Leukaemia Group B (CALGB) 9344 trial randomised women with node-positive breast cancer to receive four courses of anthracycline chemotherapy to one of three different adriamycin dose levels (60, 75 or 90 mg/m$^2$), followed by four cycles of paclitaxel or not (see below).[34] This important dose escalation trial showed no benefit for adriamycin doses above 60 mg/m$^2$ and this dose should now be considered standard.

With epirubicin, a dose effect was shown in the French Adjuvant Study Group (FASG) 05 trial that randomised lymph node-positive women with poor prognosis in favour of six cycles of FEC100 (epirubicin 100 mg/m$^2$) over six cycles of FEC50 (epirubicin 50 mg/m$^2$).[35] A significant improvement in the DFS (66.3 months vs. 54.8 months) and 5-year OS (77.4% vs. 65.3%) was seen in the FEC100 group but there were significantly more toxicities in the FEC100 group. These included neutropenia, anaemia, nausea and vomiting, stomatitis, alopecia and grade 3 infections. It is important to note that this trial did not determine that an epirubicin dose of 100 mg/m$^2$ is optimal. All that can be concluded is that 50 mg/m$^2$ is suboptimal and that some dose between the two gives the best balance between efficacy and toxicity. Further trials addressing optimal epirubicin dose are indicated.

Higher doses of anthracylines have also seemed to be related to long-term complications, including an increased incidence of acute myeloid leukaemia (AML)/myelodysplasia. In the EBC-1/MA.5 study by the NCIC CTG, which used the very high epirubicin dose of 120 mg/m$^2$, a disturbingly high incidence of AML/myelodysplasia was reported (2% at 10 years follow-up).[32]

Cardiotoxicity is a further concern with the anthracyclines. Symptomatic congestive heart failure (CHF) is a rare but very serious complication in patients receiving an anthracycline-based chemotherapy regimen, with an incidence which relates to the cumulative dose received.[36,37] As with secondary AML, there is an association between risk of cardiotoxicity and increasing age. Recent long-term data on cardiac safety in more than 40 000 early breast cancer patients treated with adjuvant anthracycline regimens at an older age have shown an increased risk of cardiotoxicity compared with a non-anthracycline chemotherapy treatment. This was statistically significant in the group of patients aged 66–70, with a 26% increased risk of developing CHF. This difference in rates of CHF continued to increase through more than 10 years of follow-up.[38]

For all these reasons, therefore, it is important to determine whether high doses (90 mg/m² and above) really are more efficacious than moderate doses of around 75 mg/m² to justify the additional toxicity and trials addressing this issue are indicated.

### Anthracyclines and HER-2-positive disease

The CALGB 8541 trial reported in 397 node-positive patients that high expression of HER-2 is associated with benefit from standard doses of doxorubicin (60 mg/m²) but not from lower doses of anthracyclines.[39] In contrast, this dose–response effect was not seen in the majority whose tumours did not overexpress HER-2. An additional cohort of 595 patients showed an even stronger correlation between HER-2 overexpression and CAF with further follow-up.[40]

In a retrospective study of 639 formalin-fixed, paraffin-embedded specimens obtained from 710 premenopausal women with node-positive breast cancer who had received either cyclophosphamide, epirubicin and fluorouracil (CEF) or CMF, *HER2* amplification or overexpression was associated with a poor prognosis regardless of the type of treatment. In patients whose tumours showed amplification of *HER2*, CEF was superior to CMF in terms of RFS (HR 0.52, 95% CI 0.34–0.80, *P* = 0.003) and OS (HR 0.65, 95% CI 0.42–1.02, *P* = 0.06).[41]

A retrospective evaluation of patients in the Southwest Oncology Group study (SWOG) 8814 trial, which randomised postmenopausal patients with node-positive, hormone receptor-positive tumours between tamoxifen and tamoxifen + CAF chemotherapy, showed that CAF offered a substantial advantage for HER-2-positive patients but little, if any, advantage for those with HER-2-negative tumours.[42]

## Taxanes

Paclitaxel (Taxol) and docetaxel (Taxotere) have emerged as two of the most active cytotoxic agents against breast cancer. In the metastatic setting, these compounds have been shown to be active in anthracyline-resistant breast cancers.[43]

A series of randomised trials have evaluated the benefit of taxanes combined with anthracyclines in the adjuvant treatment for early breast cancer,[34,44–47] but their role remains controversial. The majority but not all have shown a DFS benefit, but some have failed to show a benefit in OS[45] or in patients with four or more lymph node metastases,[46,47] or in endocrine receptor-positive tumours.[34] A recent meta-analysis of 13 randomised trials involving more than 22 000 patients assessing the addition of a taxane to an anthracycline-based regimen[48] showed an absolute improvement at 5 years of approximately 5% for recurrence and 3% for death. This benefit is present irrespective of the number of lymph nodes involved (1–3 vs. 4+), ER status (ER positive vs. ER negative) or age/menopausal status (≤50 years/premenopausal vs. >50 years/postmenopausal).

Since this publication, however, results form the largest adjuvant taxane trial, the UK Taxotere as Adjuvant Chemotherapy (TACT) trial, involving 4162 patients have been presented, so far only in abstract form. This trial compared sequential FEC-Taxotere (FEC 600/60/600 mg/m² q3w × 4 followed by docetaxel 100 mg/m² × 4) with standard UK anthracycline chemotherapy involving either FEC (600/60/600 mg/m² q3w × 8) or E-CMF (epirubicin 100 mg/m² q3w × 4 followed by CMF 100 mg/m² p.o. on days 1–14 or 600 mg/m² i.v. on days 1 and 8/40/600 mg/m² q4w × 4). First results after 5 years of follow-up showed no differences in DFS (the primary end-point; 74.7% vs. 73.9%, HR 0.97) or in OS (82% in the taxane arm and 81.8% in the anthracycline only arm, HR 0.98).[49] Neutropenia and febrile neutropenia were significantly higher in the taxane arm, as were neuropathy and lethargy.

Adjuvant docetaxel has also been tested instead of an anthracycline in patients with early breast cancer. In a provocative prospective US Oncology phase III trial, a total of 1106 patients were randomised to receive either four cycles of standard AC (doxorubicin 60 mg/m$^2$ and cyclophosphamide 600 mg/m$^2$) or four cycles of TC (docetaxel 75 mg/m$^2$ and cyclophosphamide 600 mg/m$^2$) as adjuvant treatment for early breast cancer.[50] Treatment with TC achieved a significant improvement in 5-year DFS compared with AC (86% vs. 80% respectively, HR 0.67, P = 0.015). With further follow-up a significant overall survival benefit has also emerged.[51] There was significantly more nausea and vomiting in patients receiving AC compared with TC, whereas patients receiving docetaxel experienced more oedema, myalgia, arthralgia, and a higher rate of fever and neutropenia compared with AC (5% vs. 2.5%, P = 0.07).

As with anthracyclines, there is a reported interaction between HER-2 status and benefit from taxanes based on a retrospective analysis of the CALGB 9344 trial. In this trial, in which patients with node-positive breast cancer were randomised to receive paclitaxel (175 mg/m$^2$) or observation after four cycles of AC at doses of 60, 75 and 90 mg/m$^{2,52}$ only those whose tumours showed overexpression or amplification of HER-2 showed significant benefit with paclitaxel for both risk of recurrence (HR 0.59, P = 0.01) and death (HR 0.57, P = 0.01). The greatest benefit was in those whose tumours were HER-2 positive and ER negative. In contrast those whose tumours were HER-2 negative and ER positive (by far the largest group) achieved no benefit form the addition of paclitaxel.

These results suggest that the 'one size fits all' approach to adjuvant chemotherapy may be wrong and that the benefit for taxanes and indeed for anthracyclines may be restricted to subsets of patients whose tumours overexpress HER-2.

## Duration of chemotherapy

The optimum duration of chemotherapy remains uncertain. The EBCTG meta-analysis assessed five CMF-based trials and found no survival benefit for more than 6 months treatment.[53] A French FASG-01 trial showed a significant benefit in DFS of six cycles of FEC50 over three cycles of FEC50 or 75, and improved OS with six cycles of FEC50 over

three cycles.[54] Further trials of chemotherapy duration are urgently required.

## Dose density

Recently interest has developed in accelerated (sometimes called dose-dense) chemotherapy in which treatment is given at 2-week rather than 3-week intervals with granulocyte colony-stimulating factor support to overcome the risk of neutropenic sepsis. The CALGB 9741 trial has shown that accelerated 2-weekly AC × 4 followed by accelerated Taxol × 4 has improved efficacy over the same eight courses given conventionally at 3-week intervals in women with node-positive breast cancer, with 4-year DFS of 82% and 75% respectively.[55] In addition, the accelerated arm was associated with less neutropenic sepsis.

The shortened duration of adjuvant treatment associated with accelerated chemotherapy is likely to be attractive to patients, and the reduced risk of neutropenic sepsis may save on resources. Further trials in this area are now indicated.

## Which patients really benefit from adjuvant chemotherapy?

The EBCTCG Overview shows that, overall, patients with hormone receptor-positive disease receive statistically significant improvement from chemotherapy over and above tamoxifen, with an HR of 0.64 and an absolute additional 5-year gain of 7.6% for those under 50.[3] The important question, however, is to determine those for whom the gain is large enough to be of real clinical benefit when balanced against toxicity.

In broad terms, the absolute benefit depends on the absolute risk and for this reason adjuvant chemotherapy was developed initially in women with axillary node-positive disease which remains the most powerful prognostic factor for recurrence. In recent years it has become clear that some women with high-risk node-negative disease will benefit. It is also likely that not all women with hormone receptor-positive, node-positive disease benefit from chemotherapy. Various guideline systems have been proposed, of which the most well established is perhaps the St Gallen Consensus. The most recent update (Box 12.1, Table 12.2)[56] states that for

Box 12.1 • Definition of risk categories for patients with operated breast cancer defined in St Gallen Expert Consensus Meeting 2007

**Low**

**Node negative** and **all** the following:

Tumour size ≤2 cm
Grade 1
Absence of vascular invasion
HER-2 negative
ER and/or PgR overexpressed
Age ≥35 years

**Intermediate**

**Node negative** and **at least one** of the following:

Tumour size >2 cm
Grade 2–3
Vascular invasion
HER-2 positive
ER and PgR absent
Age <35 years

**Node positive (1–3 involved nodes)** and:

ER and/or PgR expressed, **and**
HER-2 negative

**High**

**Node positive (1–3 involved nodes)** and:

ER and PgR absent, **or**
HER-2 positive

**Node positive (4 or more involved nodes)**

women with hormone receptor-positive disease 'no absolute rules can be defined' but the recommendations include women with greater than or equal to 4 involved nodes if HER-2 negative and any positive nodes if HER-2 positive. There are also recommendations to consider chemotherapy in women with node-negative disease with a tumour size greater than 2 cm, or grade 2–3, or with lymphovascular invasion, or with HER-2-positive disease, or in those aged less than 35 years.

Further insight into this question comes from an analysis of the SWOG 8814 trial in which postmenopausal women with node-positive, hormone receptor-positive tumours were randomised to tamoxifen alone or tamoxifen with anthracycline-containing chemotherapy (cyclophosphamide, adriamycin and 5-fluorouracil). Overall there was a significant benefit in favour of those receiving chemotherapy concurrently with tamoxifen but in a retrospective subset analysis, so far presented only in abstract, patients with a high ER score (Allred score 7 or 8) showed no benefit from the addition of chemotherapy even in the presence of involved nodes; likewise, women whose tumours were HER-2 negative showed no benefit from the addition of chemotherapy unless they had four or more nodes involved.[57] This analysis should be considered hypothesis-generating rather than definitive, but emphasises the need to identify molecular markers to predict which patients really benefit from chemotherapy.

For this reason, gene expression arrays and gene signatures have been developed to try to quantify more accurately the likelihood of breast cancer recurrence and predict the magnitude of chemotherapy benefit.

Table 12.2 • Treatment recommendations from St Gallen Expert Consensus Meeting 2007 based on risk categories

| | HER2/neu status: | HER-2 negative | | | | | HER-2 positive | | |
|---|---|---|---|---|---|---|---|---|---|
| | Endocrine responsive-ness: | Highly responsive* | | Incompletely responsive† | | Non-responsive‡ | Highly responsive | Incompletely responsive | Non-responsive |
| **Risk** | Menopausal status: | Pre | Post | Pre | Post | Pre and post | Pre and post | Pre and post | Pre and post |
| Low | | E | E | E | E | | | | |
| Inter-mediate | | E | E | C→E | C→E | | C→E +Tr | C→E +Tr | C +Tr |
| | | C→E | C→E | E | E | C | | | |
| High | | C→E | C→E | C→E | C→E | C | C→E +Tr | C→E +Tr | C +Tr |

*High levels of both steroid hormone receptors in a majority of cells.
†Some expression of steroid hormone receptors but at lower levels or lacking ER or PgR.
‡No detectable expression of steroid hormone receptors.
C, chemotherapy; E, endocrine therapy; Tr, trastuzumab.

Currently, the most widely used of these is a 21-gene assay now offered as a commercial reference laboratory test (Oncotype DX Genomic Health Inc.). This is based on formalin-fixed material from which the level of gene expression is used to determine a recurrence score predicting the likelihood of distant recurrence.[28] The Oncotype DX assay has been applied to a subset of patients in the NSABP B-20 trial randomising women with node-negative disease to tamoxifen and chemotherapy (CMF or MF) versus tamoxifen alone. It was found that women with a low recurrence score had virtually no benefit from chemotherapy whereas those with a high recurrence score developed very major benefit, with an absolute decrease in the 10-year rate of distant recurrence of 28% (88% vs. 60% free of distant recurence).[58] Patients with an intermediate recurrence score had a relatively small benefit and such patients are now in a trial randomising to chemotherapy or not in addition to endocrine therapy (TAILOR X).

Similarly a 70-gene signature has also shown strong correlation with outcome[29,59] and a second trial, MINDACT, is now assessing the value of this in predicting which patients with ER-positive tumours might also benefit from chemotherapy. The problem with the 70-gene signature is that it requires fresh tumour tissue, in contrast to Oncotype DX, which uses paraffin-embedded tissue.

# Bisphosphonates

Three adjuvant trials have investigated the use of bisphosphonates to prevent the appearance of bone metastases in women with early breast cancer, with conflicting results. The first trial[60] randomised 302 women with primary breast cancer and immunocytochemical evidence of cancer cells in a bone marrow aspirate to 2 years of clodronate 1600 mg/day or not. After nearly 5 years of follow-up, a reduction in the incidence of bone metastases, a trend to reduction in visceral metastases and an increase in overall survival were seen in the clodronate group. However, the effect of clodronate appeared to weaken with longer follow-up.

The second trial[61] randomised 299 women with lymph node-positive breast cancer to 3 years of clodronate 1600 mg/day or control. This showed negative results. After a minimum of 5 years follow-up, significantly more bone metastases (26% vs. 18%) and non-skeletal metastases (45% vs.

27%) were seen in the clodronate group than the placebo group. The overall survival was also significantly worse in the clodronate group (68% vs. 81%). There were, however, imbalances in lymph node positivity, tumour size and PgR status between the groups, which could account, at least in part, for these unexpected results.

The third and largest trial randomised 1079 women to receive 2 years of clodronate 1600 mg/day or placebo starting within 6 months of surgery.[62] During the 2 years of treatment, there was a significant reduction in bone metastases in the clodronate group but at 5 years this effect was lost. No differences in recurrence of visceral metastases were seen. Overall survival was significantly improved in the clodronate group.

The role of adjuvant clodronate therefore remains uncertain, although in our view the balance of evidence suggests clinical benefit. Further trials are now under way, including an NSABP study comparing 5 years of clodronate with placebo and a trial of the much more potent bisphosphonate Zoledronate (Zometa), also against placebo (AZURE).

# Trastuzumab (Herceptin)

Trastuzumab is a recombinant humanised monoclonal antibody specific to the human HER-2 receptor.

 HER-2 is amplified in around 20% of breast cancers; it plays a critical role in tumour development and is an independent marker of survival, with amplification/overexpression carrying an adverse prognosis.[63]

Trastuzumab was therefore developed in a rationalised manner to abrogate pathways downstream of this target[64] and has established efficacy, including a significantly improved survival benefit in metastatic breast cancer.[65]

Four large, multicentre randomised adjuvant trials involving more than 12 000 women have been performed to assess whether trastuzumab given concurrently with a taxane after anthracycline chemotherapy (adriamycin/cyclophosphamide, AC) (NSABP B-31, Intergroup N9831, BCIRG 006)[66,67] or concurrently with a non-anthracycline regimen of Taxotere and carboplatin (BCIRG 006),[67] or sequentially after any standard chemotherapy schedule (Herceptin in Adjuvant Breast Cancer,

HERA trial)[68,69] or sequentially after AC and a taxane (Intergroup N9831) can improve disease-free survival and survival. In all these trials trastuzumab was given for 1 year; in the HERA trial a third arm is also evaluating treatment for 2 years (**Fig. 12.3**).

 Results from these trials have been pivotal in establishing adjuvant trastuzumab as a major factor in improving survival from HER-2-positive breast cancer.[66,69]

## Trastuzumab given concurrently with chemotherapy

The combined results of the concurrent arms of the two North American studies, the NSABP B-31 and North Central Cancer Treatment Group (NCCTG) N-9831 trials reported a significant increase in DFS (85% vs. 67%) and OS (91% vs. 87%) for patients

receiving adjuvant trastuzumab compared with chemotherapy treatment alone.[66] Updated results of these trials at 2.9 years follow-up and after 619 events confirmed this benefit (HR 0.49, 95% CI 0.41–0.57, $P < 0.00001$).[70]

 Concurrent trastuzumab with docetaxel chemotherapy is also used in two of the arms of the BCIRG 006 trial.[67] The second interim analysis confirmed earlier data and reported a significant clinical benefit with trastuzumab in terms of DFS in the AC, the Taxotere combined with trastuzumab arm (HR 0.61, $P < 0.0001$), and the non-anthracycline Taxotere, carboplatin and trastuzumab arm (HR 0.67, $P = 0.0003$) compared to the AC→T arm. Overall survival was reported for the first time and was significantly improved in both the experimental arms (HR 0.59, $P = 0.004$ and HR 0.66, $P = 0.017$ respectively) compared to the control arm.

The BCIRG 006 trial therefore suggests that anthracyclines are not necessary with trastuzumab in the treatment of HER-2-positive disease, a finding that has implications in avoiding cardiotoxicity (see below).

## Sequential trastuzumab given after chemotherapy

In the HERA study, more than 5000 women with HER-2-positive breast carcinoma were randomised to undergo observation or to receive trastuzumab every 3 weeks for 1 or 2 years treatment. Only data on patients randomised to 1 year of sequential adjuvant trastuzumab have been reported. After a median of 2 years of follow-up a significant 34% reduction in the risk of death was observed for patients receiving trastuzumab after completion of chemotherapy compared with chemotherapy alone (HR 0.66, 95% CI 0.47–0.91, $P = 0.0115$).[69]

More recently, a French trial, PACS 004, also assessed trastuzumab given sequentially after chemotherapy and reported less impressive results. A total of 3010 patients <65 years with node-positive early breast carcinoma were randomised to receive six cycles of adjuvant FEC (500/100/500 mg/m$^2$) or six cycles of concomitant ED (epirubicin and doxorubicin 75 mg/m$^2$). Both regimens were administered

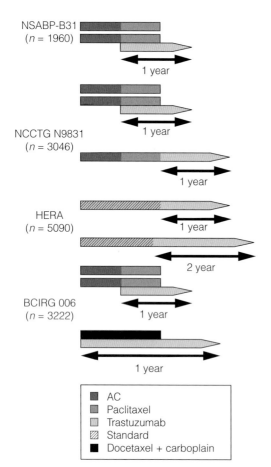

**Figure 12.3** • Schematic of the main trials testing trastuzumab in the adjuvant setting.

i.v. every 3 weeks. A total of 528 HER-2-positive patients were identified. Of those, 268 were randomised to observation only and 260 also received trastuzumab (8 mg/kg loading dose, 6 mg/kg q3w for 1 year) to start after completion of radiotherapy. No significant differences were observed between the two arms in terms of both DFS and OS.[71] The inferior results of the PACS trial raise the important issue of whether trastuzumab given sequentially after chemotherapy may be inferior to concurrent administration.

This issue is being addressed by the N9831 trial, in which patients were randomised to control (AC followed by weekly paclitaxel, arm A), versus AC followed by weekly paclitaxel with concurrent trastuzumab (arm C), versus AC followed by weekly paclitaxel and thereafter trastuzumab sequentially (arm B).

## Duration of trastuzumab

The optimal duration of adjuvant trastuzumab therapy is not known. Results of the 2-year treatment arm from the HERA trial are still awaited. Another randomised study reported similar results with just 9 weeks of treatment combined with non-anthracycline chemotherapy.[72] In the subgroup of 202 patients with HER-2-overexpressing tumours, the addition of only 9 weeks of adjuvant trastuzumab was associated with an increase in 3-year RFS compared with those receiving chemotherapy alone (89% vs. 78%; HR 0.42, $P = 0.01$).

## Cardiotoxicity with trastuzumab

The only significant toxicity associated with trastuzumab (and one that was quite unexpected from preliminary experimental studies) is that it can cause cardiotoxicity when given concurrently with or after anthracyclines. In the original pivotal trial in metastatic disease, CHF was found in 27% of patients treated concurrently with anthracyclines.[65]

This is why trastuzumab was not given concurrently with anthracyclines in the adjuvant trials. In these, the incidence of severe cardiotoxicity with CHF was low in all trials. The increased incidence compared with the control arm in the NSABP B-31 trial was 2.9%[73] and in the N9831 concurrent arm 3%.[70] The incidence was marginally lower in the HERA trial where trastuzumab was given sequen-

tially, with an increased risk of CHF of 2%,[74] and in the sequential arm of the N9831 trial where the increased risk was 2.5%.[70] The number of patients having to stop treatment because of cardiac issues, however, was much higher in the concurrent arm of the NSABP trial (15.5%) than in the HERA trial (4.3%), suggesting that trastuzumab given very shortly after anthracyclines might carry a higher risk of cardiotoxicity. Meanwhile the BCIRG trial showed a marked increase in cardiotoxicity and in particular asymptomatic reductions in left ventricular ejection fraction (LVEF), with anthracyclines followed by trastuzumab, than in the non-anthracycline-containing arm (docetaxel, carboplatin and trastuzumab, TCH). In the second interim analysis after a median follow-up of 36 months, the incidence of grade III/IV CHF was 1.9% for the AC→D + T arm, 0.4% in the TCH arm and 0.4% for patients receiving AC→D with no trastuzumab.[67]

All the trials suggest that patients are at risk only while on trastuzumab without any continuing cumulative incidence beyond 1 year. They also show some degree of recovery of LVEF once trastuzumab has stopped.

In summary, therefore, the risk of significant cardiotoxicity is low with trastuzumab but the data nevertheless encourage the search for treatments devoid of this problem, including in particular the BCIRG 006 trial approach, omitting anthracyclines completely.[75]

## Conclusion

In conclusion, adjuvant medical therapy after surgery represents the most important advance in the treatment of breast cancer for many decades and is responsible for a very significant part of the recent improvement in mortality.

Adjuvant endocrine therapy is indicated for all but the very best prognosis hormone receptor-positive tumours. Tamoxifen remains the standard endocrine therapy for premenopausal women, and current evidence suggests that there may be additional benefit with concomitant ovarian suppression. Aromatase inhibitors are now challenging tamoxifen as first-line or sequential treatment in postmenopausal women, and in particular those at higher risk. Extended adjuvant therapy with an aromatase inhibitor beyond 5 years of tamoxifen is an important new development for women at higher risk.

Adjuvant chemotherapy is likewise of major importance, particularly for women with hormone receptor-negative disease. Many patients with hormone receptor-positive disease undoubtedly also benefit, but the challenge is to define these more accurately using modern molecular marker technology.

Adjuvant trastuzumab has been a major breakthrough for patients whose tumours have amplified or overexpression of HER-2, and the likelihood is that evidence may continue to accumulate in the near future to support the use of adjuvant bisphosphonates.

## Key points

- The implementation of adjuvant treatment for breast carcinoma after surgery is responsible for an improvement in outcome.
- Endocrine treatment with tamoxifen is still the standard for premenopausal patients with hormone-responsive tumours. Additional benefit with concomitant ovarian suppression requires further investigation.
- Aromatase inhibitors now have a major role in postmenopausal patients with hormone-sensitive tumours as an initial treatment, after 2–3 years of tamoxifen or in adjuvant extended treatment.
- Adjuvant chemotherapy is particularly important in hormone receptor-negative tumours or in high-risk recurrence.
- The incorporation of taxanes into chemotherapy regimens gives some added benefit, but the best way to use these agents remains controversial.
- In tumours with overexpression and/or amplification of HER-2, adjuvant treatment with trastuzumab has been a major breakthrough and improves survival.

# References

1. Li CI, Daling JR, Malone KE. Incidence of invasive breast cancer by hormone receptor status from 1992 to 1998. J Clin Oncol 2003; 21(1):28–34.

2. Beatson G. On the treatment of inoperable cases of carcinoma of the mamma: suggestions for a new method of treatment, with illustrative cases. Lancet 1896; ii:104–7.

3. Effects of chemotherapy and hormonal therapy for early breast cancer on recurrence and 15-year survival: an overview of the randomised trials. Lancet 2005; 365(9472):1687–717.

   Fifteen-year follow-up review involving more than 33 000 women with early breast carcinoma evaluating the benefits of adjuvant treatment.

4. Fisher B, Dignam J, Bryant J et al. Five versus more than five years of tamoxifen for lymph node-negative breast cancer: updated findings from the National Surgical Adjuvant Breast and Bowel Project B-14 randomized trial. J Natl Cancer Inst 2001; 93(9):684–90.

5. Peto R, Davies C and on Behalf of the ATLAS Collaboration, ATLAS (Adjuvant Tamoxifen, Longer Against Shorter): international randomized trial of 10 versus 5 years of adjuvant tamoxifen among 11 500 women preliminary results. Breast Cancer Res Treat 2007; 106(Suppl 1):abstract, 48.

6. Coates AS, Keshaviah A, Thurlimann B et al. Five years of letrozole compared with tamoxifen as initial adjuvant therapy for postmenopausal women with endocrine-responsive early breast cancer: update of study BIG 1-98. J Clin Oncol 2007; 25(5):486–92.

7. Forbes JF, Cuzick J, Buzdar A et al. Effect of anastrozole and tamoxifen as adjuvant treatment for early-stage breast cancer: 100-month analysis of the ATAC trial. Lancet Oncol 2008; 9(1):45–53.

   These two trials demonstrate the superiority of aromatase inhibitors compared with tamoxifen as adjuvant treatment for postmenopausal patients with early breast cancer.

8. Arpino G, Weiss HL, Clark GM et al. Hormone receptor status of a contralateral breast cancer is independent of the receptor status of the first primary in patients not receiving adjuvant tamoxifen. J Clin Oncol 2005; 23(21):4687–94.

9. Dowsett M, Cuzick J, Wale C et al. Retrospective analysis of time to recurrence in the ATAC trial according to hormone receptor status: an hypothesis-generating study. J Clin Oncol 2005; 23(30):7512–17.

10. Dowsett M, Allred C and on behalf of the TransATAC Investigators. Relationship between quantitative ER and PgR expression and HER2 status with recurrence in the ATAC trial. San Antonio Breast Cancer Symp 2006; 48, abstract.

11. Viale G, Regan M, Dell'Orto P et al. Central review of ER, PgR and HER-2 in BIG 1-98 evaluating letrozole vs. tamoxifen as adjuvant endocrine therapy for postmenopausal women with receptor-positive breast cancer. San Antonio Breast Cancer Symp 2005; 44, abstract.

12. Ellis MJ, Coop A, Singh B et al. Letrozole is more effective neoadjuvant endocrine therapy than

tamoxifen for ErbB-1- and/or ErbB-2-positive, estrogen receptor-positive primary breast cancer: evidence from a phase III randomized trial. J Clin Oncol 2001; 19(18):3808–16.

13. Smith IE, Dowsett M, Ebbs SR et al. Neoadjuvant treatment of postmenopausal breast cancer with anastrozole, tamoxifen, or both in combination: the Immediate Preoperative Anastrozole, Tamoxifen, or Combined with Tamoxifen (IMPACT) multicenter double-blind randomized trial. J Clin Oncol 2005; 23(22):5108–16.

14. Duffy S, Jackson TL, Lansdown M et al. The ATAC ('Arimidex', Tamoxifen, Alone or in Combination) adjuvant breast cancer trial: first results of the endometrial sub-protocol following 2 years of treatment. Hum Reprod 2006; 21(2):545–53.

15. Thurlimann B, Keshaviah A, Coates AS et al. A comparison of letrozole and tamoxifen in postmenopausal women with early breast cancer. N Engl J Med 2005; 353(26):2747–57.

16. Coombes RC, Kilburn LS, Snowdon CF et al. Survival and safety of exemestane versus tamoxifen after 2–3 years' tamoxifen treatment (Intergroup Exemestane Study): a randomised controlled trial. Lancet 2007; 369(9561):559–70.

17. Jonat W, Gnant M, Boccardo F et al. Effectiveness of switching from adjuvant tamoxifen to anastrozole in postmenopausal women with hormone-sensitive early-stage breast cancer: a meta-analysis. Lancet Oncol 2006; 7(12):991–6.

18. Boccardo F, Rubagotti A, Puntoni M et al. Switching to anastrozole versus continued tamoxifen treatment of early breast cancer: preliminary results of the Italian Tamoxifen Anastrozole Trial. J Clin Oncol 2005; 23(22):5138–47.

19. Jakesz R, Jonat W, Gnant M et al. Switching of postmenopausal women with endocrine-responsive early breast cancer to anastrozole after 2 years' adjuvant tamoxifen: combined results of ABCSG trial 8 and ARNO 95 trial. Lancet 2005; 366(9484):455–62.

20. Jakesz R, Gnant M, Greil R et al. The benefits of sequencing adjuvant tamoxifen and anastrozole in postmenopausal women with hormone-responsive early breast cancer: 5 year-analysis of ABCSG Trial 8. San Antonio Breast Cancer Symp 2005; 13, abstract.

21. Saphner T, Tormey DC, Gray R. Annual hazard rates of recurrence for breast cancer after primary therapy. J Clin Oncol 1996; 14(10):2738–46.

22. Goss PE, Ingle JN, Martino S et al. A randomized trial of letrozole in postmenopausal women after five years of tamoxifen therapy for early-stage breast cancer. N Engl J Med 2003; 349(19):1793–802.

The first trial to demonstrate an additional benefit with the extended use of aromatase inhibitors in postmenopausal women after 5 years of adjuvant tamoxifen treatment.

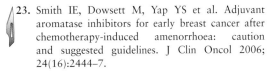

23. Smith IE, Dowsett M, Yap YS et al. Adjuvant aromatase inhibitors for early breast cancer after chemotherapy-induced amenorrhoea: caution and suggested guidelines. J Clin Oncol 2006; 24(16):2444–7.

The first retrospective review to demonstrate the risk of recovery of the ovarian function in young patients receiving aromatase inhibitors.

24. Kendall A, Dowsett M, Folkerd E et al. Caution: Vaginal estradiol appears to be contraindicated in postmenopausal women on adjuvant aromatase inhibitors. Ann Oncol 2006; 17(4):584–7.

25. Jonat W, Kaufmann M, Sauerbrei W et al. Goserelin versus cyclophosphamide, methotrexate, and fluorouracil as adjuvant therapy in premenopausal patients with node-positive breast cancer: The Zoladex Early Breast Cancer Research Association Study. J Clin Oncol 2002; 20(24):4628–35.

26. Jakesz R, Hausmaninger H, Kubista E et al. Randomized adjuvant trial of tamoxifen and goserelin versus cyclophosphamide, methotrexate, and fluorouracil: evidence for the superiority of treatment with endocrine blockade in premenopausal patients with hormone-responsive breast cancer – Austrian Breast and Colorectal Cancer Study Group Trial 5. J Clin Oncol 2002; 20(24):4621–7.

Two trials suggesting that ovarian suppression could be as effective as CMF chemotherapy treatment in premenopausal women with ER-positive tumours.

27. Dowsett M, Smith IE, Ebbs SR et al. Prognostic value of Ki67 expression after short-term presurgical endocrine therapy for primary breast cancer. J Natl Cancer Inst 2007; 99(2):167–70.

28. Paik S, Shak S, Tang G et al. A multigene assay to predict recurrence of tamoxifen-treated, node-negative breast cancer. N Engl J Med 2004; 351(27):2817–26.

29. van 't Veer LJ, Dai H, van de Vijver MJ et al. Gene expression profiling predicts clinical outcome of breast cancer. Nature 2002; 415(6871):530–6.

30. Davidson NE, O'Neill AM, Vukov AM et al. Chemoendocrine therapy for premenopausal women with axillary lymph node-positive, steroid hormone receptor-positive breast cancer: results from INT 0101 (E5188). J Clin Oncol 2005; 23(25):5973–82.

31. Hutchins LF, Green SJ, Ravdin PM et al. Randomized, controlled trial of cyclophosphamide, methotrexate, and fluorouracil versus cyclophosphamide, doxorubicin, and fluorouracil with and without tamoxifen for high-risk, node-negative breast cancer: treatment results of Intergroup Protocol INT-0102. J Clin Oncol 2005; 23(33):8313–21.

32. Levine MN, Bramwell VH, Pritchard KI et al. Randomized trial of intensive cyclophosphamide, epirubicin, and fluorouracil chemotherapy compared with cyclophosphamide, methotrexate, and fluorouracil in premenopausal women with

node-positive breast cancer. National Cancer Institute of Canada Clinical Trials Group. J Clin Oncol 1998; 16(8):2651–8.

33. Poole CJ, Earl HM, Hiller L et al. Epirubicin and cyclophosphamide, methotrexate, and fluorouracil as adjuvant therapy for early breast cancer. N Engl J Med 2006; 355(18):1851–62.

34. Henderson IC, Berry DA, Demetri GD et al. Improved outcomes from adding sequential Paclitaxel but not from escalating Doxorubicin dose in an adjuvant chemotherapy regimen for patients with node-positive primary breast cancer. J Clin Oncol 2003; 21(6):976–83.

35. Benefit of a high-dose epirubicin regimen in adjuvant chemotherapy for node-positive breast cancer patients with poor prognostic factors: 5-year follow-up results of French Adjuvant Study Group 05 randomized trial. J Clin Oncol 2001; 19(3):602–11.

36. Perez EA, Suman VJ, Davidson NE et al. Effect of doxorubicin plus cyclophosphamide on left ventricular ejection fraction in patients with breast cancer in the North Central Cancer Treatment Group N9831 Intergroup Adjuvant Trial. J Clin Oncol 2004; 22(18):3700–4.

One of the trials reviewing cardiotoxicity associated with anthracycline chemotherapy treatment in early breast carcinoma.

37. Swain SM, Whaley FS, Ewer MS. Congestive heart failure in patients treated with doxorubicin: a retrospective analysis of three trials. Cancer 2003; 97(11):2869–79.

38. Pinder MC, Duan Z, Goodwin JS et al. Congestive heart failure in older women treated with adjuvant anthracycline chemotherapy for breast cancer. J Clin Oncol 2007; 25(25):3808–15.

39. Wood WC, Budman DR, Korzun AH et al. Dose and dose intensity of adjuvant chemotherapy for stage II, node-positive breast carcinoma. N Engl J Med 1994; 330(18):1253–9.

40. Thor AD, Berry DA, Budman DR et al. erbB-2, p53, and efficacy of adjuvant therapy in lymph node-positive breast cancer. J Natl Cancer Inst 1998; 90(18):1346–60.

41. Pritchard KI, Shepherd LE, O'Malley FP et al. HER2 and responsiveness of breast cancer to adjuvant chemotherapy. N Engl J Med 2006; 354(20):2103–11.

42. Ravdin PM, Green S, Albain KS et al. Initial report of the SWOG biological correlative study of c-erbB-2 expression as a predictor of outcome in a trial comparing adjuvant CAF T with tamoxifen alone. Proc Am Soc Clin Oncol 1998; 17(97):abstract.

A retrospective study that suggests the possible superiority of an anthracycline chemotherapy regimen in patients with overexpression of HER-2.

43. Ghersi D, Wilcken N, Simes RJ. A systematic review of taxane-containing regimens for metastatic breast cancer. Br J Cancer 2005; 93(3):293–301.

44. Evans TR, Yellowlees A, Foster E et al. Phase III randomized trial of doxorubicin and docetaxel versus doxorubicin and cyclophosphamide as primary medical therapy in women with breast cancer: an Anglo-Celtic cooperative oncology group study. J Clin Oncol 2005; 23(13):2988–95.

45. Mamounas EP, Bryant J, Lembersky B et al. Paclitaxel after doxorubicin plus cyclophosphamide as adjuvant chemotherapy for node-positive breast cancer: results from NSABP B-28. J Clin Oncol 2005; 23(16):3686–96.

46. Martin M, Pienkowski T, Mackey J et al. Adjuvant docetaxel for node-positive breast cancer. N Engl J Med 2005; 352(22):2302–13.

47. Roche H, Fumoleau P, Spielmann M et al. Sequential adjuvant epirubicin-based and docetaxel chemotherapy for node-positive breast cancer patients: the FNCLCC PACS 01 Trial. J Clin Oncol 2006; 24(36):5664–71.

48. De Laurentiis M, Cancello G, D'Agostino D et al. Taxane-based combinations as adjuvant chemotherapy of early breast cancer: a meta-analysis of randomized trials. J Clin Oncol 2008; 26(1):44–53.

49. Ellis PA, Barrett-Lee PJ, Bloomfield D et al. Preliminary results of the UK Taxotere as Adjuvant Chemotherapy (TACT) Trial. San Antonio Breast Cancer Symp 2007; 78, abstract.

50. Jones SE, Savin MA, Holmes FA et al. Phase III trial comparing doxorubicin plus cyclophosphamide with docetaxel plus cyclophosphamide as adjuvant therapy for operable breast cancer. J Clin Oncol 2006; 24(34):5381–7.

51. Jones SE, Holmes F, O'Shaughnessy J et al. Extended follow-up and analysis by age of the US Oncology Adjuvant trial 9735: docetaxel/cyclophosphamide is associated with an overall survival benefit compared to doxorubicin/cyclophosphamide and is well-tolerated in women 65 or older. San Antonio Breast Cancer Symp 2007; 12, abstract.

52. Hayes DF, Thor AD, Dressler LG et al. HER2 and response to paclitaxel in node-positive breast cancer. N Engl J Med 2007; 357(15):1496–506.

53. Early Breast Cancer Trialists' Collaborative Group. Polychemotherapy for early breast cancer: an overview of the randomised trials. Lancet 1998; 352(9132):930–42.

54. Fumoleau P, Kerbrat P, Romestaing P et al. Randomized trial comparing six versus three cycles of epirubicin-based adjuvant chemotherapy in premenopausal, node-positive breast cancer patients: 10-year follow-up results of the French Adjuvant Study Group 01 trial. J Clin Oncol 2003; 21(2):298–305.

55. Citron ML, Berry DA, Cirrincione C et al. Randomized trial of dose-dense versus conventionally scheduled and sequential versus concurrent combination chemotherapy as postoperative adjuvant treatment of node-positive

primary breast cancer: first report of Intergroup Trial C9741/Cancer and Leukemia Group B Trial 9741. J Clin Oncol 2003; 21(8):1431–9.

56. Goldhirsch A, Wood WC, Gelber RD et al. Progress and promise: highlights of the international expert consensus on the primary therapy of early breast cancer 2007. Ann Oncol 2007; 18(7):1133–44.

57. Albain K, Barlow W, O'Malley FP et al. Concurrent (CAFT) versus sequetial (CAF-T) chemohormonal therapy (cyclophosphamide, doxorubicin, 5-fluorouracil, tamoxifen) versus T alone for postmenopausal, node-positive estrogen (ER) and/or progesterone (PgR) receptor-positive breast cancer: mature outcomes and new biologic correlates on phase III intergroup trial 0100 (SWOG-8814). Breast Cancer Res Treat 2004; 88(Suppl 1):37, abstract.

58. Paik S, Tang G, Shak S et al. Gene expression and benefit of chemotherapy in women with node-negative, estrogen receptor-positive breast cancer. J Clin Oncol 2006; 24(23):3726–34.

59. Van de Vijver MJ, He YD, van't Veer LJ et al. A gene-expression signature as a predictor of survival in breast cancer. N Engl J Med 2002; 347(25):1999–2009.

60. Diel IJ, Solomayer EF, Costa SD et al. Reduction in new metastases in breast cancer with adjuvant clodronate treatment. N Engl J Med 1998; 339(6):357–63.

61. Saarto T, Blomqvist C, Virkkunen P et al. Adjuvant clodronate treatment does not reduce the frequency of skeletal metastases in node-positive breast cancer patients: 5-year results of a randomized controlled trial. J Clin Oncol 2001; 19(1):10–17.

62. Powles T, Paterson S, Kanis JA et al. Randomized, placebo-controlled trial of clodronate in patients with primary operable breast cancer. J Clin Oncol 2002; 20(15):3219–24.

63. Slamon DJ, Clark GM, Wong SG et al. Human breast cancer: correlation of relapse and survival with amplification of the HER-2/neu oncogene. Science 1987; 235(4785):177–82.

Important demonstration of the role of HER-2 amplification and/or overexpression in breast cancer patients.

64. Finn RS, Slamon DJ. Monoclonal antibody therapy for breast cancer: herceptin. Cancer Chemother Biol Response Modif 2003; 21:223–33.

65. Slamon DJ, Leyland-Jones B, Shak S et al. Use of chemotherapy plus a monoclonal antibody against HER2 for metastatic breast cancer that overexpresses HER2. N Engl J Med 2001; 344(11):783–92.

66. Romond EH, Perez EA, Bryant J et al. Trastuzumab plus adjuvant chemotherapy for operable HER2-positive breast cancer. N Engl J Med 2005; 353(16):1673–84.

One of the main trials that demonstrated the benefit of adjuvant trastuzumab treatment in HER-2-positive breast carcinoma and led to the approval of the use of trastuzumab in this setting.

67. Slamon D, Eiermann W, Robert N et al. BCIRG 006: 2nd interim analysis phase III randomized trial comparing doxorubicin and cyclophosphamide followed by docetaxel (ACT) with doxorubicin and cyclophosphamide followed by docetaxel and trastuzumab (ACTH) with docetaxel, carboplatin and trastuzumab (TCH) in Her2neu positive early breast cancer patients. San Antonio Breast Cancer Symp 2006; 52, abstract.

68. Piccart-Gebhart MJ, Procter M, Leyland-Jones B et al. Trastuzumab after adjuvant chemotherapy in HER2-positive breast cancer. N Engl J Med 2005; 353(16):1659–72.

One of the main trials that demonstrated the benefit of adjuvant trastzumab treatment in HER-2-positive breast carcinoma and led to the approval of the use of trastuzumab in this setting.

69. Smith I, Procter M, Gelber RD et al. 2-year follow-up of trastuzumab after adjuvant chemotherapy in HER2-positive breast cancer: a randomised controlled trial. Lancet 2007; 369(9555):29–36.

70. Perez EA, Romond EH, Suman VJ et al. Updated results of the combined analysis of NCCTG N9831 and NSABP B-31 adjuvant chemotherapy with/without trastuzumab in patients with HER2-positive breast cancer. Proc Am Soc Clin Oncol 2007; 512, abstract.

71. Spielmann M, Roché H, Humblet Y et al. 3-year follow-up of trastuzumab following adjuvant chemotherapy in node positive HER2-positive breast cancer patients: results of the PACS-04 trial. San Antonio Breast Cancer Symp 2007; 72, abstract.

72. Joensuu H, Kellokumpu-Lehtinen PL, Bono P et al. Adjuvant docetaxel or vinorelbine with or without trastuzumab for breast cancer. N Engl J Med 2006; 354(8):809–20.

73. Rastogi P, Jeong J, Geyer CE et al. Five year update of cardiac dysfunction on NSABP B-31, a randomized trial of sequential doxorubicin/cyclophosphamide (AC)→paclitaxel (T) vs. AC→T with trastuzumab (H). Proc Am Soc Clin Oncol 2007; LBA513.

74. Suter TM, Procter M, van Veldhuisen DJ et al. Trastuzumab-associated cardiac adverse effects in the herceptin adjuvant trial. J Clin Oncol 2007; 25(25):3859–65.

75. Ewer MS, O'Shaughnessy JA. Cardiac toxicity of trastuzumab-related regimens in HER2-overexpressing breast cancer. Clin Breast Cancer 2007; 7(8):600–7.

# 13

# Locally advanced breast cancer

Douglas J.A. Adamson
Alastair M. Thompson

## Introduction

Locally advanced breast cancer (**Fig. 13.1**) defined by TNM stage includes any primary breast tumour with a diameter greater than 5 cm, breast cancers with frank skin or chest wall involvement, and any tumour with certain degrees of nodal involvement, but excludes cancers that have spread to areas other than local, supraclavicular and internal mammary chain nodes (Table 13.1). Some use a more restrictive definition and classify a T3 cancer as being locally advanced only if the axillary nodes are fixed, or if there is spread to the infra- or supraclavicular fossa or internal mammary group of lymph nodes.[1] The definition of locally advanced breast cancer includes inflammatory breast cancer (**Fig. 13.2**), which is characterised by spread of the cancer through the dermal lymphatic vessels, giving an inflamed, erythematous appearance to the whole breast. The management of this condition should be multidisciplinary in nature, and based on the stage of the disease, assessed with chest radiograph, liver ultrasound or computed tomography (CT) scanning of chest and abdomen, isotope bone scanning or whole-body magnetic resonance imaging (MRI) to detect metastatic disease (Chapter 1). There is some debate over how helpful the current TMN system is in this regard, particularly with reference to the pathological staging ('pN') rather than the clinical staging ('N') of lymph nodes.[2] Histological

confirmation of the tumour type along with appropriate immunohistochemistry for estrogen receptor and human epidermal growth factor (HER-2) receptor (supplemented by fluorescence in situ hybridisation (FISH) analysis of HER-2 status if required) is required before embarking on therapy (Chapter 2). Multimodal therapy is generally needed and the timing and nature of treatments will vary depending on whether the disease is confined to operable areas, whether there is involvement of internal mammary or supraclavicular lymph nodes, and above all the general fitness of the patient.

Locally advanced cancer may occur because of delay in presentation, and in an American population is more common in women who miss screening appointments, have a fatalistic view of life, and who rely on alternative medicines. Such women are more likely to have spouses who are passive, uninvolved in their wife's treatment, and share a fatalistic outlook on life.[3] Other patients present with cancers that have become locally advanced in a very short space of time, and patients with inflammatory breast cancer typically have a very short history.

The general principles of the oncological management of locally advanced breast cancer are similar to those for less advanced disease and draw on appropriate use of surgery, radiotherapy, chemotherapy and endocrine therapy with biological agents of

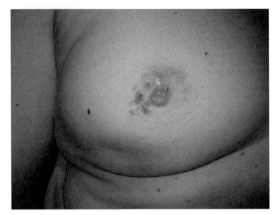

**Figure 13.1** • Locally advanced breast cancer: still operable by mastectomy.

**Table 13.1** • Locally advanced breast cancer stage and TNM

| Stage | TNM | | |
|---|---|---|---|
| IIIA | T any | N2 | M0 |
| IIIA | T3 | N1–2 | M0 |
| IIIB | T4a, b, c, d | N0–2 | M0 |
| IIIC | T any | N3 | M0 |

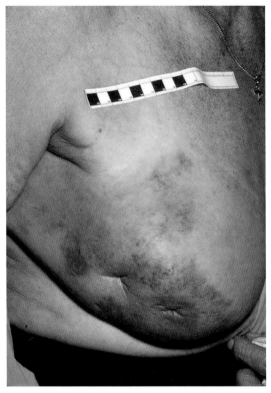

**Figure 13.2** • Inflammatory breast cancer demonstrating skin eythema (with indrawn nipple and skin tethering) and a visible axillary nodal mass.

increasing interest. The management of recurrent breast cancer in the breast, chest wall and regional nodes is also guided by these same principles.

# Surgical management

## Breast surgery

Pathological confirmation of the clinical diagnosis of locally advanced breast cancer should be made by core biopsy. If the patient is likely to be a candidate for neoadjuvant therapy, placement of a marker in the tumour immediately following the core biopsy should be considered. However, on occasion excision of a skin nodule under local anaesthetic or, rarely, incisional biopsy of a cancer where other methods have been inconclusive may be useful. Resectional surgery aims to secure clear surgical margins around the cancer. There is a balance between the completeness of excision and its link to recurrence and the known poorer cosmetic results from more extensive surgery. Radical mastectomy (including excision of pectoralis major and level III axillary clearance) does not improve survival over total mastectomy (odds

ratio of death 0.98 over 10 years[4]). Since survival following breast conservation is not significantly different from that following mastectomy, this has led some centres to favour neoadjuvant therapy for locally advanced breast cancer followed by surgery, including the option of breast conservation where appropriate. Where neoadjuvant therapy has led to a good clinical and radiological response, needle localisation biopsy may be required to pinpoint residual disease within the breast. As for all breast conservation surgery (Chapter 4), complete surgical excision with clear margins of at least 1 mm on pathology review is required to reduce disease recurrence. The term 'toilet mastectomy' has historically been applied to mastectomy performed to excise locally advanced breast cancer. While wide excision of the cancer led in the past to difficulties in skin closure with the need for split-skin grafting or application of an omental patch to the chest wall, the use of autologous flaps, particularly the latissimus dorsi flap, make this an uncommon event in modern practice.

## Axillary surgery

Many surgeons still presume that level III axillary node clearance should be the axillary surgery of choice in patients with locally advanced breast cancer due to the high probability of axillary lymph node involvement. Given the significant morbidity associated with level III axillary clearance, for patients undergoing neoadjuvant therapy with a good clinical response, this is being challenged. Sentinel lymph node biopsy of the post-treatment axilla can be used to guide therapy and is of similar efficacy to patients who have not received neoadjuvant therapy.[5]

 Sentinel lymph node biopsy after neoadjuvant chemotherapy with a good tumour response should be considered in place of axillary node clearance.[5]

## Breast reconstruction in locally advanced breast cancer

For those patients undergoing mastectomy either as primary treatment or following neoadjuvant therapy, there remains controversy regarding immediate breast reconstruction (Chapter 9). Concerns that delayed wound healing (on the chest wall or at donor sites for autologous reconstruction) may delay the timing of postoperative adjuvant chemotherapy or postoperative radiotherapy[6] and the need to avoid radiotherapy following reconstruction with prostheses has meant some surgeons do not offer immediate reconstruction to patients with locally advanced disease. Over the past 15 years US practice has swung from immediate reconstruction for patients with locally advanced breast cancer to a more conservative approach of delayed breast reconstruction.[6] There is the option for patients wishing reconstruction of a skin-sparing mastectomy and placement of a tissue expander which is deflated during radiotherapy and reflated shortly after completion of radiation. Thereafter an autologous reconstruction with a myocutaneous flap utilises the preserved skin. Autologous abdominal flap reconstruction at the time of mastectomy has been reported in the USA to produce unsatisfactory long-term outcomes, but with modern postoperative radiotherapy techniques in the UK does not appear to prejudice the cosmetic outcome nor the oncological management.[7]

## Radiotherapy

Radiotherapy is thought to work mainly by causing damage to the DNA of tumour cells, which is repaired more slowly than the damage caused in the adjacent normal tissue. Tumour tissue is therefore preferentially destroyed compared with the normal tissue over a course of radiotherapy treatment. The chance of tumour control increases with increasing total dose of radiotherapy given, but so does the chance of permanent radiotherapy-related side-effects, some of which have been implicated in treatment-related mortality[8] (Box 13.1).

Certain tissues ('late-responding tissues') such as nerves and, to some extent, lung can withstand a higher total dose of radiotherapy without giving rise to symptomatic damage, if the dose of each separate radiotherapy treatment (or 'fraction') is kept low. This means that to give a course of radiotherapy that has a chance of at least long-term tumour control, a relatively large total dose must be given over several weeks by using small daily fractions. Whilst shorter palliative courses of treatment may be considered for less fit patients, the total dose has to be reduced to minimise the toxicity of the treatment, because the fraction size for such short courses is by necessity large.[9] The reduction in the total radiotherapy dose for such short courses often means that any benefit obtained from the radiotherapy is short-lived and may not be worth the inconvenience to the patient of the treatment, and so many oncologists advocate longer courses of between 3 and 7 weeks for advanced breast cancer.

Before considering radiotherapy, it should be assessed whether the patient with locally advanced breast cancer will be able to comply with the treatment. Radiotherapy is generally given with the patient lying flat: patients with severe orthopnoea, for example (whether due to breast cancer

Box 13.1 • Side-effects of breast cancer radiotherapy

| |
| --- |
| Acute skin toxicity: erythema, dry desquamation, moist desquamation |
| Late skin toxicity: pigmentation, telangiectasia, fibrosis |
| Shoulder stiffness (if axilla treated) |
| Arm oedema (if lymphatics treated) |
| Pneumonitis (increasing likelihood with increasing lung volume in treatment field) |
| Oesophagitis (uncommon, self-limiting) |
| Bone radionecrosis (rare with modern treatments) |
| Brachial plexopathy |

metastasis or cardiorespiratory comorbidities), may not be able to cope with this treatment. During radiotherapy, the patient will be left on her own in the planning and treatment room, and will be raised off the concrete floor by several feet. If there is any chance she may fall off the treatment couch, for example if she has dementia, then the treatment cannot be given safely. If the locally advanced disease prevents abduction of the ipsilateral arm to less than 90°, then it is difficult to give conventional radiotherapy treatment to breast and axilla. In such a case, sometimes the usual treatment with photons can be changed to a chest wall treatment using electrons, so it is worth discussing this with a clinical oncologist.

## Adjuvant (postoperative) radiotherapy

Whatever surgery is performed to the breast, postoperative radiotherapy significantly reduces locoregional recurrence and improves overall survival for both premenopausal[10] and postmenopausal[11] women, and modern techniques do not have the cardiac morbidity of older treatments.[12] Postoperative radiotherapy (which may be given after adjuvant chemotherapy) reduces local recurrence from 35% without radiotherapy to 8% with radiotherapy and improves disease-free survival at 10 years from 24% to 36%.

 Postoperative radiotherapy reduces locoregional recurrence and improves survival.[10,11]

Radiotherapy following the surgical treatment of locally advanced breast cancer is given in the same way as for early breast cancer, with the aim of reducing local relapse by about two-thirds and perhaps improving survival.[13] As locally advanced breast cancer by definition has many features that predict for local relapse (large tumour size, lymph node involvement, close or positive margins despite adequate surgery), then postoperative radiotherapy is often used,[14] even if there has been a good response to neoadjuvant treatment, as the risk of local relapse in larger tumours is higher than for less advanced cancers.[15] The chest wall or breast is usually treated and the peripheral lymphatics are treated as appropriate[16] (see Chapter 15). It is unusual to specifically irradiate the internal mammary chain nodes as

evidence for the efficacy of this treatment is lacking, although much of the data relates to trials that are decades old.[17]

## Primary radical radiotherapy

If the patient is not fit for or declines surgery, and is fit for radiotherapy, then radiotherapy may be used as the principal local treatment. It is unusual to 'cure' a locally advanced cancer breast cancer without surgery, but sometimes excellent local control can be obtained (**Figs 13.3** and **13.4**) and unpleasant symptoms of the tumour, such as pain, discharge, bleeding and odour, can be partially or completely removed following radiotherapy treatment.

While there is little evidence to support the use of routine radiotherapy prior to definitive surgery, radiotherapy has been used as an alternative to surgery following neoadjuvant chemotherapy. In women with stage III disease given neoadjuvant chemotherapy, disease control, median survival

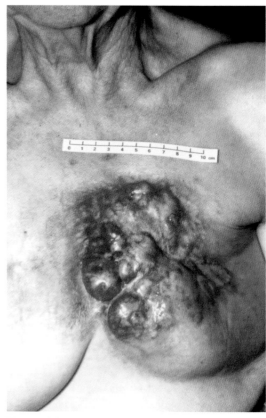

**Figure 13.3 •** Inoperable locally advanced breast cancer prior to radiotherapy.

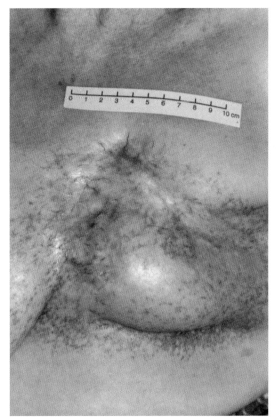

**Figure 13.4** • Locally advanced breast cancer as in Fig.13.3 following radiotherapy.

(39 months) and relapse rates appear similar in studies which randomise patients to radiotherapy or surgery.[18,19] For patients with disease operable by breast-conserving surgery, evidence does suggest that the combination of excision and radiotherapy improve local control compared to radiotherapy alone.

# Systemic treatment

If the patient has locally advanced disease and is fit for treatment, then systemic therapy is likely to be offered as the risk of relapse in locally advanced breast cancer is high. In addition, neoadjuvant treatment is often needed to 'downstage' some patients with locally advanced breast cancer to allow surgery to be completed successfully and sometimes to allow breast conservation to be achieved. Although cancer that has spread to the ipsilateral supraclavicular lymph nodes was formerly considered 'metastatic' disease, those patients with isolated supraclavicular

disease as the only site of distant disease do just as well in terms of survival as those patients with lesser stages of locally advanced breast cancer.[20]

# Neoadjuvant treatment

Treatment options include neoadjuvant chemotherapy ± trastuzumab and neoadjuvant endocrine therapy.

 Neoadjuvant chemotherapy is as effective as adjuvant chemotherapy in terms of survival benefit for locally advanced breast cancer.[21]

## Neoadjuvant chemotherapy

Neoadjuvant chemotherapy is as effective as adjuvant chemotherapy in terms of survival in locally advanced breast cancer. The choice of agents for locally advanced breast cancer is determined by emerging trial data and by local preferences, but is often similar or the same as the chemotherapy regimens given for adjuvant therapy. It has been shown that HER-2-positive tumours are more likely (by about three times) to show a complete pathological response after treatment with conventional neoadjuvant chemotherapy compared to HER-2-negative cancers, although the overall outlook for such tumours is not as good as for those which are HER-2 negative.[22] Neoadjuvant trastuzumab has been used in conjunction with chemotherapy and has shown improved rates of complete pathological response compared to chemotherapy alone, even in groups of patients which include a significant proportion of more advanced disease.[23] The primary tumour should be assessed prior to treatment with documentation of its position in the breast, accurate measurements of dimensions of the mass both clinically and on imaging and a description of the appearance of the lump and any associated changes associated with it (Figs 13.1 and 13.2). A clinical photograph is often helpful with future assessments if there is a visible mass or abnormality and helps assess response to treatment. Any palpable local lymph nodes that are thought to be involved should be carefully measured in the same way. Imaging,[24] including ultrasonography, mammography, MRI or positron emission tomography/CT scanning, is required to obtain an accurate assessment of the extent of disease before treatment and assessment of response after chemotherapy has been given if baseline images are obtained. There are some data suggesting that MRI scanning after one cycle may yield information about likely response to chemotherapy,[25] but this has not yet been proven in any large studies. There are also data to indicate that MRI is accurate in most patients at assessing response, but in a significant number can overestimate or underestimate the extent of residual disease following neoadjuvant chemotherapy.[26] Assessment is usually performed after two to four cycles of treatment and if the tumour responds, then chemotherapy should continue for up to eight cycles[27] and the patient is then assessed for definitive curative surgery.

When using adjuvant treatment, the clinician has no idea whether the chemotherapy produces an effect on micrometastatic disease (and currently there is no effective way to screen patients to select out those who have persisting disease following surgery). This is not the case for neoadjuvant chemotherapy. If the tumour fails to respond (e.g. evidence of increase in tumour size or the appearance of new areas of disease, such as malignant nodes), then the chemotherapy agents should be changed and the assessment process repeated, unless the tumour is deemed operable at that time, in which case it may be better to abandon chemotherapy and proceed directly to surgery. Lack of response to neoadjuvant chemotherapy is a poor prognostic sign.

Despite much research into markers to predict prognosis after neoadjuvant chemotherapy (Chapter 2), it appears that the degree of involvement of axillary nodes following neoadjuvant chemotherapy is the best predictor of subsequent relapse.[28] In addition, it is important to remember that both tumour grade and receptor immunohistochemistry can change following treatment[29] when pre- and post-chemotherapy pathological specimens are examined in advanced breast cancer.

## Neoadjuvant/therapeutic endocrine therapy

If the tumour is positive for estrogen or progesterone receptor immunohistochemistry, then the patient may be treated with neoadjuvant estrogen blockade instead of with chemotherapy. The side-effects are less, although time to response is generally slower. The majority of patients treated with neoadjuvant hormone therapy have been postmenopausal. The pathological changes seen following neoadjuvant treatment with an aromatase inhibitor such as letrozole appear to be different from those seen with neodjuvant chemotherapy, with more 'central scarring' with this type of estrogen blockade, compared with more cancers showing diffuse changes and a complete pathological response rate with chemotherapy.[30] Neoadjuvant therapy can potentially increase anxiety in patients (and clinicians) and could potentially lead to delay in switching to an effective treatment should the first agent used be ineffective, as about 3 months of treatment is needed before a true impression of response can be obtained. Progression during treatment is rare with hormone therapy and affects less than 5% of patients. The relative lack of side-effects, and the potential for excellent tumour response,[31] makes neoadjuvant endocrine treatment an attractive prospect. Primary endocrine blockade also acts as a chemotherapy-sparing treatment strategy, allowing more options in the future as the patient is chemotherapy naive. Some work has been done comparing neoadjuvant estrogen blockade with neoadjuvant chemotherapy in older women with hormone-sensitive breast cancers; the results of the two treatments, in this one small study, appeared to be equivalent for outcomes such as response rate and time to response,[32] with a suggestion of a greater rate of conversion to breast-conserving surgery with endocrine therapy.

 Aromatase inhibitors appear more effective than tamoxifen in the neoadjuvant treatment of locally advanced breast cancer.[36]

For many years, it has been clear that postmenopausal women with advanced disease, including metastatic disease, respond to an aromatase inhibitor at least as well[33] or better[34] than to tamoxifen. In the treatment of locally advanced and metastatic breast cancer in postmenopausal women, treatment failure rate is lower with anastrozole (79%) compared with tamoxifen (84%), with a median time to progression of 11.1 months for anastrozole and 5.6 months for tamoxifen.[35] Letrozole is superior to tamoxifen in terms of objective response rate (30% vs. 20%) and treatment failure (85% vs. 75%).[36] The difference could be related to a genuine difference between different classes of estrogen blocking drugs. In addition, it is known that tamoxifen metabolism by the cytochrome P450 system varies in different individuals according to genotype and because of the influence of other medication,[37] but the influence of individual variation in the metabolism of tamoxifen (and indeed aromatase inhibitors) and their subsequent efficacy is unclear. The pure estrogen antagonist, fulvestrant, is as effective as anastrozole in postmenopausal women with advanced breast cancer progressing after prior endocrine treatment,[38] but the place of this drug, which must be given parenterally, in the treatment of locally advanced breast cancer is still being evaluated.

## Adjuvant systemic treatment

Adjuvant systemic treatment for advanced breast cancer that has been treated successfully by surgery is very similar to that given for early-stage breast cancer. Locally advanced breast cancer has a higher risk of relapse than early-stage breast cancer, and so it is likely that following surgery the patient will be offered adjuvant estrogen blockade, local radiotherapy and therapies targeting specific signalling pathways such as the HER-2/neu transmembrane receptor, assuming that the tumour is found to be of the correct biological type for the patient to potentially benefit from such treatments (Chapter 2). Certainly, adding chemotherapy or endocrine therapy or both with radiotherapy for stage IIIB disease reduces locoregional recurrence from 60% to 50% but may not secure a long-term survival advantage.

## Problems of locally recurrent disease after previous treatment

It is vital to know what treatment a patient has received in the past to be able to advise them on future treatment for a recurrent cancer. For example, if the patient has only had an axillary sampling procedure done in the past, and further breast surgery is required to treat recurrent disease, then an axillary clearance should be considered.

The patient who has already been treated with radiotherapy and who develops disease recurrence in the treated area poses a problem. For the reasons given above, there is a limit to how much radiotherapy can be delivered to one area of the body. If the tolerance dose is exceeded, then severe side-effects such as central or peripheral nervous system, lung, bone and skin damage may occur. The results of such treatment may occasionally be worse than the disease. Accurate written information on previous radiotherapy prescriptions is therefore vital before further treatment can be administered safely. Previous permanent skin marks (if still visible) tattooed at the time of the first radiotherapy treatment can accurately delineate what areas may be irradiated in the event of recurrence. If the lymphatics have been omitted from the original treatment and the recurrence is nodal, then sometimes a radical course of radiotherapy can be given to these areas, avoiding the previous treatment field. Re-treatment with radiotherapy for chest wall disease in a patient with terminal disease may occasionally be used to aid palliation of particularly offensive fungating lesions.

The use of systemic treatment for advanced, recurrent disease will depend on what was given as adjuvant therapy at the time of the original diagnosis. In general, different chemotherapy agents are used to treat the recurrent disease, on the basis that the ones used originally did not sterilise the tumour completely, and also because some, notably the anthracyclines, have cumulative side-effects which can be serious. Likewise, there may be some gain from rotating estrogen-blocking agents to palliate locally advanced cancers when there are no other treatment options. Tamoxifen may work when aromatase inhibitors start to fail and vice versa. Sometimes older agents such as megestrol acetate or newer agents such as fulvestrant are effective when other agents fail to control the cancer.

The use of biological agents continues to evolve. The use of trastuzumab in locally advanced disease typically mimics its use in metastatic disease (for inoperable locally advanced cancers) or as adjuvant treatment (in those advanced cancers amenable to more radical treatment). Trastuzumab is seldom used as a single agent, as the response rates in combination with chemotherapy are much better.[39]

There remains considerable uncertainty around the management of locally advanced breast cancer. The accuracy of detecting systemic disease, the value of data 20–30 years old and the relevance of agents and regimens in old trials to the new endocrine agents, chemotherapy agents, biological therapies and current radiotherapy fractionation are currently unclear and, in many regards, for operable locally advanced breast cancer surgery remains a good treatment option.

## Key points

- Locally advanced breast cancer should be treated by a multidisciplinary team.
- The surgeon removing the primary tumour as primary therapy or after neoadjuvant therapy should aim for clear resection margins.
- Sentinel node biopsy may be as good after successful neoadjuvant therapy as axillary clearance.
- Immediate breast reconstruction should be considered.
- Postoperative radiotherapy significantly reduces local recurrence and improves survival in locally advanced breast cancer.
- After neoadjuvant chemotherapy, radical radiotherapy or surgery have a similar efficacy.
- Neoadjuvant chemotherapy is as effective as adjuvant chemotherapy in prolonging survival for patients with locally advanced breast cancer.
- Neoadjuvant therapy with aromatase inhibitors is more effective than tamoxifen.
- Surgery remains a good option for operable locally advanced breast cancer.

# References

1. Ahern V, Brennan M, Ung O et al. Locally advanced and metastatic breast cancer. Aust Fam Physician 2005; 34(12):1027–32.

2. Verma S, Clemons M, Fitzgerald B et al. Treatment of locally advanced breast cancer/three of the authors respond. Can Med Assoc J 2004; 171(3):219–22.

3. Mohamed IE, Williams KS, Tamburrino MB et al. Understanding locally advanced breast cancer: what influences a woman's decision to delay treatment? Prevent Med 2005; 41:399–405.

4. Early Breast Cancer Trialist's Collaborative Group. Effects of radiotherapy and surgery in early breast cancer: an overview of the randomised trials. N Engl J Med 1995; 333:1444–55.

5. Xing Y, Foy M, Cox DD et al. Meta-analysis of sentinel lymph node biopsy after preoperative chemotherapy in patients with breast cancer. Br J Surg 2006; 93(5):539–46.

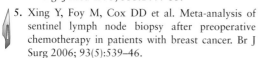

Sentinel lymph node biopsy of the post-treatment axilla may be used to guide therapy.

6. Motwani SB, Strom EA, Schechter NR et al. The impact of immediate breast reconstruction on the technical delivery of postmastectomy radiotherapy. Int J Radiat Oncol Biol Phys 2006; 66(1):76–82.

7. Chatterjee J, Lee A, Baker L et al. Postoperative radiotherapy does not adversely affect the outcome of autologous free abdominal flap reconstruction. Breast Cancer Res Treat 2007; S195:4084.

8. Early Breast Cancer Trialists' Collaborative Group. Radiotherapy for early breast cancer (Cochrane Review). In: The Cochrane Library, Issue 2. Oxford: Update Software, 2002.

9. Adamson DJA. The radiobiological basis of radiation side effects. In: Faithfull S, Wells M (eds) Supportive care in radiotherapy. Edinburgh: Churchill Livingstone, 2003; pp. 71–96.

10. Overgaard M, Hansen PS, Overgaard J et al. Postoperative radiotherapy in high-risk premenopausal women with breast cancer who receive adjuvant radiotherapy. N Engl J Med 1997; 337:949–55.

11. Overgaard M, Jensen MB, Overgaard J et al. Postoperative radiotherapy in high-risk postmenopausal women with breast cancer given adjuvant tamoxifen: Danish Breast Cancer Cooperative Group DBCG 82c randomised trial. Lancet 1999; 353: 1641–8.

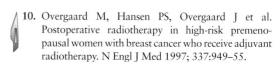

The above two papers show that postoperative radiotherapy reduces locoregional recurrence and improves survival

12. Hojris I, Overgaard M, Christensen JJ et al. Morbidity and mortality of ischaemic heart disease in high-risk breast-cancer patients after adjuvant postmastectomy systemic treatment with or without radiotherapy: analysis of DBCG 82b and 82c randomised trials. Radiotherapy Committee of the Danish Breast Cancer Cooperative Group. Lancet 1999; 354(9188):1425–30.

13. Whelan TJ, Julian J, Wright J et al. Does locoregional radiation therapy improve survival in breast cancer? A meta-analysis. J Clin Oncol 2000; 18(6):1220–9.

14. Chua B, Olivotto IA, Weir L et al. Increased use of adjuvant regional radiotherapy for node-positive breast cancer in British Columbia. Breast J 2004; 10(1):38–44.

15. Rouzier R, Extra J-M, Carton M et al. Primary chemotherapy for operable breast cancer: incidence and prognostic significance of ipsilateral breast tumour recurrence after breast-conserving surgery. J Clin Oncol 2001; 19(18):3828–35.

16. Recht A, Edge SB, Solin LJ et al. Postmastectomy radiotherapy: clinical practice guidelines of the American Society of Clinical Oncology. J Clin Oncol 2001; 19(5):1539–69.

17. SIGN clinical guideline number 84. Management of breast cancer in women. Edinburgh: Scottish Intercollegiate Guidelines Network, 2005.

18. Perloff M, Lesnick GJ, Korzun A et al. Combination chemotherapy with mastectomy or radiotherapy for stage III breast carcinoma: a Cancer and Leukaemia Group B Study. J Clin Oncol 1988; 6:261–9.

19. De Lena M, Varini M, Zucali R et al. Multimodality treatment for locally advanced breast cancer. Results of chemotherapy–radiotherapy versus chemotherapy–surgery. Cancer Clin Trials 1981; 4:229–36.

    After neoadjuvant chemotherapy, radical radiotherapy may have equivalent relapse and survival to surgical resection.

20. Wolff AC. Systemic therapy. Curr Opin Oncol 2001; 13:436–49.

21. Deo SV, Bhutani M, Shukla NK et al. Randomized trial comparing neo-adjuvant versus adjuvant chemotherapy in operable locally advanced breast cancer (T4b N0–2 M0). J Surg Oncol 2003; 84(4):192–7.

    Paper showing equivalence of neoadjuvant chemotherapy compared with adjuvant in terms of survival.

22. Penault-Llorca F, Abrial C, Mouret-Reynier M-A et al. Achieving higher pathological complete response rates in HER-2-positive patients with induction chemotherapy without trastuzumab in operable breast cancer. Oncologist 2007; 12:390–6.

23. Limentani SA, Brufsky AM, Erban JK et al. Phase II study of neoadjuvant docetexel, vinorelbine, and trastuzumab followed by surgery and adjuvant doxorubicin plus cyclophosphamide in women with human epidermal growth factor receptor 2-overexpressing locally advanced breast cancer. J Clin Oncol 2007; 25(10):1232–8.

24. Hsiang DJ, Yamamoto M, Mehta RS et al. Predicting nodal status using dynamic contrast-enhanced magnetic resonance imaging in patients with locally advanced breast cancer undergoing neoadjuvant chemotherapy with and without sequential trastuzumab. Arch Surg 2007; 142(9):855–61.

25. Melsamy S, Bolan PJ, Baker EH et al. Neoadjuvant chemotherapy of locally advanced breast cancer: predicting response with in vivo 1H MR spectroscopy – a pilot study at 4 T. Radiology 2004; 233:424–31.

26. Kwong MS, Chung GC, Horvath LJ et al. Postchemotherapy MRI overestimates residual disease compared with histopathology in responders to neoadjuvant therapy for locally advanced breast cancer. Cancer J 2006; 12(3):212–21.

27. Rastogi P, Anderson SJ, Bear HD et al. Preoperative chemotherapy: updates of National Surgical Adjuvant Breast and Bowel Project Protocols B-18 and B-27. J Clin Oncol 2008; 26(5):778–85.

28. Escobare PF, Patrick RJ, Rybicki LA et al. Prognostic significance of residual breast disease and axillary node involvement for patients who had primary induction chemotherapy for advanced breast cancer. Ann Surg Oncol 2006; 13(6):783–7.

29. Shet T, Agrawal A, Chinoy R et al. Changes in the tumor grade and biological markers in locally advanced breast cancer after chemotherapy – implications for a pathologist. Breast J 2007; 13(5):457–64.

30. Thomas JSJ, Julian HS, Green RV et al. Histopathology of breast carcinoma following neo-adjuvant systemic therapy: a common association between letrozole therapy and central scarring. Histopathology 2007; 51:219–26.

31. Dixon JM, Love CDB, Bellamy COC et al. Letrozole as primary medical therapy for locally advanced and large operable breast cancer. Breast Cancer Res Treat 2001; 66(3):191–9.

32. Semiglazov VF, Semiglazov VV, Dashyan GA et al. Phase 2 randomized trial of primary endocrine therapy versus chemotherapy in postmenopausal patients with estrogen receptor-positive breast cancer. Cancer 2007; 110(2):244–54.

33. Bonneterre J, Thürlimann B, Robertson JFR et al. Anastrozole versus tamoxifen as first-line therapy for advanced breast cancer in 668 postmenopausal women: results of the tamoxifen or arimidex randomized group efficacy and tolerability study. J Clin Oncol 2000; 18(22):3748–57.

34. Macaskill EJ, Renshaw L, Dixon JM. Neoadjuvant use of hormonal therapy in elderly patients with early or locally advanced hormone receptor-positive breast cancer. Oncologist 2006; 11:1081–8.

35. Nabholtz JM, Buzdar A, Pollak M et al. Anastrozole is superior to tamoxifen as first-line therapy for advanced breast cancer in postmenopausal women: results of a north American multicenter randomized trial. J Clin Oncol 2000; 18(22):3758–67.

36. Mouridsen H, Gershanovich M, Sun Y et al. Superior efficacy of letrozole (Femara) versus tamoxifen as first-line therapy for postmenopausal women with advanced breast cancer: results of a phase III study of the International Breast Cancer Group. J Clin Oncol 2001; 19(10):2596–606.

    Aromatase inhibitors may be more effective than tamoxifen in the neoadjuvant treatment of locally advanced breast cancer.

37. Jin Y, Desta Z, Stearns V et al. CYP2D6 genotype, antidepressant use, and tamoxifen metabolism during adjuvant breast cancer treatment. J Natl Cancer Inst 2005; 97(1):30–9.

38. Osborne CK, Pippen J, Jones SE et al. Double-blind, randomized trial comparing the efficacy and tolerability of fulvestrant versus anastrozole in postmenopausal women with advanced breast cancer progressing on prior endocrine therapy: results of a North American trial. J Clin Oncol 2002; 20(16):3386–95.

39. Lewis R, Bagnall A-M, Forbes C et al. The clinical effectiveness of trastuzumab for breast cancer: a systemic review. Health Technol Assess 2002; 6(13).

# 14

# Metastatic disease and palliative care

John Dewar
Pamela Levack

## Introduction

Metastatic spread is defined as spread of breast cancer beyond the breast and ipsilateral axillary and/or internal mammary lymph nodes. With current therapies, metastatic disease is incurable and treatment is, by definition, palliative. It cannot be overemphasised, however, that such patients may benefit considerably from treatment. The purpose of this chapter is to outline the principles and practice of treatment, which is best provided by a combination of active disease management, active symptom management and appropriate support for patient and family.

Historically, palliative care and terminal care were one and the same. However, modern palliative care includes symptom and supportive care for patients 'upstream' in their illness. As cancer advances, patients' symptom burden increases, and they need the best of symptom control as well as the best of cancer treatment. All surgeons should be able to provide high-quality basic palliative care for their patients, and specialist palliative care staff should be available to support staff to manage the most complex and persisting problems.

A frequent dilemma is how much and how intensively to treat, and how much and how intensively to provide care aimed at comfort. The issues faced by staff working at this interface between intensive palliative surgical (or medical) treatment and intensive symptom control are demanding and complex.

To help the doctor decide how aggressive treatment and/or investigations should be, we need to know what patients understand about their illness and prognosis, and what their concerns and wishes are.

## Presentation and prognosis

A minority of breast cancer patients (<10%) present initially with metastatic disease.[1] Most metastatic patients, however, present months or years after their primary treatment (surgery and appropriate adjuvant therapy). The natural history of breast cancer can be very long – patients still die from breast cancer 20 years and more after their initial treatment.[2]

Most patients present with symptoms of metastatic disease between follow-up visits;[3] screening asymptomatic patients is not worthwhile.[4,5] The common sites of metastatic spread are listed in Table 14.1; among other sites is the peritoneum, to which breast cancer of lobular histology can spread and present with non-specific abdominal symptoms and/or obstruction.

## Staging

All patients presenting with locally advanced, or inoperable, or locally recurrent breast cancer should undergo a series of investigations to adequately stage their disease. In addition, patients presenting with

Table 14.1 • Symptoms commonly associated with metastatic spread to different organs

| Site | Common symptoms |
|------|-----------------|
| Pleura | Dyspnoea (due to effusion) |
| Bone | Pain<br>Pathological fracture<br>Nausea and thirst (due to associated hypercalcaemia) |
| Lung | Dyspnoea<br>Cough (dry cough is often seen with lymphangitis carcinomatosa) |
| Liver | Fatigue<br>Nausea<br>Anorexia<br>Pain over liver |
| Brain | Headache (often worse first thing in the morning)<br>Unilateral weakness<br>Unsteady gait |

metastatic disease at one site (e.g. bone) should have investigations to assess the extent of spread to other organs. The principal sites of spread are the thorax, bone and liver. Thus tests may include a full blood count, clinical chemistry (urea and electrolytes, bone chemistry and liver function tests), tumour markers (carcinoembryonic antigen and carbohydrate antigen 15-3, which can be useful to assess response[6]), bone scintigram and computed tomography (CT) scan of thorax and abdomen. Alternatives are a liver ultrasound or magnetic resonance imaging (MRI). Increased long bone activity identified on bone scintigraphy should be further visualised by plain X-ray, supplemented by MRI if necessary, to assess degree of destruction and risk of pathological fracture. The brain should be assessed (CT or MRI) if the patient has symptoms suggestive of intracranial metastases. Urgent MRI of the whole spine is required if the patient has symptoms of spinal cord compression.

Clinicians need to understand the limitations of these investigations. Although bone scintigraphy is more sensitive than plain X-ray, it will not detect all metastases. If a patient has persistent bony symptoms and a negative bone scan (or negative in the symptomatic area) then an MRI should be requested since it is more sensitive than bone scintigraphy. Discrete liver metastases are well visualised by most techniques, but diffuse infiltration may not be apparent on liver ultrasound.

# Treatment

Management is palliative and the aim of treatment is to give the patient the best quality of life with the minimum of side-effects. Successful management of symptoms will tend to prolong survival, but the emphasis of treatment is on the quality of the life lived rather than only its length. Patients need to understand from their clinician the nature of their illness and the aims of treatment before discussing treatment options, likely side-effects and potential benefits.

Broadly speaking, systemic therapies control breast cancer and specific therapies control specific symptoms. The two are not mutually exclusive and most patients will need both.

## Systemic therapy

In general, a durable response to systemic therapy offers the best quality of life (see guidance in **Fig. 14.1**).

 Most patients with estrogen receptor (ER)-positive tumours will be initially treated with hormone therapy: it is generally less toxic than chemotherapy, responses are of longer duration and there is no evidence that patients with ER-positive metastatic disease do better with chemotherapy first.[7]

Exceptions are patients with lymphangitis carcinomatosa or extensive liver metastases – hormone-induced response rates at both these sites are low, and one may not be able to wait the 6–8 weeks for a response, hence chemotherapy is preferable. Endocrine therapy is ineffective in ER-negative breast cancer. If patients respond well to either endocrine or chemotherapy, then they may respond to second-line agents on relapse.

## Endocrine therapy

### Premenopausal women

In 1896, Beatson[8] demonstrated the endocrine sensitivity of breast cancer for the first time, by undertaking surgical oophorectomy for advanced breast cancer. Current therapy (Table 14.2) aims to either decrease levels of circulating estrogen (ovarian ablation) or block its effect on the estrogen receptor (antiestrogens). Ovarian ablation can be performed either by surgical removal (usually laparoscopically), by a short course of radiotherapy to the pelvis (infrequent – because of gastrointestinal side-effects),

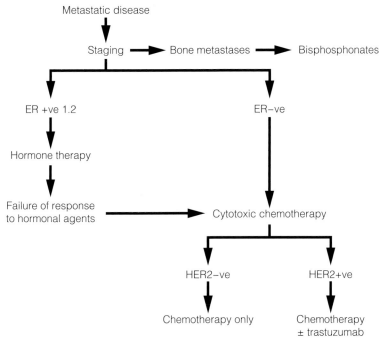

Metastatic disease

Staging → Bone metastases → Bisphosphonates

ER +ve 1.2

Hormone therapy

Failure of response
to hormonal agents → Cytotoxic chemotherapy

ER−ve

HER2−ve

HER2+ve

Chemotherapy only

Chemotherapy
± trastuzumab

**Figure 14.1** • Outline of systemic therapy. Estrogen receptor positive (ER +ve) includes all ER-positive and/or progesterone receptor-positive patients. ER-positive patients with lymphangitis carcinomatosa or liver metastases would normally be considered for chemotherapy in preference to hormone therapy.

Table 14.2 • Endocrine agents used in breast cancer

| Class of agent | Examples | Main side-effects |
|---|---|---|
| Ovarian ablation | Surgical oophorectomy Radiation menopause LH-RH agonists | Menopausal symptoms |
| Antiestrogens | Tamoxifen Fulvestrant | Menopausal symptoms Thromboembolism |
| Aromatase inhibitors | Anastrozole Letrozole Exemestane | Menopausal symptoms Arthralgia Osteoporosis |
| Progestagens | Megesterol acetate Medroxyprogesterone | Weight gain Increased appetite Thomboembolism Glucocorticoid suppression |

 Response to ovarian ablation is improved if tamoxifen is added.[9]

Aromatase inhibitors (AIs; see next section) work in postmenopausal but not in premenopausal women. Particular caution should be taken with women who have chemotherapy-induced amenorrhoea, as they may still have some ovarian function, making AIs ineffective.[10] In premenopausal women, a combination of LH-RH agonist plus AI has shown responses.[11]

Progestagens (e.g. megesterol acetate, medroxyprogesterone) at high dose have been used for many years, for their antiestrogenic action. Their main side-effects are significant weight gain and increased risk of thromboembolic disease. Suppression of glucocorticoid production has been reported,[12] so patients may need hydrocortisone to cover physiological stress (e.g. pinning of pathological fractures, infections, etc.).

Thus, first-line therapy would be tamoxifen with or without ovarian ablation, with an AI/LH-RH agonist as second line and progestagens as third line. Choice will, however, be influenced by prior adjuvant therapy, though if it is >1 year since the last endocrine therapy (e.g. tamoxifen) it may be worth retrying it.

or the use of a luteinising hormone-releasing hormone (LH-RH) agonist, e.g. goserelin. The latter is given by monthly injection into the anterior abdominal wall and is reversible; thus, if there is no tumour response, the patient's periods can be restored and menopausal symptoms abolished.

## Postmenopausal patients

Ovarian ablation has no role. Estrogen in post-menopausal women is produced by conversion of androstenedione to estrone by aromatase,[13] mostly in peripheral fat but also in liver, normal breast tissue and some breast cancers. AIs (Table 14.2) reduce circulating estrogen to nearly immeasurable levels.

There are two types of AI: non-steroidal (anastrozole and letrozole) and steroidal (exemestane). Their side-effects are, however, similar (Table 14.2), implying that they are due to reduced circulating estrogen.

 AIs are more effective[14] than tamoxifen (appropriate second-line agent) and progestagens (third line).

Fulvestrant is relatively newer and unlike tamoxifen has no agonist action. It binds to, blocks and degrades the estrogen receptor. Clinical trials in postmenopausal women have shown it to be as active as anastrozole.[15] It is given monthly by intramuscular injection – a potential advantage where oral compliance is a problem.

# Chemotherapy

Chemotherapy is used to treat ER-negative breast cancer, ER-positive breast cancer that is no longer sensitive to endocrine agents, and advanced ER-positive or ER-negative visceral disease. The main classes of drugs and their side-effects are listed in Table 14.3. These drugs are toxic and should only be prescribed by clinicians (usually oncologists) experienced in their use.

 Drug combinations are more effective than single agents partly because combinations of drugs with different modes of action increase efficacy and reduce the risk of drug resistance but are associated with more toxicity.[16]

The drug groups with the highest activity are the anthracyclines and the taxanes. The major limitation to anthracycline use is cardiomyopathy – the risk increasing as cumulative dose increases. A course of anthracyclines cannot, therefore, usually be repeated. Taxanes are active and more effective than some other regimes.[17] Capecitabine is an oral prodrug of 5-fluorouracil. It is metabolised into the active component in the liver and possibly in the tumour itself.

Table 14.3 • Main cytotoxic chemotherapy drugs used in breast cancer

| Group of drugs | Examples | Main side-effects* |
|---|---|---|
| Anthracyclines | Doxorubicin Epirubicin | Mouth ulcers Cardiomyopathy |
| Alkylating agents | Cyclophosphamide | |
| Antimetabolites | 5-Fluorouracil (capcitabine) Methotrexate Gemcitabine | Coronary spasm Hand–foot symdrome |
| Taxanes | Docetaxel Paclitaxel | Peripheral and autonomic neuropathy Mouth ulcers |
| Vinca alkaloids | Vinorelbine | Neuropathy |
| Platinum | Carboplatinum Cis-platinum | Neuropathy Renal impairment |

*Nearly all these drugs can cause fatigue, nausea, vomiting, myelosuppression, cessation of periods (premenopausal women) and alopecia, so they are not listed individually.

As more agents are used in the adjuvant (or neo-adjuvant) setting, the use of other active drugs such as vinorelbine, gemcitabine and platinum agents in metastatic disease is likely to increase. Platinum salts may have particular activity in the treatment of patients with basal-type tumours[18] and are currently being studied in clinical trials.

The choice of chemotherapy agents is influenced by prior therapy, the general health of the patient, and what agent is most likely to produce useful palliation with minimal side-effects.

## Trastuzumab

A growth factor receptor gene, human epidermal growth factor (HER-2), is amplified in about 25% of breast cancers and is associated with a poorer prognosis.[19] Trastuzumab is a humanised monoclonal antibody that targets the HER-2 receptor in patients whose tumours overexpress HER-2 as assessed by immunohistochemistry and /or fluorescence in situ hybridisation (FISH) testing.

 Whilst it has some activity as a single agent (response rates of 20–50% partly depending on previous treatments), it increases the response rate and survival of patients when added to taxane chemotherapy.[20]

Trastuzumab is generally well tolerated except for cardiac toxicity so should not be given with anthracyclines. It should be used with caution in patients with prior anthracycline exposure or significant cardiac disease; patients require cardiac monitoring by MUGA scan or echocardiogram.

With these provisos, trastuzumab can be used in HER-2-positive patients. It is generally given with a taxane and continued as a single agent whilst response is maintained. Response may last months and even years. Trastuzumab is a large molecule and does not pass the blood–brain barrier, so patients who respond may develop brain metastases as the sole site of active disease. The brain metastases should be treated actively (see later), trastuzumab continued and the patient may regain remission.

Lapatininab inhibits the tyrosine kinases of HER-2 and has been shown to be active in combination with capecitabine in patients who have relapsed on trastuzumab.[21]

## Assessment of response

The most important measure is whether the patient's symptoms have improved. Nevertheless, symptoms can improve independently of systemic therapy (e.g. analgesics for pain). Thus, it is important to assess objectively response to systemic therapy. Locally recurrent disease can be assessed by regular photography and compared with previous clinical photographs of the lesions. Similarly, monitoring measurable lesions on CT provides objective evidence of response. Assessment of bony metastases can be difficult. Plain X-ray changes are slow to develop with response, and responding sclerotic lesions will show little change. Bone scintigraphy can be misleading; 3 months after starting therapy, there may be increased uptake at sites of disease ('flare') indicating response – indistinguishable from progression. Scans at 6 months or later are more reliable. Changes in the levels of tumour markers at 3 months can predict response at 6 months.[22]

### Surgery

For patients presenting with metastatic disease, surgery to the primary site is not usually part of the initial management because it does not help symptoms and is likely to influence prognosis. There are, however, some patients with limited bulk metastatic disease that is responding to treatment in whom surgery should be considered – it provides improved local control and may even improve survival, although results are from retrospective series[23] and are thus subject to selection bias.

## Control of symptoms

 Patients with advanced malignancy can carry a high burden of distressing symptoms, which is frequently under-reported by patients, in some reports by a factor of 10.[24]

Nonetheless patients expect their symptoms to be taken seriously. Intractable pain and nausea affect quality of life and interfere with patients' ability to make considered treatment decisions. Meticulous symptom control should therefore be rapidly available.

Staff, patients and families may be concerned that intensive symptom management will have adverse effects on physiology, including hastening death, despite the lack of supporting data. There is also the fear that appropriate analgesia and symptom control may prevent further palliative treatment of underlying cancer. Intensive symptom control is part of overall cancer management.

### Pain

Sixty-five percent of patients with advanced cancer suffer pain[25] and they expect it to be treated vigorously. One-third of those with pain have one pain, another third have two different types of pain and the remaining third have three or more types of pain, and the presence of both neuropathic and nociceptive pain is common. Approximately 90% of pain is due to the underlying cancer or its treatment.[26] A structured pain history is necessary – the 'NOPQRST' (Box 14.1) is short and simple. Patients and professionals frequently disagree about severity; hence this should be routinely measured – a simple 0–10 analogue scale is widely used.

Analgesic requirements are likely to increase with time. The standard analgesic in severe pain is a strong opioid.

 Morphine is the most commonly used, but newer agents with improved risk–benefit profiles are available.[27]

Box 14.1 • NOPQRST tool for effective pain history taking

N: number of pains

O: origin of pain

P: palliate and potentiate

Q: quality, e.g. is it neuropathic

R: radiation

S: severity *or* suffering – 7–10 is a serious problem, >10 overwhelming

*Suffering is the impact pain has on the patient*

T: timing, including incident pain, for example moving or dressing changes

Box 14.2 • Three questions to ask patient suspected of being opioid toxic

It is important to specifically ask these as the patient may not volunteer it – for fear they are going a little mad.

1. Have you experienced any vivid dreams recently?

2. Have you woken suddenly with a start or had sudden jerky movements?

3. Have you ever imagined that someone was sitting on your bed and you came to with a start and found you had imagined it?

The doses, if switching from morphine, need careful calculation. Hydromorphone, for example, is useful in older patients experiencing opioid toxicity but the oral preparation is eight times as strong as morphine.

Non-oral routes (e.g. by a subcutaneous syringe driver) are preferable when nausea is a major problem. It should be explained that this does not mean that the patient is dying, merely that it is a means to deliver drugs (especially combinations) when absorption is poor – for example, in a patient with pain but who is also vomiting due to hypercalcaemia and constipation. Morphine (10 mg given by intermittent intravenous boluses) may lead to erratic pain control and sleepiness, which can be avoided by using lower doses by subcutaneous infusion, until the situation has resolved and oral medications are appropriate.

Common concerns over opioid analgesics

Whilst morphine is the drug of first choice, side-effects or inadequate pain relief (10–30%) may limit benefit in some patients. Switching opioids may reduce side-effects (Box 14.2) and although this has become accepted practice, the evidence in support is derived from uncontrolled or observational trials. If pain is not opioid sensitive and toxicity is not a problem, switching from one to the other alone will not solve uncontrolled pain.

Specific pains

 Incident pain (e.g. with weight bearing or coughing, etc.) occurs in two-thirds of patients with pain.[28]

Analgesia may be sufficient to manage a pain peak, but may cause toxicity in relation to background pain. It is common in patients with bone metastases.

Severe root pain, particularly on movement, may indicate malignant epidural disease. The aim is to find an effective rescue dose.

Fentanyl, which is 75–200 times more potent than morphine, is very rapidly absorbed in transmucosal form ('actiq') and can give fast, short-acting analgesia, e.g. pre-emptively before severe movement-related pain.

**Liver capsule** pain from liver metastases usually responds to dexamethasone 4–12 mg p.o. daily or, for a fast result or if pain is associated with nausea or vomiting, 12 mg over 24 hours by subcutaneous syringe driver (CSCI), for a few days until the symptoms are resolved. The dose should be then be reduced to the smallest effective maintenance dose.

Neuropathic pain

Patients often find it difficult to accurately describe nerve pain – the descriptors burning, shooting, stabbing, knife-like or tingling are regularly used and patients frequently accompany their description by rubbing the dermatome where the pain is felt. It has a distressing quality, which may not be adequately reflected in a simple 0–10 scale, but a simple neuropathic pain-screening tool has been recently developed.[29] It is critical to recognise neuropathic pain and to diagnose the underlying pathology, as it usually represents new (treatable) metastatic disease.

Neuropathic pain is responsive to opioids in approximately one-third of patients, but the remaining two-thirds may be difficult to treat. Nerve root involvement is most likely to result from brachial plexus involvement or epidural disease as a result of vertebral metastases and subsequent bony collapse. Drugs used primarily for reasons other than analgesia may help,[30] e.g. low doses of antidepressants (amitriptyline or nortrip-tyline[31]), anticonvulsants (gabapentin[32]) or specific *N*-methyl-D-aspartate antagonists (ketamine[33]). Methadone (specialist use only) is helpful when pain consists of a mixture of neuropathic and non-neuropathic pain but there is insufficient published evidence.[34] Finally interventional procedures – cordotomy (unilateral nerve root pain) or epidural followed by an intrathecal implant – may be considered following consultation with the local pain or anaesthetic service.

## Spinal cord compression

Patients with severe increasing back pain plus neuropathic pain referred around the chest wall, abdomen or down one or both legs should be assessed for the risk of spinal cord compression.

 Waiting until the patient has neurological signs of compression (loss of power and/or a sensory level) may be too late to institute appropriate treatment.[35]

If spinal cord compression is suspected, patients should have an urgent MRI scan of the whole spine. If the diagnosis is confirmed they should be referred for radiotherapy or surgical intervention.[36]

## Bony metastases

This is the commonest site of metastatic disease and can cause significant pain and morbidity.

 Specific treatment guidelines have been published.[22]

### Bisphosphonates

Bisphosphonates inhibit osteoclast activity, leading to decreased bone absorption.

 There is good evidence[37,38] that regular treatment with bisphosphonates for 6 months or longer reduces 'skeletal morbidity', namely reduction in pathological fractures, need for palliative radiotherapy and hypercalcaemia.

The drugs used are clodronate, pamidronate and increasingly the third-generation drugs zelendronate and ibandronate. Pamidronate and zoledronate are given intravenously every 4 weeks (or 3-weekly with chemotherapy); ibandronate can be given orally (on an empty stomach 1 hour before food). They are usually reasonably well tolerated but can cause flu-like symptoms, gastrointestinal disturbance and rarely osteonecrosis of the jaw.[39] They should be given with caution in patients with renal impairment. Intravenous bisphosphonates can also reduce pain in patients with widespread bony metastases.[40]

## Bone pain

Non-steroidal analgesics are helpful and are opioid sparing. The most commonly used by palliative medicine physicians is diclofenac 75 mg slow release twice daily. A slow-release preparation reduces early morning pain due to overnight immobility. When pain is severe and distressing, immediate relief may need a non-oral prescription, e.g. 48-hour syringe driver with, for example, opioid and a non-steroidal such as ketorolac, before returning to oral medication. Patients with very advanced disease often have 'symptom clusters', e.g. patients with widespread bony metastases may have pain, nausea, vomiting and constipation due to hypercalcaemia, and patients who are very constipated or nauseated absorb medication poorly.

 Palliative radiotherapy to painful bony metastases can be very helpful in reducing pain and single fractions are as effective as multiple fractions.[41]

## Fractures

Pathological fractures cause severe bony pain. Orthopaedic interventions can stabilise fractures of long bones (commonly femur or humerus). The results of orthopaedic interventions are usually better if done prophylactically rather than as an emergency. In either case, surgery will normally be followed by palliative radiotherapy. Most vertebral fractures will be managed by palliative radiotherapy but selected cases may benefit from surgical stabilisation and/or decompression, especially where there is a risk of spinal cord compression.[22]

## Effusions

Pleural spread is common, especially on the ipsilateral side. The patient usually presents with dyspnoea, and drainage with pleurodesis (using talc[42]) gives good symptomatic relief. Ascites is less common than pleural spread and is managed by drainage.

### Cerebral metastases

This is typically a relatively late site of metastases. Occasionally, it may be the sole site of metastases. Presentation is usually with headache (characteristically worst in the morning if the patient has raised intracranial pressure), weakness and/or altered sensation, difficulty walking or severe persisting nausea. Diagnosis is confirmed by CT or MRI. A short course (five fractions) of palliative radiotherapy to the whole brain may provide useful palliation for patients whose clinical condition is reasonably well preserved. A patient who is in good general condition and has a single cerebral metastasis may get a more prolonged remission from neurosurgical removal followed by radiotherapy.

### Nausea, vomiting and retching

These are common, distressing symptoms and are reported in 50–60% of patients suffering from advanced cancer. Numerous neurotransmitters and receptor types are involved; thus, antiemetics are mainly neurotransmitter blockers (Table 14.4).[43]

### Constipation

Constipation is present in half of all patients with advanced cancer. It causes pain, distension, anorexia, nausea, malaise and embarrassment, and diagnostic confusion if it results in 'overflow' diarrhoea. Contributory factors include opioid use, reduced fluid and fibre intake, and reduced mobility. A recent Cochrane systematic review[44] concluded that all laxatives assessed were ineffective for a significant proportion of patients, and some patients required multiple 'rescue' laxatives. Patients on opiates should be routinely prescribed a stimulant and a softener.

# Overall care of the patient approaching death

On approaching the terminal phase, patient and clinicians need to recognise that active treatment becomes less appropriate, although active symptom palliation remains paramount. The primary care team and the hospital specialists involved in the care of the patient will often have known the patient for some considerable time and have some knowledge of the family circumstances. But if the patient does not understand the reality of their situation, then important issues may not have been discussed. For example, the young single mother will need to address the future care of her children, an older woman the care of a frail elderly spouse.

Table 14.4 • Management of nausea/vomiting due to cancer or its treatment

| | Antiemetic |
|---|---|
| Metabolic, e.g. hypercalcaemia | Haloperidol 1.5 mg nocte/b.d. |
| Drug/toxin induced, e.g. opioid | Levomepromazine 6 mg tab nocte |
| | Haloperidol 1.5 mg nocte/bd |
| | Levomepromazine 6 mg nocte |
| Chemotherapy | Ondansetron |
| | Dexamethasone |
| Radiotherapy | Ondansetron 8 mg p.o. b.d. |
| Raised intracranial pressure (cerebral metastases, brainstem or meningeal disease) | Cyclizine 50 mg t.d.s. or 150 mg/24 h s.c. |
| | Dexamethasone 4–16 mg in the morning |
| Bowel obstruction (if surgery inappropriate) | Cyclizine 50 mg p.o. t.d.s./150 mg/24 h s.c. |
| | Hyoscine butyl bromide 40–100 mg/24 h s.c. |
| | Octreotide 300–1000 mg/24 h s.c. |
| | Ondansetron 8–24 mg/24 h p.o., i.v., s.c. |
| Gastric stasis/outlet obstruction | Metoclopramide or domperidone 10–20 mg q.d.s. or |
| | Metoclopramide 30–100 mg /24 h s.c. |
| Vestibular disease (base skull tumour) | Cyclizine 50 mg p.o. t.d.s. |
| | Levomepromazine 6 mg p.o. |
| | Haloperidol 1.5 mg b.d. |
| | Trial dexamethasone |

Patients may have survived many relapses over the years, and they and their families may believe that they will recover from the current episode. Clinical staff need to recognise the patient's likely prognosis – is she ill with very advanced metastatic breast cancer, is she maybe dying or is she actively dying?

What does the patient understand? Although clinical prediction of survival is a useful independent predictor for survival, it tends to be over-optimistic and for many patients it will be inaccurate. Broadly speaking, when deterioration in health has been noted over months, survival is likely to be months; when it has been over weeks, survival is likely to be weeks; and when it has been over days, survival is likely to be days.

In advanced malignancy, symptoms rather than test results may be more useful in predicting survival. Patients with low performance status (Palliative or Karnofsky Performance Scales) have a poorer survival, although higher performance status does not necessarily predict for longer survival. Certain symptoms such as nausea, breathlessness and weakness have independent value as prognostic factors. Combining clinical prediction with other factors to produce a prognostic score (Table 14.5) gives simple and clinically more accurate useful bedside prognostic information.[45]

# Recognition and communication that the patient may be dying

## 'Is this a patient who could die during this admission?'

Making and communicating a diagnosis that 'this patient may be dying' is the key to good end-of-life care, but it is a difficult skill. It is not exclusively a nursing responsibility – the doctor's role in diagnosis and prognostication is vital. If there is no gap between aggressive or interventional palliative treatments and terminal care, the patient and family will be unprepared – a change from 'doing everything' to 'doing nothing'.

## 'The physician does and does not want to pronounce a death sentence and the patient does and does not want to hear it'

The patient and the family value communication for information and support – it will come from a variety of sources (e.g. doctors, specialist and general nurses, palliative care staff) at different times and stages. Patients, families and professionals need to understand that death is a possibility before they

Table 14.5 • Palliative Prognostic Index (PPI; palliative.info/teaching_material/Prognosis.pdf)

| | Maximum possible | | |
|---|---|---|---|
| Palliative Performance Scale | 10–20 | 4 | 4 |
| | 30–50 | 2.5 | |
| | ≥60 | 0 | |
| Oral intake | Severely reduced (≤ mouthfuls) | 2.5 | 2.5 |
| | Moderately reduced (> mouthfuls) | 1 | |
| | Normal | 0 | |
| Oedema | Present | 1 | 1 |
| | Absent | 0 | |
| Dyspnoea at rest | Present | 3.5 | 3.5 |
| | Absent | 0 | |
| Delirium | Present | 4 | 4 |
| | Absent | 0 | |
| | Total | | 15 |

If PPI >6, survival is less than 3 weeks.

can discuss management options. Several consultations may need to take place over a few days as people psychologically edit what they are told.

Communication in difficult situations is difficult, and easy for professionals to avoid. Some patients prefer not to discuss these matters, as do some professionals. Both patient and professional may collude to limit such discussion.[46]

There is usually more agreement about the most appropriate approach when a patient is actively dying, i.e. the last few days or hours. Requests for transfer to hospice are common during this time, even when the patient is comfortable and their needs are being met. A number of comprehensive, evidence-based pathways have been developed for the last 48 hours, to ensure high-quality end-of-life care can be provided by generalists.[47] Two criteria need to be confirmed for such pathways to be implemented: (1) all possible reversible causes for the current condition have been considered; (2) the responsible team have agreed and accepted that the patient is dying.

## Key points

- Metatastic breast cancer can be actively treated and many patients will survive with a good quality of life for months and often years.
- Most of this time the patients will be in the community and care will be shared between primary and secondary care. Good communication between the two is vital.
- The patient will need considerable support from a multidisciplinary team during this illness and the needs for the help of different members of the team will vary over time.
- Care will be a combination of active oncological management and meticulous symptom control.
- Metastatic breast cancer is an ultimately fatal condition and it is the duty of the staff looking after the patient to optimise survival but also to recognise that the final phase of life needs to be actively and sympathetically managed in line with the wishes of the patient and their family.

# References

1. Scottish Breast Cancer Focus Group and Scottish Cancer Therapy Network. Scottish Breast Cancer Audit 1987 and 1993: report to the Chief Scientist and CRAG. Edinburgh: SCTN, ISD, 1996.

2. Brinkley D, Haybittle JL. The curability of breast cancer. Lancet 1975; ii:95–7.

3. Dewar JA, Kerr GR. Value of routine follow up of women treated for early carcinoma of the breast. BMJ 1985; 291:1464–7.

4. Givio Investigators. Impact of follow-up testing on survival and health-related quality of life in breast cancer patients: a multicentre randomized controlled trial. JAMA 1994; 271:1567–92.

5. Rosselli Del Turci M, Palli D, Cariddi A et al. Intensive diagnostic follow-up after treatment of primary breast cancer: A randomized trial. National Research Council Project on Breast Cancer follow-up. JAMA 1994; 271:1593–7.

6. Harris L, Fritsche H, Mennel R et al. American Society of Clinical Oncology 2007 update of recommendations for the use of tumour markers in breast cancer. J Clin Oncol 2007; 25(33):5287–312.

7. Wilcken N, Hornbuckle J, Ghersi D. Chemotherapy alone versus endocrine therapy alone for metastatic breast cancer. Cochrane Database Syst Rev 2003; 2:CD002747.

8. Beatson GT. On the treatment of inoperable cases of carcinoma of the mamma: suggestions for a new method of treatment, with illustrative cases. Lancet 1896; ii:104–7, 162–5.

9. Robertson JF, Blamey R. The use of gonadotrophin-releasing hormone (GnRH) agonists in early and advanced breast cancer in pre- and perimenopausal women. Eur J Cancer 2003; 7:861–9.

10. Smith IE, Dowsett M, Yap YS et al. Adjuvant aromatase inhibitors for early breast cancer after chemotherapy induced amenorrhoea: caution and suggested guidelines. J Clin Oncol 2006; 24:2444–7.

11. Forward DP, Cheung KL, Jackson L et al. Clinical and endocrine data for goserilin plus anastrozole as second-line endocrine therapy for premenopausal advanced breast cancer. Br J Cancer 2005; 92:416–17.

12. Naing KK, Dewar JA, Leese GP. Megesterol acetate (Megace) therapy and secondary adrenal suppression. Cancer 1999; 86(6):1044–9.

13. Miller WR. Aromatase inhibitors: mechanism of action and role in the treatment of breast cancer. Semin Oncol 2003; 30(4, Suppl 14):3–11.

14. Gibson LJ, Dawson CK, Lawrence DH et al. Aromatase inhibitors for the treatment of advanced breast cancer in postmenopausal women. Cochrane Database Syst Rev 2007; 1:CD003370.

This meta-analysis of all the trials comparing AIs with other endocrine therapies confirms the advantages of AIs.

15. Howell A, Pippen J, Elledge RM et al. Fulvestrant versus anastrozole for the treatment of advanced breast cancer: a prospectively planned combined analysis of two multicentre trials. Cancer 2005; 104:236–9.

16. Carrick S, Parker S, Wilcken N et al. Single agent versus combination chemotherapy for metastatic breast cancer. Cochrane Database Syst Rev 2005; 2: CD003372.

A systematic review of 37 trials and although the results are summarised in the text, there is heterogeneity between the trials reflecting differences in efficacy of the drugs used.

17. Ghersi D, Wilcken N, Simes J et al. Taxane containing regimes for metastatic breast cancer. Cochrane Database Syst Rev 2005; 2:CD003366.

18. Brody LC. Treating cancer by targeting a weakness. N Engl J Med 2005; 253:949–50.

19. Slamon DJ, Clark GM, Wong SG et al. Human breast cancer: correlation of relapse and survival with amplification of the HER2/neu oncogene. Science 1987; 235:177–82.

20. Slamon DJ, Leyland-Jones B, Shak S et al. Use of chemotherapy plus a monoclonal antibody against HER2 for metastatic breast cancer that overexpresses HER2. N Engl J Med 2001; 344:783–92.

The first randomised trial to demonstrate the activity of a monoclonal antibody in human breast cancer.

21. Geyer CE, Forster J, Lindquist D et al. Lapatininib plus capcitabine for HER2-positive advanced breast cancer. N Engl J Med 2006; 355:2733–43.

22. Breast Speciality Group of the British Association of Surgical Oncology. Guidelines for the management of metatastic bone disease in breast cancer in the United Kingdom. Eur J Surg Oncol 1999; 25:3–23.

23. Rapiti E, Verkooijen HM, Vlastos G et al. Complete excision of primary breast tumor improves survival of patients with metastatic breast cancer at diagnosis. J Clin Oncol 2006; 24:2743–9.

24. Grossman SA, Sheidler VR, Swedeen K et al. Correlation of patient and caregiver ratings of cancer pain. J Pain Symptom Mgmt 1991; 6:53–57.

25. van den Beuken, van Everdingen MHJ, de Rijke JM et al. Prevalence of pain in patients with cancer: a systematic review of the past 40 years. Ann Oncol 2007; 18:143749.

26. Twycross R. Pain relief in advanced cancer. New York: Churchill Livingstone, 1994; pp. 55–61.

27. Hanks GW. Morphine and alternative opioids in cancer pain: the EAPC recommendations. Br J Cancer 2001; 84(5):587–93.

28. Caraceni A, Martini C, Zecca E. Breakthrough pain characteristics and syndromes in patients with cancer pain. An international survey. Pall Med 2004; 18:177–83.

29. Portenoy R. Development and testing of a neuropathic pain screening questionnaire. ID Pain Curr Med Res Opin 2006; 22(8):1555–65.

30. Dworkin RH, O'Connor AB, Backonja M et al. Pharmacologic management of neuropathic pain: evidence-based recommendations. Pain 2007; 132(3):237–51.

31. Saarto T, Wiffin PJ. Antidepressants for neuropathic pain. Cochrane Database Syst Rev 2005; 3: CD005454.

32. Wiffen PJ, McQuay HJ, Edwards JE et al. Gabapentin for acute and chronic pain. Cochrane Database Syst Rev 2005; 3:CD005452.

33. Bell RF, Ecclestone C, Kalso E. Ketamine as an adjuvant to opioids for cancer pain. Cochrane Database Syst Rev 2003; 1:CD003351.

34. Nicholson AB. Methadone for cancer pain. Cochrane Database Syst Rev 2004; 2:CD003971.

35. Levack P, Graham J, Collie D et al. Don't wait for a sensory level – listen to the symptoms: a prospective audit of the delays in the diagnosis of malignant spinal cord compression. Clin Oncol 2002; 14:472–80.

36. Loblaw DA, Perry J, Chambers A et al. Systematic review of the diagnosis and management of malignant cord compression: the cancer care Ontario practice guidelines initiative's neuro-oncology disease site group. J Clin Oncol 2005; 23(9):2028–37.

37. Pavlakis N, Schmidt R, Stockler M. Bisphosphonates for breast cancer. Cochrane Database Syst Rev 2005; 3:CD003474.

38. Ross JR, Saunders Y, Edmonds PM et al. Systematic review of role of bisphosphonates on skeletal morbidity in metastatic cancer. BMJ 2003; 327:469–72.

Both of these reviews confirm, from large randomised studies in women with advanced breast cancer, that bisphosphonates when given in addition to systemic endocrine therapy or chemotherapy reduce the risk of skeletal morbidity.

39. Marx RE, Sawatari Y, Fortin M et al. Bisphosphonate-induced exposed bone (osteonecrosis/osteopetrosis) of the jaws: risk factors, recognition, prevention and treatment. J Oral Maxillofac Surg 2005; 63:1567–75.

40. Wong R, Wiffen PJ. Bisphosphonates for the relief of pain secondary to bone metastastases (Cochrane review). In: The Cochrane Library, Issue 2. Chichester: John Wiley & Sons, 2004.

41. Chow E, Harris K, Fan G et al. Palliative radiotherapy trials for bone metastases: a systematic review. J Clin Oncol 2007; 25(11):1423–36.

A systematic review of 16 trials comparing single fractions vs. multiple fractions confirms that both are as effective in relieving pain, but patients who had a single fraction are more likely to be re-treated.

42. Tan C, Sedrakyan A, Browne J et al. The evidence on the effectiveness of management for malignant pleural effusion: a systematic review. Eur J Cardiothorac Surg 2006; 29:829–38.

# Chapter 14

43. Hallenbeck JL. Palliative care perspectives. Oxford University Press, 2003.

44. Miles CL, Fellowes D, Goodman ML et al. Laxatives for the management of constipation in palliative care patients. Cochrane Database Syst Rev 2006; 4:CD003448.

45. Lau F, Cloutier-Fischer D, Kuziemsky C et al. A systematic review of prognostic tools for estimating survival time in palliative care. J Pall Care 2007; 23(2):93–112.

46. The A-M, Hak T, Koeter G et al. Collusion in doctor–patient communication about imminent death: an ethnographic study. BMJ 2000; 321:1376–81.

47. http://www.mcpcil.org.uk/files/hospital_pathway.pdf

# 15

# Adjuvant radiotherapy in the management of breast cancer

Gillian Ross
Virginia Wolstenholme

## Introduction

Radiotherapy has a key role in the reduction of risk of breast cancer recurrence. Importantly, results of recent clinical trials also suggest that successful locoregional tumour control may impact on overall survival. This chapter reviews the evidence base for current recommendations for adjuvant radiotherapy and highlights areas of developments in practice.

## What is radiotherapy?

Radiotherapy is the use of ionising radiation to kill cancer cells. When beams of X-rays pass through human tissue, the packets of energy (called photons) interact with tissue atoms and gradually lose momentum. The energy released within tissue damages critical molecules like DNA, producing strand breaks. Normal cells activate cell-cycle checkpoints, slowing progression to S phase, or mitosis, to enable DNA repair to occur. Most malignant cells are mutated in key cell-cycle genes (e.g. *p53*) and do not activate arrest of the cell cycle in the presence of radiotherapy-induced DNA damage. Tumour cells therefore pass on damaged DNA to daughter cells, usually activating apoptosis. Radiotherapy therefore exploits these key differences between normal and cancer cells.[1]

## How is radiotherapy delivered?

Patients attend a treatment planning session before radiotherapy can begin. At this visit, the clinician marks the margins of the breast where radiation beams will be directed. Increasingly, computed tomography (CT) scans are used to plan the treatment (**Fig. 15.1**). Treatment beams pass across the chest and through the breast tissue, efforts usually being made to minimise the amount of lung tissue included in the beam. This is important for avoiding radiation pneumonitis or long-term fibrosis. In the case of left-sided cancers, avoidance of cardiac irradiation is also important.

The unit of dose for radiotherapy is the gray (Gy). Treatment courses vary between departments, but a commonly used schedule comprises 50 Gy given as daily treatments of 2 Gy over 5 weeks to the whole breast. In order to minimise patient attendance, especially in areas where geographical access to cancer centres is difficult, an alternative schedule of 40 Gy given in 15 treatments over 3 weeks is also commonly used.

Recent data have shown 40 Gy delivered over 3 weeks is at least as favourable in terms of local control and late effects as 50 Gy given over a 5-week schedule.[2]

Minor variations on these dosing schedules are common, but treatment intensity is selected to give a high probability of inactivating microscopic cancer

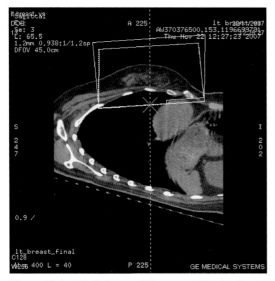

**Figure 15.1** • Radiotherapy CT scan used to plan breast radiotherapy.

cells while minimising adverse effects. To increase treatment intensity in the index quadrant of the tumour, it is common practice to deliver a 'boost' dose with electrons very focally.

 Additional boost radiation to the tumour bed reduces the risk of local recurrence in all age groups, with the greatest absolute benefit being in patients younger than 50 years.[3]

Electrons have the property of depositing their energy (i.e. DNA damage) within a few centimetres, and are used to increase the radiotherapy dose to the tumour bed. Typical boost doses range from 10 Gy in five fractions to 16 Gy in eight fractions.

## Adverse effects

A principal effect of radiotherapy is to halt the process of division in dividing cells. In the breast area the overlying normal epidermis is affected by the radiotherapy, which suppresses cell proliferation throughout the course of treatment resulting in thinning, dryness and, in some cases, temporary moist desquamation of the skin. Blood vessels become more leaky and a varying degree of erythema develops. These effects usually resolve within 10–14 days of completing treatment. Increased pigmentation due to stimulation of melanocytes may last months. Simple skin-care advice by an experienced radiographer or nurse is valuable during treatment. It is extremely uncommon for patients to feel unwell, and fatigue is not a problem unless the patient has had prior cytotoxic chemotherapy. Irradiation of lymph glands is recommended if there is nodal involvement on sampling, sentinel node biopsy and level I dissection, and no further axillary surgery is planned.

 A completion axillary clearance is usually recommended following a positive sentinel node biopsy or axillary sampling in order to acquire prognostic information and as definitive axillary therapy.[4]

 Radiotherapy is also an option for treating involved axillary nodes after sentinel node biopsy or axillary sampling.

Irradiation of the supraclavicular fossa is indicated in patients with more than four involved axillary lymph glands. If the axilla has been cleared, supraclavicular glands alone are treated. Irradiation of a fully dissected axilla should be avoided unless there is extensive extracapsular tumour extension into fat. In these circumstances, axillary and supraclavicular nodes are treated to maximise chances of achieving local tumour control, counselling the patient that postoperative irradiation in this circumstance increases the risk of treatment-related lymphoedema to approximately 40%.

## Radiotherapy and breast conservation

The aims of breast conservation therapy which incorporates wide local excision of the cancer and adjuvant radiotherapy are to ensure survival equivalent to mastectomy, while optimising the cosmetic outcome and minimising risks of disease recurrence in the conserved breast. Since the 1970s, there have been six prospective randomised trials in which breast-conserving surgery (BCS) has been compared with mastectomy. The results are summarised in Table 15.1.

Randomised studies have confirmed the equivalence of BCS plus radiotherapy and mastectomy with respect to survival (**Fig. 15.2**).

Table 15.1 • Local recurrence rates in randomised trials comparing breast-conserving surgery (BCS) and radiotherapy (RT) with mastectomy

| Reference | Trial | Follow-up (years) | Local recurrence (%) | | |
| --- | --- | --- | --- | --- | --- |
| | | | Mastectomy | BCS + RT | Type of BCS |
| Sarrazin et al.[5] | Gustave-Roussy | 10 | 9 | 7 | 2-cm margin |
| Veronesi et al.[6] | Milan | 10 | 2 | 4 | Quadrantectomy |
| Fisher et al.[7] | NSABP B-06 | 8 | 8 | 10 | Lumpectomy |
| Poggi et al.[8] | NCI | 8 | 6 | 20 | Gross excision |
| Van Dongen et al.[9] | EORTC | 8 | 9 | 13 | 1-cm margin |
| Blichert-Toft et al.[10] | Danish Breast Group | 6 | 4 | 3 | Wide excision |

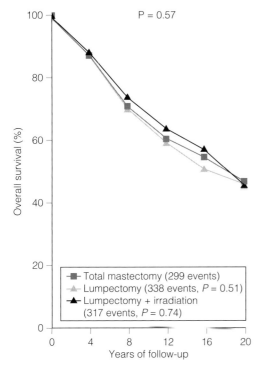

Figure 15.2 • Overall survival among 589 women treated with total mastectomy, 634 treated with lumpectomy alone and 628 treated with lumpectomy plus radiotherapy.

Differing surgical and radiotherapy techniques have different rates of recurrence in the breast that vary from 4% to 20% at 10 years. Although mastectomy is a more radical surgical procedure which results in significant rates of psychosexual morbidity, mastectomy is still associated with a significant risk of local recurrence of 2–9%.

Efforts have focused on refining and improving outcomes. There is now a greater understanding of factors affecting risk of local recurrence, as well as quality of cosmesis, and greater awareness of techniques that help minimise treatment-related complications.

## Risk factors for recurrence following BCS

The local recurrence rates observed in both randomised and retrospective studies range from 8% to 20% at 10 years. However, some of the longest follow-up has been obtained in retrospective studies. Kurtz et al.[11] documented an incidence of recurrence that increased from 7% at 5 years to 14% at 10 years, rising to 20% at 20 years. The study group comprised 1593 women with stage I or II breast cancer that had been completely excised. Of the recurrences, 79% were in the vicinity of the tumour bed, but as time from treatment increased so the percentage of recurrences located elsewhere in the breast also increased. The majority of recurrences after 10 years were considered new tumours. Locoregional control was 88% at 5 years after salvage mastectomy and 64% after breast-conserving salvage procedures.

Factors that influence local recurrence include patient factors (e.g. young age), tumour factors (e.g. extensive intraductal component, lymphovascular invasion and grade) and treatment factors (e.g. resection margins, intensity of radiotherapy and adjuvant systemic treatment) (see Chapter 4). Although tumour size and lymph node positivity are the most important predictive factors for overall survival, neither has an impact on local failure in the breast;[12,13] however, this may be difficult to ascertain due to competing risks of systemic failure in high-risk patients.

Pathological studies of the extent of microscopic invasive and in situ carcinoma that surrounds the macroscopic tumour in mastectomy specimens indicate that microscopic tumour extends some distance from the gross tumour. In T1 and T2 invasive cancers, microscopic extension may be present more than 2 cm from the tumour in more than 40% of patients.[14,15] This accords with the 42% probability of breast recurrence seen in the lumpectomy without radiotherapy treatment arm of the National Surgical Adjuvant Breast and Bowel Project (NSABP) B-06 trial.[7,16] The principles behind modern BCS/radiotherapy are the surgical removal of enough breast tissue to ensure that the residual microscopic tumour burden is sufficiently low to be sterilised by moderate-dose adjuvant radiotherapy (**Fig. 15.3**). In all epithelial malignancies the total radiation dose required to control disease increases as tumour clonogen bulk increases. At the high radiation doses required to sterilise macroscopic disease or even large quantities of microscopic disease, there is very little therapeutic ratio in favour of tumour control over normal tissue damage. This leads to unacceptable late radiation effects in the breast and underlying chest wall. The 12% probability of ipsilateral breast recurrence in the adjuvant radiotherapy arm compared with 8% in the mastectomy arm of NSABP B-06 suggests that moderate-dose radiotherapy can achieve acceptable

local control when the margins of excision are microscopically free of tumour cells.[7,16] Modern randomised controlled comparisons of BCS/radiotherapy and adjuvant radiotherapy with mastectomy indicate that breast preservation is not associated with any detriment to overall survival. However, local recurrence within the treated breast (3–20%) has generally been reported to be more common than chest wall recurrence after mastectomy (4–9%) (see Table 15.1).[5–7,9,10,16,17] Local recurrence rates are however falling (see Chapter 4).

## Natural history of, and risk factors for, local recurrence

The natural history of local recurrence is protracted, with recurrence risks previously reported at 1–2% per year over at least 10 years following BCS/radiotherapy, most recurrences within the first 5 years occurring within the index quadrant.[11,18] In contrast, postmastectomy recurrence tends to occur within 3 years of surgery.

The selection of patients for a BCS/radiotherapy strategy should take into account factors known to increase the risk of breast recurrence. Young patient age (<35–40 years) has been found to be a risk factor by several authors;[18–21] although youth correlates with the presence of adverse histopathological factors,[21] it independently signifies increased risk.[18] Retrospective analyses indicate that patients younger than 35 years also have an increased risk of recurrence following

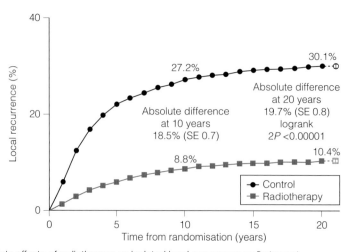

**Figure 15.3** • Absolute effects of radiotherapy on isolated local recurrence as first event.

mastectomy.[22,23] The prospective trials of BCS/radiotherapy compared with mastectomy do not show any survival advantage for mastectomy in the subgroup of young patients. Youth is therefore not considered a contraindication to BCS/radiotherapy and adjuvant radiotherapy. Tumour multifocality, increasing tumour grade, vascular invasion, the presence of an extensive intraduct component (EIC) and the inadequacy of the surgical margins of excision have also been shown to be risk factors for breast recurrence on multivariate analyses. The increased risk of local recurrence associated with EIC is lost in multivariate analysis controlled for the presence of a tumour-free margin of excision.[18,24–27] The only one of these factors that is considered a definite contraindication to BCS/radiotherapy is macroscopic multifocality, although even this is being re-examined.

## Importance of local recurrence

The effect of breast recurrence on overall survival is controversial. The apparent lack of detriment to survival of BCS/radiotherapy, despite an increased risk of ipsilateral breast recurrence, argues against any detrimental effect of local recurrence on survival.[5–7,9,10,16,17] More recently, the effect of prevention of local or regional recurrence on survival has been demonstrated in the 15-year follow-up results of two trials of postmastectomy radiotherapy[28,29] on long-term follow-up of BCS trials. This highlights the very long follow-up required to see differences in survival attributable to improvement in local disease control. This is especially the case in the context of BCS/radiotherapy, as local recurrence occurs later than that seen after mastectomy and this risk of recurrence continues for at least 10 years after treatment.[11,18] NSABP B-06 has shown that patients with local recurrence following BCS without radiotherapy have an increased risk of metastatic disease.[16] Touboul et al.[30] found isolated local recurrence an independent risk factor for metastatic disease, with a relative risk of 9.9 (95% CI 5.5–18) after a mean follow-up of 7 years. It can be argued that these results may simply represent the effect of lead-time bias, as those with local recurrence may have early metastatic disease detected when they are restaged. However, others argue that it is intuitive that local recurrence can metastasise and compromise survival. The observed increases in distant metastasis associated with high rates of local

recurrence may precede reductions in overall survival as observed in trials with 15-year follow-up.[31] Despite the controversy, it seems sensible to minimise the risk of local recurrence associated with breast conservation if this can be achieved with good cosmetic outcome. If not, one should consider mastectomy and breast reconstruction in those whose risk factors indicate a risk of local recurrence unacceptable to the individual patient.

## Balance between optimal local control and cosmesis

Quadrantectomy was associated with a risk of local recurrence of 5.3% and lumpectomy of 13.3% in the Milan II trial, despite both being followed by radiotherapy. Microscopic involvement of the surgical margin by tumour occurred in 3% of the quadrantectomy group and 16% of the lumpectomy group, accounting for the excess local recurrence rate with lumpectomy. Cosmesis was significantly worse following quadrantectomy.[6] There is thus a balance between minimising the volume of breast tissue excised in order to maintain a good cosmetic result and removing sufficient tissue to allow maintenance of the radiation dose below that which leads to unacceptable late radiation damage, which itself compromises cosmesis.[32] This is discussed in more detail in Chapter 4.

## Margin status and local recurrence risk

The final surgical margin is a critical determinant of local recurrence risk, with actuarial recurrence rates of 2–5% for margin-negative groups and 16–21% for margin-positive groups.[21,21,25,27,33] More recent publications have suggested that although diffuse involvement of the margin is associated with an increased recurrence rate, focal involvement of the margin is not.[34–37]

## Influence of systemic therapy on local recurrence following BCS

Chemotherapy alone without radiotherapy does not reduce local recurrence risk after BCS.[7,16] Data on the effect of systemic therapy in addition to adjuvant radiotherapy on local recurrence are scarce.

Retrospective series are confounded by competing risks, with those selected for systemic therapy more likely to develop distant disease before local recurrence. Treatment with adjuvant chemotherapy did seem to be associated with reduced risk of local failure following BCS/radiotherapy and radiotherapy in one study.[37] The analysis did not take into account the status of the surgical margin. Randomised data from NSABP B-13 indicate that in patients with clear margins adjuvant chemotherapy does appear to reduce risk of ipsilateral breast recurrence from 13.4% to 2.6% at 8 years.[38]

For patients with involved margins, a multivariate analysis of the Stanford series found the use of concurrent adjuvant chemotherapy to be independently associated with better local control in those with margins that were not more than 2 mm clear.[35] Other series including patients with involved margins have not found use of adjuvant chemotherapy to be associated with reduced risk of local recurrence.[21,27,30,33,39] Tamoxifen does reduce the risk of local recurrence, and in postmenopausal women the new aromatase inhibitors appear to be better than tamoxifen in maintaining local control and reducing both local recurrences and new primary cancers in the treated breast.

## Optimising breast conservation with adjuvant radiotherapy

Current research is now focusing on optimising the physical delivery of radiotherapy to maintain benefits of treatment, with reduced late toxicity. Active studies are now addressing technical issues such as optimal dose fractionation and improved homogeneity of dose delivery by intensity modulation of beams. Given the increasing proportion of women receiving both adjuvant chemotherapy and radiotherapy, we need to define the most efficacious sequencing based on evidence. Finally, as the UK Breast Screening Programme has identified a significant proportion of women with ductal carcinoma in situ or small (<2 cm), low-grade, node-negative cancers, there is a need to carefully examine the role of adjuvant radiotherapy in such good-prognosis patients to be certain that such treatment is necessary.

## Postmastectomy radiotherapy

Despite the widespread use of BCS in the management of early breast cancer, a significant number of patients are unsuitable for this approach and are offered mastectomy. Many women who are offered mastectomy rather than breast conservation tend to have larger tumours with adverse histopathological prognostic features. Many such patients are candidates for neoadjuvant therapy. Despite the near complete removal of breast tissue that occurs at mastectomy, locoregional recurrence occurs in 30–40% of women with these adverse prognostic features. The chest wall is the commonest site of locoregional recurrence and it is thought that recurrence arises from tumour that has involved dermal lymphatics. Unsurprisingly, the presence of tumour in axillary lymph nodes is the strongest indicator of risk of locoregional recurrence. High-grade cancers within a tumour diameter over 4 cm and direct invasion of skin or pectoral fascia are also risk factors. Unlike breast recurrence following BCS, chest wall recurrence can only be controlled in about half of patients. Uncontrolled chest wall recurrence, which can progress to encase the hemithorax, is one of the most distressing manifestations of advanced breast cancer and is difficult to palliate satisfactorily.

Adjuvant radiotherapy may be used following radiotherapy with two potential benefits: reduction in risk of locoregional recurrence and improved overall survival. A number of trials over the past 30 years have examined the effect of postoperative radiotherapy on these two end-points. Many of the early trials were conducted before adjuvant systemic therapy had been shown to eradicate micrometastatic disease in some patients and before modern radiotherapy techniques that minimise normal tissue irradiation effects were used widely.

A meta-analysis published in 1987 of all randomised controlled trials started before 1975 showed that postmastectomy radiotherapy was associated with a 66% reduction in risk of locoregional recurrence. However, radiotherapy was associated with an excess mortality in those surviving more than 10 years after randomisation. In this group the 25-year survival was 42% following radiotherapy and 51% following surgery alone. The excess mortality in the radiotherapy group was due to cardiac deaths (**Fig. 15.4**) and was balanced by a reduction in breast cancer mortality (**Fig. 15.5**). In 2005, the Early Breast Cancer Trialists' Collaborative Group[40] published a meta-analysis of randomised controlled trials started before 1985. This included 8500 women randomised in trials where surgery involved some form of mastectomy and 7300 women randomised in trials where surgery involved BCS.

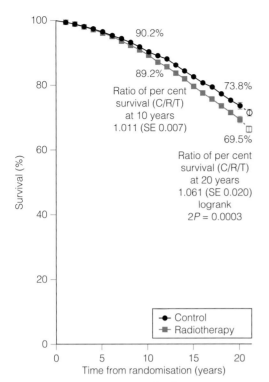

**Figure 15.4** • Absolute effects of radiotherapy on non-breast cancer deaths.

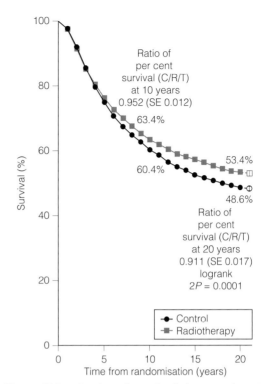

**Figure 15.5** • Absolute effects of radiotherapy on breast cancer deaths.

The additional use of radiotherapy was associated with a 17% and 19% reduction in risk of local recurrence in the two respective groups. For women with node-negative disease, the 5-year local recurrence risk after mastectomy and axillary clearance was only 6%, even in the absence of radiotherapy. After chest wall radiotherapy, this risk is reduced to 2%. There was no significant reduction in 15-year mortality in this group. Node-positive disease, however, had a 5-year local recurrence rate of 23% in the absence of radiotherapy. This figure was reduced to 6% with radiation. With regard to mortality, there was a 5.4% absolute reduction in risk of death at 15 years with the addition of chest wall radiation ($P - 0.0002$).

The effects of radiotherapy on non-breast cancer deaths can be seen at 15 years (15.9% vs. 14.6% in radiotherapy-treated and non-radiotherapy-treated groups respectively). These figures are confounded by differences in laterality (effecting cardiac dose), dose to lung and vascular structures, in addition to patient age and smoking habits. There are significant separate differences seen in cancer mortality at

different time periods following the completion of radiotherapy. This is likely to reflect the time when patients were randomised with early trials using radiotherapy techniques which were less sophisticated and less able to reduce normal tissue irradiation. The differences are significant in patient ages both under and over 50 years.

Modern radiotherapy techniques recognise the importance of minimising the cardiac volume irradiated and use fractionated radiotherapy regimens that reduce late normal tissue radiation effects.

Three large randomised trials have recently reported long-term results of postoperative radiotherapy after mastectomy in high-risk premenopausal women treated with cyclophosphamide, methotrexate and 5-fluorouracil (CMF) chemotherapy and high-risk postmenopausal women treated with tamoxifen. The Danish trial[28] included 1789 premenopausal women with pathologically positive axillary lymph nodes, tumour greater than 5 cm in diameter or invasion of the skin or the pectoral fascia. Following total mastectomy with stripping of the pectoral fascia and level I/II axillary dissection, patients received eight to nine cycles of CMF chemotherapy. Adjuvant radiotherapy was the randomised treatment and was delivered to the chest wall, axilla, supraclavicular and infraclavicular nodes and the internal mammary nodes using a cardiac-sparing technique. After a median follow-up of 114 months, the use of radiotherapy was associated with a 21% absolute reduction in risk of local recurrence (9% vs. 32%, $P < 0.001$) and a 9% absolute increase in overall survival ($P < 0.001$). The effect of radiotherapy on overall survival was irrespective of tumour size, node status, number of positive nodes or the histopathological grade.

The British Columbia trial[41] also examined the effect of postoperative radiotherapy in premenopausal women with pathologically involved axillary lymph nodes treated with modified radical mastectomy, including level I/II axillary dissection and six cycles of CMF chemotherapy. This group also irradiated the axilla, supraclavicular fossa and internal mammary chain (IMC). After 15-years follow-up the use of radiotherapy was associated with a 20% absolute reduction in risk of locoregional recurrence (13% vs. 33%, $P = 0.003$) and a 17% absolute increase in disease-free survival (50% vs. 33%, $P = 0.007$) and metastasis-free survival (51% vs. 34%, $P = 0.006$). Overall survival was improved by 8% at 15 years (54% vs. 46%, $P = 0.007$). These trials have received some criticism because the management of the axilla and the chemotherapy used was suboptimal, 3-weekly intravenous CMF being considered not as good as more modern anthracycline-containing regimens. Many patients in these studies had small numbers of axillary nodes retrieved and so residual axillary nodal disease will have been left untreated. In the absence of data showing a reduction of risk of death of equivalent magnitude for anthracycline-containing adjuvant regimens over CMF, it seems unlikely that the use of these regimens would negate the 30% reduction of risk of death gained by use of radiotherapy seen in these trials. Both of these trials demonstrate that prevention of locoregional recurrence reduces metastatic disease and death.

The effect of postmastectomy radiotherapy in postmenopausal women under 70 years of age treated with adjuvant tamoxifen has recently been reported by the Danish Breast Cancer Cooperative Group;[42] 1460 women were treated with total mastectomy and level I/II axillary dissection. All had pathologically positive axillary lymph nodes, tumours greater than 5 cm in diameter or involvement of skin or

pectoral fascia. All received 30 mg tamoxifen daily for a year. Radiotherapy to the chest wall, axilla, supraclavicular/infraclavicular fossa and IMC was randomised. After a median follow-up of 119 months for survivors and 46 months for those that died, locoregional recurrence had occurred in 8% of the radiotherapy arm and 35% of the no radiotherapy arm. Radiotherapy was associated with a 9% absolute overall survival advantage at 10 years (45% vs. 36%, $P = 0.03$). There was no difference in proportionate benefit of radiotherapy in those with large or small tumours or with few or many positive nodes. The median number of nodes removed was seven, which is small, fuelling concerns that some women with multiple node involvement will have been left with untreated residual axillary nodal disease. The proportionate benefit of radiotherapy, however, was identical in those who had more or less than eight nodes removed. The benefit of radiotherapy on overall survival only became apparent more than 4 years after randomisation. There was no evidence of increased cardiac morbidity or mortality after 10 years of follow-up.

The duration of tamoxifen treatment and the absence of adjuvant chemotherapy would now be considered suboptimal. Whether the reduction in risk of local recurrence and subsequent improval in overall survival associated with radiotherapy would be nullified by use of tamoxifen for 5 years is unknown. One would have to demonstrate a sustained 27% absolute improvement in locoregional recurrence and 9% absolute improvement in survival compared with 1 year of tamoxifen alone to negate the observed advantage of radiotherapy.

 Numerous consensus reports[43,44] recommend that patients with four or more positive axillary nodes are offered postmastectomy chest wall radiotherapy.

A subgroup analysis of patients with one to three positive lymph nodes has recently been reported, suggesting other patients groups may also benefit from postmastectomy radiation.[45] This study included high-risk pre- and postmenopausal women who were randomised to postmastectomy radiation followed by adjuvant systemic therapy. The overall 15-year survival rate was 39% and 29% ($P = 0.0015$) after radiotherapy and no radiotherapy respectively. Radiotherapy reduced 15-year locoregional failure rate from 51% to 10% in the 4+ positive node group and from 27% to 4% in the 1–3 positive node group. This has stimulated further interest in the use of radiotherapy for such patients and is now the subject of a national trial in the UK (SUPREMO trial, www. supremo-trial.com), which randomises intermediate-risk patients to postmastectomy radiotherapy.

These three randomised trials comprising 3500 women treated with more modern radiotherapy techniques and with adjuvant systemic therapy demonstrate very similar absolute improvements in locoregional recurrence and overall survival. Based on these data, postmastectomy radiotherapy will prevent one death for every 11 women treated, and one locoregional recurrence for every three to five women treated.

# Radiotherapy and post-mastectomy reconstruction

Despite the success of conservative therapy for early breast cancer, many patients still require or choose mastectomy. For these patients the option of breast reconstruction offers improved cosmesis, body image and quality of life. The indications for postoperative radiotherapy are no different to those previously described for postmastectomy patients. It is clearly important to know how radiotherapy might impact on the success of the reconstruction. This will have implications for the advice and information given to such patients regarding the best timing and techniques for, and likely outcome of, the procedure. The target volume for radiotherapy after mastectomy should include the skin of the chest wall and the superficial fascia of the underlying muscles.

Implant reconstruction usually involves either prosthesis implantation only or a latissimus dorsi myocutaneous flap with an underlying implant. When surgery is followed by radiotherapy, there is often worsening of cosmesis and capsule formation around the implant. Implant removal is frequently recorded; overall surgical revision rates increase after radiotherapy and include capsulotomy, wound debridement and adjustment of implant position. Most implants that are removed because of capsule formation are successfully replaced, with a good outcome. In general, even with radiotherapy the proportion of patients with good or excellent cosmesis scores (albeit with various methods of assessment) is satisfyingly high.

Transverse rectus abdominis myocutaneous flap reconstruction is usually performed without prosthesis implantation. A number of studies have reported significantly increased complication rates (mostly flap failure and fat necrosis) in patients with a history of prior radiotherapy and a worse cosmetic outcome. There is little doubt that radiotherapy impacts on the outcome of implant reconstructions following mastectomy. It is likely that, despite this, the benefits of immediate reconstruction to the patient's overall quality of life are still significant and substantial. Furthermore, there is no evidence that delayed reconstruction improves the outcome. On this background it seems reasonable to advocate a policy of immediate reconstruction, with a myocutaneous flap rather than an implant/expander alone even if the patient is likely to require radiotherapy. Another option is to perform a skin-sparing mastectomy and insert a tissue expander to maintain the skin envelope, expand immediately but deflate during radiotherapy, re-inflating 2 weeks after completion. A myocutaneous flap with or without implant is then performed 6–12 months later using the skin envelope to minimise the size of the skin paddle needed from the abdomen or back. Clearly, the surgeon and the radiotherapist must do everything possible to lower the morbidity. The increased risk of capsule formation and implant removal must be made clear to the patient.

# Partial breast and intraoperative radiotherapy

With screening identifying increasing numbers of patients with in situ or small cancers, there is an increasing interest in evaluating whether the positive effects of radiotherapy can be maintained by focusing treatment on the index breast quadrant alone, so-called partial breast radiotherapy. Techniques for partial breast radiotherapy include standard linear accelerator-based three-dimensional external beam therapy, radioactive implants (so-called 'brachytherapy') and intraoperative single-fraction treatment. A variety of devices are being evaluated in the USA to deliver the local radiotherapy and these are implanted either at the time of surgery or later under image guidance. Partial breast radiotherapy using the two approaches is being evaluated in two randomised studies against whole-breast radiotherapy in Europe and in numerous studies in the USA.[46,47]

# Palliative radiotherapy in breast cancer

Radiotherapy has a major role in symptom control in locally advanced breast cancer and metastatic disease. Women with locally advanced cancers unsuitable for surgery can have significant reduction in size of fungating or bleeding tumours by radiotherapy. Although low-dose treatments (e.g. 20 Gy in five fractions) can help achieve some tumour control, if the patient's life expectancy is longer than 6 months, then it is worth offering standard adjuvant therapy as 'high-dose' palliation, for example 50 Gy in 25 fractions (or its approximate biological equivalent) can gain long-term local control of bulk disease, especially if a boost dose to a smaller region of disease can be increased to 60–70 Gy.

Radiotherapy often produces rapid relief of bone pain in women with metastatic disease. Doses such as 8-Gy single treatments are appropriate for non-weight-bearing bones. Higher doses are required to achieve enough tumour regression to permit some bone remodelling and are more appropriate in disease involving vertebrae, major pelvic bones or femur. Treatment can impact significantly on fracture rate or progression to overt spinal cord compression. It can be combined with early systemic therapy with bisphosphonates to reduce morbidity of bone metastases.

## Summary

Adjuvant radiotherapy has an established role in the reduction of risk of locoregional breast cancer recurrence, after both mastectomy and BCS. It may also impact on overall survival, adding to the benefits accrued by systemic adjuvant therapy. New developments include assessing the efficacy of partial breast irradiation in small cancers, and improving standard breast radiotherapy by intensity-modulated techniques.

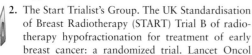

**Key points**

- Radiotherapy after wide local excision confers survival equivalent to mastectomy, with improved body image, and is the standard of care for women wishing to preserve the breast.
- With proper attention to surgical margins, adjuvant radiotherapy should give local control rates of 95% or better at 5 years.
- Postmastectomy chest wall and nodal radiotherapy is offered routinely to women with high risk of locoregional relapse; risk factors include grade 3 cancers, involvement of four or more nodes and dermal or pectoral infiltration.
- Future directions in breast radiotherapy research include adopting techniques aimed at minimising cardiac irradiation, defining the place of partial breast treatment and identifying those in whom radiotherapy can be safely omitted.

## References

1. Perez CA, Brady LW. Principles and practice of radiation oncology, 4th edn. Philadelphia: Lippincott, Williams & Wilkins.

2. The Start Trialist's Group. The UK Standardisation of Breast Radiotherapy (START) Trial B of radiotherapy hypofractionation for treatment of early breast cancer: a randomized trial. Lancet Oncol 2008; 9:331–41.

   This randomised trial of 2215 women suggests that a radiation schedule delivering 40 Gy in 15 fractions seems to offer rates of locoregional tumour relapse and late adverse effects at least as favourable as the standard schedule of 50 Gy in 25 fractions.

3. Bartelink K, Horiot JC, Poortmans P et al. Recurrence rates after treatment of breast cancer with standard radiotherapy with or without additional radiation. N Engl J Med 2001; 345:1378–87.

   This trial randomised patients to receive tumour bed boost of 16 Gy or no additional radiation. Local recurrences were reduced in the boost arm and reduction in local recurrence was greatest in the under 40 year group.

4. Lyman GH, Giuilano AE, Somerfield MR et al. American Guideline Recommendation for sentinel lymph node biopsy in early stage breast cancer. J Clin Oncol 2005; 23(30):7703–20.

   Sentinel node sampling is a safe and effective way of identifying non-involvement of the nodes in early breast cancer, although there are no data to prove any survival benefit to date.

5. Sarrazin D, Lê MG, Arriagada R et al. Ten-year results of a randomized trial comparing a conservative treatment to mastectomy in early breast cancer. Radiother Oncol 1989; 14:177–84.

6. Veronesi U, Banfi A, Salvador B et al. Breast conservation is the treatment of choice in small breast cancer: long-term results of a randomized trial. Eur J Cancer 1990; 26:668–70.

7. Fisher B, Redmond C, Poisson R et al. Eight-year results of a randomized clinical trial comparing total mastectomy and lumpectomy with or without irradiation in the treatment of breast cancer. N Engl J Med 1989; 320:822–8.

8. Poggi MM, Danforth DN, Sciuto LC et al. Eighteen-year results in the treatment of early breast carcinoma with mastectomy versus breast conservation therapy: the National Cancer Institute Randomised Trial. Cancer 2003; 98:697–702.

9. Van Dongen JA, Bartelink H, Fentiman IS et al. Randomized clinical trial to assess the value of breast-conserving therapy in stage I and II breast cancer, EORTC 10801 trial. J Natl Cancer Inst Monogr 1992; 11:15–18.

10. Blichert-Toft M, Brincker H, Andersen JA et al. A Danish randomized trial comparing breast-preserving therapy with mastectomy in mammary carcinoma. Preliminary results. Acta Oncol 1988; 27:671–7.

11. Kurtz JM, Almaric R, Brandone H et al. Local recurrence after breast conserving surgery and radiotherapy: frequency, time course and prognosis. Cancer 1989; 63:1912–17.

12. Clarke DH, Lê MG, Sarrazin D et al. Analysis of local–regional relapses in patients with early breast cancers treated by excision and radiotherapy: experience of the Institut Gustave-Roussy. Int J Radiat Oncol Biol Phys 1985; 11:137–45.

13. Halverson KJ, Perez CA, Taylor ME. Age as a prognostic factor for breast and regional nodal recurrence following breast conserving surgery and irradiation in stage I and II breast cancer. Int J Radiat Oncol Biol Phys 1993; 27:1045–50.

14. Ohtake T, Abe R, Kimijima I et al. Intraductal extension of primary invasive breast cancer treated by breast-conservative surgery: computer graphic three dimensional reconstruction of the mammary duct–lobular system. Cancer 1995; 76:32–45.

15. Holland R, Veling SH, Mravunac M et al. Histologic multifocality of Tis, T1–2 breast carcinomas: implications for clinical trials of breast-conserving surgery. Cancer 1985; 56:979–90.

16. Fisher B, Anderson S, Redmond CK et al. Reanalysis and results after 12 years of follow-up in a randomized clinical trial comparing total mastectomy with lumpectomy with or without irradiation in the treatment of breast cancer. N Engl J Med 1995; 333:1456–61.

17. Straus K, Lichter A, Lippman M et al. Results of the National Cancer Institute early breast cancer trial. J Natl Cancer Inst Monogr 1992; 11:27–32.

18. Fourquet A, Campana F, Zafrani B et al. Prognostic factors of breast recurrence in the conservative management of early breast cancer: a 25-year follow-up. Int J Radiat Oncol Biol Phys 1989; 17:719–25.

19. Kurtz JM, Spitalier JM, Amalric R et al. Mammary recurrences in women younger than forty. Int J Radiat Oncol Biol Phys 1988; 15:271–6.

20. Boyages J, Recht A, Connolly JL et al. Early breast cancer: predictors of breast recurrence for patients treated with conservative surgery and radiation therapy. Radiother Oncol 1990; 19:29–41.

21. Kurtz JM, Jacquemier J, Amalric R et al. Why are local recurrences after breast-conserving therapy more frequent in younger patients? J Clin Oncol 1990; 8:591–8.

22. Donegan W, Perez-Mesa C, Watson F. A biostatistical study of locally recurrent breast carcinoma. Surg Gynecol Obstet 1966; 122:529.

23. Matthews RH, McNeese MD, Montague RH et al. Prognostic implications of age in breast cancer patients treated with tumorectomy and irradiation or with mastectomy. Int J Radiat Oncol Biol Phys 1988; 14:659–63.

24. Anscher MS, Jones P, Prosnitz LR et al. Local failure and margin status in early-stage breast carcinoma treated with conservation surgery and radiation therapy. Ann Surg 1993; 218:22–8.

25. Gage I, Schnitt SJ, Nixon AJ et al. Pathologic margin involvement and the risk of recurrence in patients treated with breast-conserving therapy. Cancer 1996; 78:1921–8.

26. Solin LJ, Fowble BL, Schultz DJ et al. The significance of the pathology margins of the tumor excision on the outcome of patients treated with definitive irradiation for early stage breast cancer. Int J Radiat Oncol Biol Phys 1991; 21:279–87.

27. Borger J, Kemperman H, Hart A et al. Risk factors in breast-conservation therapy. J Clin Oncol 1994; 12:653–60.

28. Overgaard M, Hansen PS, Overgaard J et al. Postoperative radiotherapy in high-risk premenopausal women with breast cancer who receive adjuvant chemotherapy. Danish Breast Cancer Cooperative Group 82c Trial. N Engl J Med 1997; 337:949–55.

29. Ragaz J, Jackson SM, Le N et al. Adjuvant radiotherapy and chemotherapy in node-positive premenopausal women with breast cancer N Engl J Med 1997; 337:956–62.

30. Touboul E, Buffat L, Belkacemi Y et al. Local recurrences and distant metastases after breast conserving surgery and radiation therapy for early breast cancer. Int J Radiat Oncol Biol Phys 1999; 43:25–38.

31. Hellman S. Stopping metastases at their source. N Engl J Med 1997; 337:996–7.

32. Wazer DE, DiPetrillo T, Schmidt-Ullrich R et al. Factors influencing cosmetic outcome and complication risk after conservative surgery and radiotherapy for early-stage breast carcinoma. J Clin Oncol 1992; 10:356–63.

33. Spivack B, Khanna MM, Tafra L et al. Margin status and local recurrence after breast-conserving surgery. Arch Surg 1994; 129:952–6; discussion 956–7.

34. Di Biase SJ, Komarnicky LT, Schwartz GF et al. The number of positive margins influences the outcome of women treated with breast preservation for early stage breast carcinoma. Cancer 1998; 82: 2212–20.

35. Smitt MC, Nowels KW, Zdeblick MJ et al. The importance of the lumpectomy surgical margin status in long-term results of breast conservation. Cancer 1995; 76:259–67.

36. Peterson ME, Schultz DJ, Reynolds C et al. Outcomes in breast cancer patients relative to margin status after treatment with breast conserving surgery and radiation therapy. Int J Radiat Oncol Biol Phys 1999; 43:1029–35.

37. Rose MA, Henderson IC, Gelman R et al. Premenopausal breast cancer patients treated with conservative surgery, radiotherapy and adjuvant chemotherapy have a low risk of local failure. Int J Radiat Oncol Biol Phys 1989; 17:711–17.

38. Fisher B, Dignam J, Mamounas HP et al. Sequential methotrexate and fluorouracil for the treatment of node-negative breast cancer patients with oestrogen-receptor negative tumours: eight-year results from NSAPB B-13 and first report of findings from NSABP B-10 comparing methotrexate and fluorouracil. J Clin Oncol 1996; 14:1982.

39. Ryoo MC, Kagan AR, Wollin M et al. Prognostic factors for recurrence and cosmesis in 393 patients after radiation therapy for early mammary carcinoma. Radiology 1989; 172:555–9.

40. Early Breast Cancer Trialists' Collaborative Group. Effects of radiotherapy and surgery in early breast cancer: an overview of the randomized trials. Lancet 2005; 366:2087–106.

41. Overgaard M, Jensen MB, Overgaard J et al. Postoperative radiotherapy in high-risk postmenopausal breast-cancer patients given adjuvant tamoxifen: Danish Breast Cancer Cooperative Group DBGG 82c randomised trial. Lancet 1999; 353:1641–8.

42. Harris JR, Halpin-Murphy P, McNeese M et al. Consensus statement on post mastectomy radiation therapy. Int J Radiat Oncol Biol Phys 1999; 44:989–90.

This statement is based on a meta-analysis of randomised trials and has shown reduction in local recurrence rates and improved survival following chest wall radiation for patients with four or more positive lymph nodes.

43. Recht A, Edge SB, Solin LJ et al. American Society of Clinical Oncology post mastectomy radiation: clinical practice guidelines of the American Society of Clinical Oncologists. J Clin Oncol 2001; 19:1539–69.

44. Overgaard M, Nielsen HM, Overgaard J. Is the benefit of post mastectomy irradiation limited to patients with four or more positive nodes, as recommended in international consensus reports? A subgroup analysis of the DBCG 82 b&c randomized trials. Radiother Oncol 2007; 82(3):247–53.

45. Keisch M. Partial breast radiotherapy. Breast Cancer Res 2005; 7(3):110–2.

46. Ross GM. Partial breast radiotherapy: technically feasible but who will benefit? Breast Cancer Res 2005; 7(4):106–9.

# 16

# Psychosocial issues in breast cancer

Lesley Fallowfield
Valerie A. Jenkins

## Introduction

Despite the many advances made in the management of breast cancer over the past 20 years, its diagnosis and treatment remains a source of considerable psychological, social, physical and sexual dysfunction for women, exerting a deleterious impact on the quality of their lives. The number of women who develop psychological problems has barely changed, with a significant minority (25–30%) experiencing affective and adjustment disorders. But what of those who do not merit a diagnosis of clinical depression or anxiety. Are the many changes in diagnostic techniques, service delivery, information and support provision helping women to cope better with their disease? This chapter outlines some of the main sources of psychological, social, physical and sexual problems in breast cancer that impact on quality of life, and examines the existing evidence base, assessing the efficacy of interventions aimed at preventing or ameliorating problems.

## Psychological morbidity

### Mastectomy versus breast conservation

Despite the advances made, with more surgeons performing breast-conserving surgery wherever possible, women still have to confront the fact that they have a potentially life-threatening disease and fear of this often predominates initially rather than anxiety about breast loss. Although there are benefits from less mutilating surgery, in particular some advantages in preserving body image and sparing women the nuisance factor of wearing an external prosthesis, this does not always translate into measurable reductions in psychological morbidity. A meta-analysis summarising the findings of 40 publications suggests that better techniques and improved specialist medical and nursing care for women are starting to show some benefits. The mean weighted effect sizes calculated for psychosocial outcomes, which included psychological morbidity, partnership/sexual and social adjustment, body/self-image and cancer fears, demonstrated modest advantages for those women who had breast-conserving surgery.[1]

## Choice and decision-making about surgical option

Some have suggested that psychological morbidity could be prevented if only women were allowed to choose their preferred surgical treatments. Although the proponents of more consumerist approaches strongly assert the putative benefits of active participation by women with breast cancer in treatment decision-making, these benefits are rarely supported by firm data. In one study the decision-making preferences of 150 women with newly diagnosed breast cancer were established and compared with those of 200 women with benign breast disease. The majority of women with breast cancer preferred a more passive role, whereas the majority of the benign disease group wished for a more collaborative role.[2] In another study of 269 women treated by surgeons who either favoured one approach (i.e. mastectomy or breast-conserving surgery) or who offered choice between options whenever possible, psychological morbidity was lowest for the women treated by surgeons who offered the choice. However, benefits to those treated by 'choice' doctors were observed irrespective of whether the choice could in fact be offered.[3] What helped women adapt and adjust to their disease and treatment had less to do with choice than satisfaction with the communication they had with their doctors about the rationale for one treatment rather than another. Those satisfied with the communication at the time that diagnosis was given and the treatment options discussed experienced less psychological morbidity at 12, 24 and 36 months follow-up compared with those who felt that communication had been inadequate.

More recent data from the USA examined decision-making in 1884 women with ductal carcinoma in situ (DCIS) and invasive breast cancer. Results showed that 11.5% had clinical contra-indications to breast-conserving surgery but 30% had mastectomy as their initial surgical treatment. The majority of the women (41%) reported that they had been the primary decision-maker, 37% felt that the decision was shared with the surgeon and 22% felt that the decision had been made by their surgeon.[4] Intriguingly, the greater the patient involvement in decision-making the more likely that mastectomy was the preferred surgery. After adjusting for clinical and demographic variables, significant correlations were found. Only 5.8% of women whose surgeon made the decision had a mastectomy compared with 16.8% of the women who shared decision-making and 27% of those who made the decision themselves ($P = 0.003$). The primary reason for a mastectomy preference was fear about recurrence. Although 80% expressed a high degree of confidence about their decisions, fewer than 50% were able to answer correctly a true/false question about the lack of a survival difference between surgical treatments.

In another publication on a subgroup of this sample ($n = 1028$), the concordance between decision control and patients' preferences was examined.[5] The mismatch between that desired and the actual involvement was 31%, with 20% claiming to have been more involved than they wished and 11% less involved. The latter, who felt their involvement insufficient, tended to be younger; they felt that only one option had been discussed and were more likely to have been seen by surgeons treating high volumes of patients.

A further important issue was satisfaction. Just over one-third (37%) of women were dissatisfied with the decision-making process, 23% dissatisfied with the doctor/patient relationship and 24% with the communication.[6] Satisfaction did not appear to correlate with sex of surgeon, seniority or treatment centre, but increased satisfaction was associated with high-volume breast cancer surgeons.

When all the literature on decision-making is reviewed, it shows the importance of good communication. If women are to be offered opportunities to be more involved in determining their treatment then they need time and good quality information on which to base those decisions. The USA studies showed that many patients thought themselves well informed about options and were confident about the decisions they made, but that they were often basing their choices on inaccurate information. Furthermore, there were significant mismatches between preferred involvement and what actually happened.[7]

## Impact of axillary surgery on quality of life

Management of the axilla in breast cancer surgery is a controversial area. Arm morbidity following both clearance and sampling is well documented. Extensive surgery aimed at clearing the axilla of positive nodes might well reduce recurrence and improve survival but comes at considerable cost to the patient in terms of arm morbidity. Complications such as muscle weakness, numbness, pain and lymphoedema are common, and can have a deleterious impact on a woman's quality of life even if she is cured of her breast cancer. Research has shown that up to 83% of women will experience at least one arm problem following surgery.[8] Assessment of arm morbidity using traditional objective methods rather than patient self-report has often proved inconsistent and may fail to capture the extent of patients' problems.

More recently, a robust and validated patient self-report measure (FACT-B+4) has been developed that may prove useful in monitoring the presence and longevity of arm morbidity in trials of new techniques aimed at minimising problems.[9] This was used in the UK-based Axillary Lymphatic Mapping Against Nodal Axillary Clearance (ALMANAC) trial, a multicentre randomised clinical trial comparing sentinel node biopsy with conventional axillary surgical techniques in women presenting with clinically node-negative breast cancer. ALMANAC showed that the benefits of sentinel node biopsy are not only reduction of unnecessary resection of the axilla but also a marked reduction in unwanted sequelae such as arm morbidity, thus permitting a better quality of life, without sacrificing any staging accuracy.[10,11] A total of 829 women returned completed questionnaires; 405 patients were randomised to standard treatment and 424 to sentinel node biopsy. Response remained high throughout the trial: 93% patients returned questionnaires up to 6 months following surgery, 91% at 12 months and 88% at 18 months; 80% (662/829) of patients returned all six questionnaires. These return rates permit a greater confidence in the results than is usual in many similar types of study. One important finding at each postal follow-up was that, irrespective of randomised group, arm functioning was worse and the deterioration in functioning greater for patients whose intercostobrachial nerve (ICBN) was divided ($P < 0.001$) than for those whose nerve was preserved.

## Interventions to reduce psychological morbidity

The large numbers of women who still experience considerable psychological morbidity, despite improvements in service provision, is puzzling and needs some explanation. The almost obsessional, often sensational and excessive preoccupation with breast cancer by the media surely has some responsibility. Women are bombarded by mixed messages about things such as the risks and benefits of screening, the value of self-examination and breast awareness. They are also surrounded by misleading and often inaccurate claims about the causes of breast cancer, ranging from dietary factors to the use of deodorants. Campaigns to promote breast awareness often use young women, perpetuating

unreasonable fears among the very age groups least at risk of developing the disease. Not surprisingly, women overestimate their risk of getting breast cancer, especially when figures such as 1 in 10 or 12 are bandied about, failing to convey the fact that this is a woman's lifetime risk of developing breast cancer.[12] So at a time when there has never been quite so much information available or so many resources directed at trying to prevent or ameliorate psychological stress, we appear to have created as much if not more anxiety than was discernible previously. The key is to help guide women through reliable information sources and to ensure that verbal communication and support provided by healthcare professionals is congruent with information accessed through other media. As a group, the needs of women with breast cancer are probably better served than many other cancers. Charities such as Cancerbackup, Breakthrough Breast Cancer, Breast Cancer Care, and Cancer Care, to name but a few, provide some excellent websites and materials.

## Counselling/specialist nurses

Despite its prevalence, patients with cancer experience psychological dysfunction that is rarely documented during routine clinic visits.[13] This is unfortunate as evidence is growing that if psychological morbidity is recognised, then a number of different psychosocial interventions of proven efficacy can be offered.[14] In busy clinics some surgeons feel that they do not have time, even if they possess the skills needed, to enquire into the psychological functioning of patients. Responsibility for this often falls on specialist breast cancer nurses.

Despite the equivocal evidence of efficacy, the high prevalence of psychological and sexual dysfunction associated with breast cancer has led to the creation of many posts for specialist nurses with counselling skills. Their role is now firmly established in breast cancer clinics; indeed, it seems difficult to recall a time when clinics were organised without them. Initially, the specialist nurse doubled up as a stoma nurse, as one of her primary roles was to offer advice about breast prostheses. However, the modern specialist nurse now has to undergo considerable training in the skills required to recognise and treat some of the psychological problems found in women with breast cancer. Although there is not a substantial methodologically sound research base demonstrating the efficacy of specialist nurse counsellors, many women and clinicians attest to the benefits of their work. An Australian study examined the implementation of an evidence-based model of care using specialist breast cancer nurses and reported improvements in many areas of care, in particular information and support for women and more appropriate referrals.[15]

Another source of help for women with breast cancer comes from support groups and there are many different types available. There is a large body of research suggesting strong associations between emotional distress and immunological and neuroendocrine responses in women with breast cancer. This link has been responsible for a burgeoning interest in support groups that putatively lead to improved psychological and physiological outcomes, and is an area full of controversy.[16] In 1989, the *Lancet* published an important paper by Spiegel et al.[17] reporting the results from the 10-year follow-up of a prospective randomised trial of supportive–expressive group therapy in women with metastatic breast cancer. An earlier report by this group had shown that this intervention, which included professionally led peer group support encouraging emotional expression, relaxation therapy and autohypnosis, produced significant psychological benefits. Those women randomised to group support compared with the control group reported better mood states, fewer maladaptive coping responses and fewer phobic reactions.[18] Although the study was designed to establish the potential benefits on psychological well-being, Spiegel et al. examined post hoc the death records to determine the impact of the intervention on disease progression and mortality. This showed a statistically significant difference in mean survival that favoured the intervention group (36.6 months vs. 18.9 months for the control). This work has been criticised by many[19,20] and others have failed to replicate Spiegel et al.'s findings of an effect on survival,[20,21] but it did stimulate an interesting and important body of research aimed at establishing plausible psychoendocrine and psychoneuroimmunological explanations for improved survival.[22] Spiegel et al.'s original research was never designed to test the impact support groups would have on survival but rather its overall impact on quality of life, and they always cautioned against over-interpretation of the research. However, more recent work evaluating quality of life in women with metastatic breast cancer,

who were randomised to supportive–expressive group therapy or a control arm, failed to show any benefits of the intervention.[23] In studies that have shown a modest impact on survival, advantages are probably due to psychotherapeutic benefits improving such things as compliance, better nutrition and physical activity.[24] It could be argued that one of the most important aspects of supportive–expressive group therapy is to help patients to face the fact of their breast cancer and to confront the reality of death.

# Psychosexual morbidity

Although much has been written about the effects that treatments have on body image and self-esteem, one quality-of-life issue that has received rather less attention is the effect that diagnosis and treatment for breast cancer has on a woman's psychosexual functioning. Often it is towards the end of cancer treatment that most sexual dysfunction caused by therapy occurs, when a woman has completed her main hospital treatments and the initial threat of death and dying is slowly replaced with trying to get back to a normal life. In a review of sexual dysfunction, Schover et al.[25] note that although sexuality in breast cancer patients was studied as an aspect of quality of life over 40 years ago, little progress has been made since then. Early research focused on the initial impact of mastectomy versus breast-conserving surgery and the benefits of reconstruction, but less was known about the effects of chemotherapy and different hormone therapies on sexuality. There is still relatively little systematic research into the effect that different treatments have on a woman's feelings of altered body image and loss of sexual desire, and even fewer interventions in place to help these women. Much of the available data on sexuality following breast cancer treatment is too general, and it is rare for women to be assessed before, during and after treatment in order to determine when problems begin and how long they last, let alone develop and examine ameliorative interventions.

Different treatments undoubtedly affect a woman's psychosexual well-being. Surgery can leave a woman with feelings of mutilation and a loss of sense of femininity. The introduction of better surgical techniques, including immediate reconstructive surgery, may help patients retain a more intact sense of body image and self-esteem and thus adjust more easily. An early study by Schain et al.[26]

reported that those patients who had immediate reconstructive surgery had significantly less recalled distress about their mastectomy at 1 year than those who had delayed reconstruction, although initial differences in adjustment disappeared over time. However, another report assessing psychosocial morbidity in 254 patients who had undergone breast-conserving surgery for primary breast cancer showed that the final cosmetic result had a marked bearing on the subsequent psychological outcome. Al-Ghazal et al.[27] reported significant correlations between cosmesis and levels of anxiety and depression, and between cosmesis and body image, sexuality and self-esteem. In another study of patients receiving either immediate reconstructive surgery or breast-conserving treatment, no differences were found between the groups in self-reported quality of life or changes in body image. Interestingly, significant differences were found in cosmetic outcomes favouring immediate reconstruction over breast-conserving surgery as rated by the surgical team.[28] However, objective assessment of cosmesis does not always correlate with patients' perceptions about body image.

Harcourt et al.[29] showed in a prospective study that breast reconstruction is not a universal panacea for the emotional and psychological consequences of mastectomy. Women in this study chose whether to have reconstructive surgery (immediate or delayed) and completed self-assessments of anxiety, depression, body image and quality of life preoperatively and postoperatively at 6 and 12 months. Psychological distress decreased following surgery in all groups, but women still reported feeling conscious of altered body image 12 months later regardless of whether or not they had breast reconstruction. This finding should alert healthcare professionals not to assume that breast reconstructive surgery necessarily confers psychological benefits compared with mastectomy alone.

## Surgery for women at high genetic risk

Another group of women with issues about eventual cosmesis and its impact on sexuality are those at high genetic risk who are contemplating prophylactic surgery in order to reduce their chance of developing breast cancer later in life. Hatcher et al.[30] assessed the psychosocial impact of either

accepting or declining bilateral prophylactic surgery in 143 women with increased risk of breast cancer. Quality of life, psychiatric morbidity, body image and sexual activity were measured at baseline and at 6 and 18 months. Results showed a significant decrease in psychological morbidity in those women who chose surgery, whereas those who opted for regular surveillance and declined surgery experienced anxiety and depression that did not decrease significantly over an 18-month period. There was no significant difference between the groups in the degree of sexual pleasure experienced over time. Women who opted for surgery (most of whom had immediate reconstruction) maintained a positive body image. There were some interesting personality differences between women who pursued prophylactic surgery and those who declined. The decliners had significantly higher anxiety personality traits than those who had surgery and tended to use detachment as a coping strategy rather than the problem-focused approach used more frequently by those who had surgery. Thus, regular surveillance for an at-risk woman who had a predisposition to worry and who usually coped with anxiety by trying to ignore it only made these women more anxious. Women clearly need careful preoperative counselling and assessment prior to embarking on any prophylactic management policy.[31]

## Psychosexual impact of adjuvant therapies

Increasing numbers of women are receiving neo-adjuvant or adjuvant hormonal and chemotherapy treatments for breast cancer, yet the impact of these on psychosocial and sexual well-being is less well explored. Chemotherapy can produce overtly disfiguring side-effects, for example alopecia and weight gain, and other debilitating problems such as nausea and fatigue. On top of this, most premenopausal women will experience a premature menopause, with all its associated adverse effects including hot flushes, cold sweats, vaginal dryness or discharge, and dyspareunia.

Berglund et al.[32] examined the effects of different adjuvant treatments on sexuality in a prospective study. The women were all premenopausal and taking part in a European clinical trial in which they were randomised to tamoxifen or goserelin, a combination of tamoxifen and goserelin or no adjuvant endocrine therapy. Results indicated that women who received chemotherapy had a higher level of sexual dysfunction than patients who had not. The addition of endocrine treatment did not alter this result; however, in those women who did not receive chemotherapy, goserelin alone and combined with tamoxifen produced a significantly higher level of sexual dysfunction from 1 to 2 years compared with those who received tamoxifen alone or no endocrine therapy.

The effect that tamoxifen has on psychological and sexual functioning has been studied closely in chemoprevention studies for women at high risk of developing breast cancer.[33] Almost 500 women have participated in these double-blind trials, 254 randomised to the tamoxifen arm and 234 to the placebo arm. Psychological morbidity was assessed using standardised anxiety and depression tools, and sexual functioning was measured using Fallowfield's Sexual Activity Questionnaire,[34] a self-report questionnaire that describes sexual functioning in terms of activity, pleasure and discomfort. Changes in anxiety, mood state and sexual functioning were not associated with treatment group. Nor were there differences in the proportions of women experiencing vaginal dryness, pain or discomfort during penetration.[33] However, the women taking tamoxifen were more likely to report vaginal discharge. This may be a reason why sexual activity was not impaired. The 2- and 5-year quality-of-life data from the Arimidex or Tamoxifen, Alone, Combined (ATAC) trial and the Intergroup Exemestane trial show that patients receiving an aromatase inhibitor experienced significantly more vaginal dryness, pain on intercourse and loss of sexual interest than women receiving tamoxifen.[35–37] Although it is evident that most treatments for breast cancer impact in some way on a woman's psychosexual functioning, few are informed that these problems can occur and how to ameliorate adverse effects before they become a problem.[38] One reason may be that health professionals feel embarrassed or inadequate about dealing with such issues. However, sexuality and intimacy are important concerns, particularly for patients with breast cancer, and need to be addressed.

Although much literature exists on the need for intervention for sexual dysfunction in patients with cancer, few results are available from randomised controlled clinical trials.[39] One study from the USA evaluated a nurse-led intervention for postmenopausal women with breast cancer that aimed to provide relief of menopausal symptoms, improvement in sexual functioning and quality of life.[40] The intervention took place over a 4-month period and focused on symptom assessment, education, counselling, and specific pharmacological and behavioural interventions; 72 women completed the study, half receiving the usual care and half the intervention. Results revealed a significant improvement in sexual functioning and menopausal symptoms but no difference in quality of life between the groups.

Although there are guidelines available for health professionals on assessment and treatment of sexual dysfunction in breast cancer patients, encouragement and support to attend educational programmes is required. Too few recognise that counselling patients about sexual issues is an important aspect of patient care.

# Psychological aspects of service delivery

## Delay in presentation with breast cancer

Anxiety about the disease and fears about treatment can lead women to delay seeking advice. Delay can be described in terms of patient or provider delay. Patient delay refers to the interval between first detection of symptoms and first medical consultation. The period that most authors accept as prolonged delay is 12 weeks or more,[41] although Nosarti et al.[42] regard patient delay as 4 weeks or more. Provider or system delay is defined as the interval between first presentation to the GP and initial treatment, and is not easy to define. Although guidelines in the UK now suggest no longer than 2 weeks should elapse between first presentation to the GP with a suspicious lump and referral to a specialist, surgical treatment can be delayed for a wide variety of reasons. Delayed presentation of symptomatic breast cancer is associated with lower survival, particularly delays of 3–6 months or longer.[43] Therefore it is important to identify which factors influence patient delay and also whether provider delay contributes to poorer outcomes that may affect survival.

A systematic review of risk and delay in presentation by Ramirez et al.[41] found 86 studies in patients and 28 in providers. Only 23 studies were of adequate quality to include in the assessment. The authors generated hypotheses about the relationship between putative risk factors for patient and provider delay, and assigned strength of evidence according to a combination of the number and size of studies that supported, failed to support or refuted their hypotheses. The risk factors for patient delay were grouped under the following headings: sociodemographic, clinical, psychological and social. The results showed strong evidence for an association between older age and delay and strong evidence that marital status was unrelated to delay by patients. Provider delay was associated with younger age and presentation with a breast symptom other than a lump.

Ramirez's group and others have examined delay from a number of perspectives, involving both quantitative and qualitative research. In one study they interviewed 185 women with breast cancer 2 months after their diagnosis in order to examine the incidence and effects of patient and provider delay;[44] 19% of women delayed 12 weeks or more and a number of factors predicted delay, including initial breast symptoms other than a lump and not disclosing discovery of the breast lump immediately to somebody close. Patient delay was also related to a clinical tumour size of 4 cm or more and a higher incidence of metastatic disease.

Of these women, 46 (15 non-delayers and 31 delayers) were also interviewed to determine any differences between the groups.[45] Results suggested that those who recognised the seriousness of their symptoms presented promptly to the GP. The perceived seriousness was influenced by the nature of the symptom and how far it matched the individual's expectations of breast cancer as a painless lump. Other factors that influenced the seeking of help included beliefs about the consequences of treatment for breast cancer and attitudes to GP attendance. These results showed that women's knowledge about the symptoms and treatments of breast cancer was very limited despite the fact that it is a high-profile topic.

## One-stop clinics

Since the early 1990s there have been many patient demands for a comprehensive cancer service and an increasing professional requirement on the part of clinicians for improved healthcare delivery in breast cancer through published guidelines such as BASO, SIGN and the Patient's Charter. The guidelines have suggested the establishment of organised specialist breast clinics with the aim of providing rapid diagnosis for patients with malignant disease and reassurance for symptomatic patients who do not have breast cancer. Requests for fast results, quicker throughput of patients and a decrease in unnecessary outpatient follow-up has led to the introduction of one-stop clinics within these centres. Alongside this came the 2-week referral rule for a woman reporting a breast lump to her GP. These were seen as potentially helpful developments, as 'waiting for results' is perceived by many women as one of the most traumatic periods during the whole breast cancer experience. However, there are increasing concerns that all these changes might not be providing the beneficial outcomes that were expected. In particular, the increase in demand for immediate referral reinforces the idea that breast cancer is a dire medical emergency, which it is not; rather it is an emotional emergency.

One-stop clinics have become a double-edged sword. The primary healthcare sector is referring more and more women and does not always follow published guidelines, leading to a huge increase in patient numbers but not the staff to deal with them. In one prospective audit of 321 referrals to a Glasgow one-stop clinic,[46] 10% of women had breast cancer and 90% had benign disease or no pathology. The authors highlighted the fact that over one-third of referrals from the primary healthcare sector were inappropriate and inevitably reduced the efficiency of the service provided for patients. Another audit in London[47] examined whether the service to women had improved since the original audit 5 years previously. This was a prospective audit of four consecutive clinics and a total of 300 patients were seen. Forty women had one-stop investigations and 86% of these had benign disease, demonstrating yet again that the majority of women referred to a breast clinic and those attending post-screening assessment have benign breast disease.

What does attendance at one-stop clinics do to a woman's psychological condition, be it a benign or malignant result? Most patients with benign disease will be in a state of heightened anxiety until they have undergone specialist assessment, the necessary investigations and eventual reassurance. In contrast, women who receive a diagnosis of breast cancer will still have heightened anxiety for many months during and following their treatment.[3] One study[48] examined the costs and benefits of a one-stop clinic compared with a dedicated breast clinic. As part of the assessment, anxiety was measured at baseline, 24 hours, 3 weeks and 3 months in the 478 women who participated (267 at the one-stop clinic and 211 at the standard clinic). Results showed that in both groups mean anxiety scores at all time points were lower than at baseline. Reduction in mean anxiety was significantly greater for one-stop clinic patients at 24 hours but not for other time points. Harcourt et al.[49] showed a similar initial reduction in anxiety in one-stop clinic patients. Another study[50] reported the psychological distress associated with waiting for results in a delayed-results breast clinic. The findings from 126 women showed that the waiting sustained but did not exacerbate psychological distress. The qualitative aspect of this study also suggested that the structure of the delayed-results clinic might facilitate psychological preparation for test results.

## Psychological aspects of mammographic screening

In 2002 the World Health Organisation concluded that trials have provided sufficient evidence to show that mammographic screening reduces deaths from breast cancer in women aged 55–69 years. However, there have been some vociferous debates about the true value of screening and even whether breast screening is associated with health benefits; it also has financial, physical and emotional costs for patients. Women who attend for screening have to offset potential health gains against such things as work time lost, fears of radiation, pain of the mammographic procedure, and the physical and psychological consequences of recall for further examinations where the initial mammogram was interpreted as indeterminate or abnormal.

The existing literature is inconsistent in its conclusions as to whether recall has short- or long-term psychological consequences. Some researchers have reported that women who receive false-positive results experience elevated anxiety after receiving a letter recalling them for further mammography,[51] and that increased levels of anxiety and concern can last from 1 month[52] up to 6 months.[53,54] The effect can last even longer, as shown in a UK study of women who had initially been recalled with false-positive results.[53] Three years later, just before being invited for their next routine breast screening despite having received a final clear result 3 years previously, women who had undergone fine-needle aspiration, surgical biopsy or had been placed on early recall had significantly greater adverse psychological consequences at 1 month before their next screening appointment than women who had received a clear result after their initial mammogram at their last routine breast screening. In contrast, others have shown that although recalled women are more likely to have borderline or clinically significant anxiety than at baseline or screening, this effect lasts less than 5 weeks.[55] Similar findings of moderate negative short-term distress have been reported in other studies.[56] However, one of these, a large Finnish study[56] of 1718 patients, noted that women who received false-positive findings experienced intrusive thoughts and worry about breast cancer at 2 months which still prevailed at 12 months. Similarly, Sandin et al.[57] examined differences between 597 women attending a second-stage breast cancer screening and 598 women attending routine screening with regard to affective cognitive distress and psychopathology and whether the psychological impact was temporary or longer-lasting. Results showed that women recalled for further assessment had higher levels of affective cognitive impact, specifically worry, fear and thinking about getting breast cancer. However, this distress did not persist following notification of the benign result.

Research is needed to characterise optimal support services for women who undergo screening, but good communication is a key requirement throughout the entire mammography process.

## Newer research issues associated with treatments

### Cognition and chemotherapy/ endocrine therapy

The increased and widespread use of treatments for breast cancer has produced a new aspect of research, namely the possible harmful effects that these treatments have on memory and attention. Anecdotal reports from patients of changes in their memory and concentration (forgetfulness and inattention) following chemotherapy have been supported by results from cross-sectional studies. However, results from recent prospective studies, which include pretreatment cognitive testing, have questioned the veracity of the proposition.

The argument is that chemotherapy and/or endocrine treatments may disrupt the functioning of the brain processes in a variety of ways, resulting in subtle changes in cognition. Chemotherapy may have a direct toxic effect on the brain, produce metabolic changes, increase the levels of cytokines and cause cerebral microinfarcts. Similarly, both chemotherapy and hormone treatments for breast cancer disrupt the bioavailability of estrogen, which may contribute to the cognitive problems experienced by some but not all patients. In addition, there are factors that are known to affect memory and must always be accounted for when an assessment is made, including a person's age, level of intelligence, and mood.

On one side of the coin there is compelling evidence from both animal and clinical research that estrogen is important in memory and cognition (for overview see Ref. 58). Early laboratory work has shown that estrogen treatment reverses the learning deficits seen in ovarectomised rats on a variety of tests such as T maze avoidance, radial, water maze and place discrimination tasks.[59,60] Clinical evidence comes from a series of early experiments conducted by Barbara Sherwin and colleagues that assessed cognitive functioning in premenopausal women pre- and postoophorectomy for benign disease. They reported that scores on a short-term verbal memory task were maintained in women who received estrogen treatment postoperatively compared to those who were randomly assigned placebo.[61,62] In contrast, data from studies examining the effects of chemotherapy and endocrine therapy on cognition are not as compelling. One of the early problems was the snowballing effect caused by the results from small cross-sectional studies. In these studies patients had received chemotherapy and/or endocrine treatments several months or even years prior to cognitive assessment.[63–67] Making sense of the results from any of the cross-sectional studies is difficult due to the different assessment time points and type of statistical analysis.[68] Results are also compounded by many other factors associated with cancer diagnosis and treatment. These include the stress, anxiety and depression that can negatively affect a patient's ability to focus, concentrate and organise, together with the effect that fatigue and pain has on multitasking and processing speed.

There are probably more reviews, opinions and commentaries published about the cognitive effects of breast cancer treatments than original prospective studies. However, recently three longitudinal studies have been conducted in Europe, and all included pretreatment assessments.[69–71] In the Jenkins study 85 women with breast cancer received chemotherapy (mainly 5-fluorouracil, epirubicin and cyclophosphamide, FEC), 43 did not receive chemotherapy and 49 were healthy age-matched controls. Assessments were made at baseline (pretreatment), 6 months and 18 months. Repeated measures analysis found no significant interactions or effect of group after controlling for age and intelligence. Using a calculation to examine performance at an individual level, reliable decline on multiple tasks was seen in 20% of chemotherapy patients, 26% of non-chemotherapy patients and 18% of controls at 6 months (18%, 14% and 11% at 18 months). These results showed that few women experienced objective measurable decline in their concentration and memory, and the majority were either unaffected or improved over time. As mentioned earlier, chemotherapy may have a direct toxic effect on the brain; if this is correct then one may predict that those women who receive high-dose therapy might experience worse problems. Schagen et al.'s earlier work[64] suggested high-dose chemotherapy produced more impairment and in 2006 published results from a prospective study. In this study 28 women received high-dose chemotherapy (cyclophosphamide thiotepa carboplatin), 39 received standard-dose 5-fluorouracil epirubicin cyclophosphamide (FEC), 57 had no chemotherapy and there was a group of 60 healthy subjects. All participants were tested twice, before treatment and 12 months later; control subjects were tested 6 months later. Results showed no differences at baseline between the four groups but at the second assessment more of those who received high-dose chemotherapy experienced deterioration over time compared to the healthy controls (25% vs. 6.7%). No such difference was observed for the FEC or no chemotherapy groups. The third study worth mentioning assessed 101 women prior to and toward the end of receiving neoadjuvant chemotherapy (anthracycline and taxanes). The authors showed that at baseline a subgroup of patients with breast cancer showed cognitive impairments unrelated to measures of anxiety or depression. During chemotherapy cognitive function remained stable for the majority of patients, improved in one subgroup (28%) and deteriorated in another (27%). They suggest that the finding of cognitive compromise at baseline is related to a stress response – rather like post-traumatic stress disorder that is associated with memory and concentration problems.[72]

However, there is one consistent finding throughout the literature and that is the relatively high subjective perception of a decline in cognitive performance following chemotherapy.[67,73,74] Despite this fact, the association between objective neuropsychological changes and self-reported cognitive deficits is weak but correlates strongly with increased levels of anxiety. It is of note that not all women demonstrate objective decline, and preliminary studies suggest that there may be a genetic predisposition, in particular the e4 allele of apolipoprotein E (ApoE), which has been associated with reduced neuropsychological performance. In one study carriers of the e4 allele with breast cancer or lymphoma who were treated with chemotherapy tended to score lower on tests of visual memory, spatial ability and psychomotor functioning than survivors with other alleles of APoE.[75]

Finally, emerging studies using neuroimaging tools and techniques such as functional magnetic resonance imaging and positron emission tomography will hopefully illuminate the mechanisms for putative chemotherapy-related changes in brain function.

# Summary

Despite the many advances made in treating breast cancer, improvements in the delivery of care and provision of support services, the diagnosis of breast cancer still causes considerable distress. Women cope in many different ways with the knowledge that they have a potentially life-threatening disease requiring unpleasant treatments. For some it is a major emotional and social catastrophe, whereas others approach it with a degree of equanimity or stoicism. It is sometimes difficult to predict how women will react, adapt and adjust to what lies ahead. Greater awareness of some of the psychosocial, sexual and cognitive dysfunction associated with different treatments should enable us to design interventions to prevent or ameliorate their problems, but the importance of good clear information delivered in a supportive, honest and empathic manner should not be overlooked. The communication skills of a surgeon can exert a surprisingly useful psychotherapeutic impact on a woman and her ability to cope with the disease and its treatment.

## Key points

- The majority of patients do want to be involved in the discussion about which type of breast surgery they are to receive but do not necessarily wish to choose the treatment. Clear communication helps patients to adapt to the choice of surgery and their disease.
- Sentinal node biopsy results in reduced axillary surgery and consequently less arm morbidity and significantly better arm functioning.
- Much information is now available to patients and many resources directed at trying to prevent or ameliorate psychological stress. Anxiety is just as high, however; some of this might be ameliorated by guiding patients to well-established websites and information resource centres. Misinformation is as psychonoxious as no information.
- Women need careful preoperative counselling and assessment prior to embarking on any prophylactic management policy.
- Adjuvant therapies can cause unpleasant side-effects for patients that compromise their quality of life. Clinicians and their specialist breast care nurses need to explain the side-effects associated with treatments and offer interventions to deal with them. More research is needed in this area.
- There is strong evidence that patient delay is associated with older age, and provider delay is associated with younger age and presentation with a breast symptom other than a lump. Better education and awareness of guidelines for referral are needed for patients and their GPs.
- There is no clear evidence that chemotherapy and/or endocrine therapy produce long-lasting cognitive impairement. Prospective studies show that few women are affected; future randomised trials investigating this phenomena might include prospective studies using imaging techniques (functional magnetic resonance imaging and positron emission tomography) to identify putative mechanisms and pathways.

# References

1. Moyer A. Psychosocial outcomes of breast-conserving surgery versus mastectomy: a meta-analytic review. Health Psychol 1997; 16(3):284–98.

2. Beaver K, Luker KA, Owens RG et al. Treatment decision making in women newly diagnosed with breast cancer. Cancer Nurs 1996; 19(1):8–19.

3. Fallowfield LJ, Hall A, Maguire P et al. Psychological effects of being offered choice of surgery for breast cancer. BMJ 1994; 309(6952):448.

4. Katz SJ, Lantz PM, Janz NK et al. Patient involvement in surgery treatment decisions for breast cancer. J Clin Oncol 2005; 23(24):5526–33.

5. Hawley ST, Lantz PM, Janz NK et al. Factors associated with patient involvement in surgical treatment decision making for breast cancer. Patient Educ Couns 2007; 65(3):387–95.

6. Waljee JF, Hawley S, Alderman AK et al. Patient satisfaction with treatment of breast cancer: does surgeon specialization matter? J Clin Oncol 2007; 25(24):3694–8.

7. Morrow M. Decision making in local therapy for breast cancer. Breast Cancer Res 2007; 9 (Suppl 2) 58 (doi 10.1186/bcr 1806).

8. Poole K, Fallowfield LJ. The psychological impact of post-operative arm morbidity following axillary surgery for breast cancer: a critical review. Breast 2002; 11(1):81–7.

9. Coster S, Poole K, Fallowfield LJ. The validation of a quality of life scale to assess the impact of arm morbidity in breast cancer patients post-operatively. Breast Cancer Res Treat 2001; 68(3):273–82.

10. Mansel RE, Fallowfield L, Kissin M et al. Randomized multicenter trial of sentinel node biopsy versus standard axillary treatment in operable breast cancer: the ALMANAC Trial. J Natl Cancer Inst 2006; 98(9):599–609.

11. Fleissig A, Fallowfield LJ, Langridge CI et al. Post-operative arm morbidity and quality of life. Results of the ALMANAC randomised trial comparing sentinel node biopsy with standard axillary treatment in the management of patients with early breast cancer. Breast Cancer Res Treat 2006; 95(3):279–93.

12. Baum M. Epidemiology versus scare mongering: the case for the humane interpretation of statistics and breast cancer. Breast J 2000; 6(5):331–4.

13. Fallowfield L, Ratcliffe D, Jenkins V et al. Psychiatric morbidity and its recognition by doctors in patients with cancer. Br J Cancer 2001; 84(8):1011–5.

14. Fallowfield L. Psychosocial interventions in cancer. BMJ 1995; 311(7016):1316–7.

15. Liebert B, Parle M, Roberts C et al. An evidence-based specialist breast nurse role in practice: a multicentre implementation study. Eur J Cancer Care (Engl) 2003; 12(1):91–7.

16. Luecken LJ, Compas BE. Stress, coping, and immune function in breast cancer. Ann Behav Med 2002; 24(4):336–44.

17. Spiegel D, Bloom JR, Kraemer HC et al. Effect of psychosocial treatment on survival of patients with metastatic breast cancer. Lancet 1989; 2(8668):888–91.

18. Spiegel D, Bloom JR, Yalom I. Group support for patients with metastatic cancer. A randomized outcome study. Arch Gen Psychiat 1981; 38(5):527–33.

19. Fox BH. A hypothesis about Spiegel et al.'s 1989 paper on psychosocial intervention and breast cancer survival. Psychooncology 1998; 7(5):361–70.

20. Cunningham AJ, Edmonds CV, Jenkins GP et al. A randomized controlled trial of the effects of group psychological therapy on survival in women with metastatic breast cancer. Psychooncology 1998; 7(6):508–17.

21. Goodwin PJ, Leszcz M, Ennis M et al. The effect of group psychosocial support on survival in metastatic breast cancer. N Engl J Med 2001; 345(24):1719–26.

22. Temoshok LR, Wald RL. Change is complex: rethinking research on psychosocial interventions and cancer. Integr Cancer Ther 2002; 1(2):135–45.

23. Bordeleau L, Szalai JP, Ennis M et al. Quality of life in a randomized trial of group psychosocial support in metastatic breast cancer: overall effects of the intervention and an exploration of missing data. J Clin Oncol 2003; 21(10):1944–51.

24. Kogon MM, Biswas A, Pearl D et al. Effects of medical and psychotherapeutic treatment on the survival of women with metastatic breast carcinoma. Cancer 1997; 80(2):225–30.

25. Schover LR, Yetman RJ, Tuason LJ et al. Partial mastectomy and breast reconstruction. A comparison of their effects on psychosocial adjustment, body image, and sexuality. Cancer 1995; 75(1):54–64.

26. Schain WS, Wellisch DK, Pasnau RO et al. The sooner the better: a study of psychological factors in women undergoing immediate versus delayed breast reconstruction. Am J Psychiat 1985; 142(1):40–6.

27. Al-Ghazal SK, Fallowfield L, Blamey RW. Does cosmetic outcome from treatment of primary breast cancer influence psychosocial morbidity? Eur J Surg Oncol 1999; 25(6):571–3.

28. Cocquyt VF, Blondeel PN, Depypere HT et al. Better cosmetic results and comparable quality of life after skin-sparing mastectomy and immediate autologous breast reconstruction compared to breast conservative treatment. Br J Plast Surg 2003; 56(5):462–70.

29. Harcourt DM, Rumsey NJ, Ambler NR et al. The psychological effect of mastectomy with or without

breast reconstruction: a prospective, multicenter study. Plast Reconstr Surg 2003; 111(3):1060–8.

30. Hatcher MB, Fallowfield L, A'Hern R. The psychosocial impact of bilateral prophylactic mastectomy: prospective study using questionnaires and semistructured interviews. BMJ 2001; 322(7278):76.

31. McAllister M, O'Malley K, Hopwood P et al. Management of women with a family history of breast cancer in the North West Region of England: training for implementing a vision of the future. J Med Genet 2002; 39(7):531–5.

32. Berglund G, Nystedt M, Bolund C et al. Effect of endocrine treatment on sexuality in premenopausal breast cancer patients: a prospective randomized study. J Clin Oncol 2001; 19(11):2788–96.

33. Fallowfield L, Fleissig A, Edwards R et al. Tamoxifen for the prevention of breast cancer: psychosocial impact on women participating in two randomized controlled trials. J Clin Oncol 2001; 19(7):1885–92.

34. Thirlaway K, Fallowfield L, Cuzick J. The Sexual Activity Questionnaire: a measure of women's sexual functioning. Qual Life Res 1996; 5(1):81–90.

35. Fallowfield L, Cella D, Cuzick J et al. Quality of life of postmenopausal women in the Arimidex, Tamoxifen, Alone or in Combination (ATAC) Adjuvant Breast Cancer Trial. J Clin Oncol 2004; 22(21):4261–71.

36. Cella D, Fallowfield L, Barker P et al. Quality of life of postmenopausal women in the ATAC ("Arimidex", tamoxifen, alone or in combination) trial after completion of 5 years' adjuvant treatment for early breast cancer. Breast Cancer Res Treat 2006; 100(3):273–84.

37. Fallowfield LJ, Bliss JM, Porter LS et al. Quality of life in the intergroup exemestane study: a randomized trial of exemestane versus continued tamoxifen after 2 to 3 years of tamoxifen in postmenopausal women with primary breast cancer. J Clin Oncol 2006; 24(6):910–7.

38. Cella D, Fallowfield LJ. Recognition and management of treatment-related side effects for breast cancer patients receiving adjuvant endocrine therapy. Breast Cancer Res Treat 2008; 107(2):167–80.

39. Shell JA. Evidence-based practice for symptom management in adults with cancer: sexual dysfunction. Oncol Nurs Forum 2002; 29(1): 53–66; quiz 67–9.

40. Ganz PA, Greendale GA, Petersen L et al. Managing menopausal symptoms in breast cancer survivors: results of a randomized controlled trial. J Natl Cancer Inst 2000; 92(13):1054–64.

41. Ramirez AJ, Westcombe AM, Burgess CC et al. Factors predicting delayed presentation of symptomatic breast cancer: a systematic review. Lancet 1999; 353(9159):1127–31.

42. Nosarti C, Crayford T, Roberts J et al. Delay in diagnosis in breast cancer. Lancet 1999; 353(9170):2154; author reply 2155.

43. Richards MA, Smith P, Ramirez AJ et al. The influence on survival of delay in the presentation and treatment of symptomatic breast cancer. Br J Cancer 1999; 79(5–6):858–64.

44. Burgess CC, Ramirez AJ, Richards MA et al. Who and what influences delayed presentation in breast cancer? Br J Cancer 1998; 77(8):1343–8.

45. Burgess C, Hunter MS, Ramirez AJ. A qualitative study of delay among women reporting symptoms of breast cancer. Br J Gen Pract 2001; 51(473):967–71.

46. Patel RS, Smith DC, Reid I. One stop breast clinics – victims of their own success? A prospective audit of referrals to a specialist breast clinic. Eur J Surg Oncol 2000; 26(5):452–4.

47. Chan SY, Berry MG, Engledow AH et al. Audit of a one-stop breast clinic – revisited. Breast Cancer 2000; 7(3):191–4.

48. Dey P, Bundred N, Gibbs A et al. Costs and benefits of a one stop clinic compared with a dedicated breast clinic: randomised controlled trial. BMJ 2002; 324(7336):507.

49. Harcourt D, Ambler N, Rumsey N et al. Evaluation of a one stop breast clinic: a randomised controlled trial. Breast 1998; 7:314–9.

50. Poole K, Hood K, Davis BD et al. Psychological distress associated with waiting for results of diagnostic investigations for breast disease. Breast 1999; 8(6):334–8.

51. Sutton S, Saidi G, Bickler G et al. Does routine screening for breast cancer raise anxiety? Results from a three wave prospective study in England. J Epidemiol Community Health 1995; 49(4): 413–8.

52. Lowe JB, Balanda KP, Del Mar C et al. Psychologic distress in women with abnormal findings in mass mammography screening. Cancer 1999; 85(5): 1114–18.

53. Brett J, Austoker J. Women who are recalled for further investigation for breast screening: psychological consequences 3 years after recall and factors affecting re-attendance. J Public Health Med 2001; 23(4):292–300.

54. Olsson P, Armelius K, Nordahl G et al. Women with false positive screening mammograms: how do they cope? J Med Screen 1999; 6(2):89–93.

55. Gilbert FJ, Cordiner CM, Affleck IR et al. Breast screening: the psychological sequelae of false-positive recall in women with and without a family history of breast cancer. Eur J Cancer 1998; 34(13):2010–4.

56. Aro AR, Pilvikki Absetz S, van Elderen TM et al. False-positive findings in mammography screening induces short-term distress – breast cancer-specific concern prevails longer. Eur J Cancer 2000; 36(9):1089–97.

57. Sandin B, Chorot P, Valiente RM et al. Adverse psychological effects in women attending a second-stage breast cancer screening. J Psychosom Res 2002; 52(5):303–9.

58. Jenkins V, Atkins L, Fallowfield L. Does endocrine therapy for the treatment and prevention of breast cancer affect memory and cognition? Eur J Cancer 2007; 43(9):1342–7.

59. Singh M, Meyer EM, Millard WJ et al. Ovarian steroid deprivation results in a reversible learning impairment and compromised cholinergic function in female Sprague–Dawley rats. Brain Res 1994; 644(2):305–12.

60. O'Neal MF, Means LW, Poole MC et al. Estrogen affects performance of ovariectomized rats in a two-choice water-escape working memory task. Psychoneuroendocrinology 1996; 21(1):51–65.

61. Sherwin BB. Estrogen and/or androgen replacement therapy and cognitive functioning in surgically menopausal women. Psychoneuroendocrinology 1988; 13(4):345–57.

62. Phillips SM, Sherwin BB. Effects of estrogen on memory function in surgically menopausal women. Psychoneuroendocrinology 1992; 17(5):485–95.

63. Wieneke M, Dienst ER. Neuropsychological assessment of cognitive functioning following chemotherapy for breast cancer. Psychooncology 1995; 4:61–66.

64. van Dam FS, Schagen SB, Muller MJ et al. Impairment of cognitive function in women receiving adjuvant treatment for high-risk breast cancer: high-dose versus standard-dose chemotherapy. J Natl Cancer Inst 1998; 90(3):210–8.

65. Brezden CB, Phillips KA, Abdolell M et al. Cognitive function in breast cancer patients receiving adjuvant chemotherapy. J Clin Oncol 2000; 18(14):2695–701.

66. Ferguson RJ, McDonald BC, Saykin AJ et al. Brain structure and function differences in monozygotic twins: possible effects of breast cancer chemotherapy. J Clin Oncol 2007; 25(25):3866–70.

67. Castellon S, Ganz P, Bower J et al. Neurocognitive performance in breast cancer survivors exposed to adjuvant chemotherapy and tamoxifen. J Clin Exp Neuropsychol 2004; 26(7):955–69.

68. Shilling V, Jenkins V, Trapala IS. The (mis)classification of chemo-fog – methodological inconsistencies in the investigation of cognitive impairment after chemotherapy. Breast Cancer Res Treat 2006; 95(2):125–9.

69. Jenkins V, Shilling V, Deutsch G et al. A 3-year prospective study of the effects of adjuvant treatments on cognition in women with early stage breast cancer. Br J Cancer 2006; 94(6):828–34.

70. Hermelink K, Untch M, Lux MP et al. Cognitive function during neoadjuvant chemotherapy for breast cancer: results of a prospective, multicenter, longitudinal study. Cancer 2007; 109(9):1905–13.

71. Schagen SB, Muller MJ, Boogerd W et al. Change in cognitive function after chemotherapy: a prospective longitudinal study in breast cancer patients. J Natl Cancer Inst 2006; 98(23):1742–5.

72. Horner MD, Hamner MB. Neurocognitive functioning in posttraumatic stress disorder. Neuropsychol Rev 2002; 12(1):15–30.

73. Schagen SB, van Dam FS, Muller MJ et al. Cognitive deficits after postoperative adjuvant chemotherapy for breast carcinoma. Cancer 1999; 85(3):640–50.

74. Shilling V, Jenkins V. Self-reported cognitive problems in women receiving adjuvant therapy for breast cancer. Eur J Oncol Nurs 2007; 11(1):6–15.

75. Ahles TA, Saykin AJ, Noll WW et al. The relationship of APOE genotype to neuropsychological performance in long-term cancer survivors treated with standard dose chemotherapy. Psychooncology 2003; 12(6):612–9.

# 17

# Benign breast disease

Steven Thrush
J. Michael Dixon

## Introduction

Over 90% of patients presenting to a breast clinic have normal breasts or benign breast disease.[1] An understanding of the aetiology, symptoms and management will ensure correct treatment and patient satisfaction. The expectation that the breast surgeon's role is simply to diagnose or exclude breast cancer has long disappeared. Benign breast disease causes considerable morbidity and anxiety, and with increasing patient awareness and expectations, the number of such patients attending clinics is likely to increase. Effective treatment includes accurate diagnosis followed by adequate explanation of the condition and how it is best managed This is a rewarding part of a breast specialist's workload.

Benign breast disease can be divided into congenital abnormalities, aberrations of normal breast development and involution (ANDI) and conditions secondary to some extrinsic precipitatory factors (non-ANDI).

## Congenital abnormalities

Although not diseases as such, developmental abnormalities of the breast can cause considerable concern and are not uncommon reasons for referral to a breast clinic.

## Supernumerary nipples and accessory breast tissue

Accessory breast tissue is usually found in the axilla and supernumerary or *accessory* nipples are usually seen below the breast and above the umbilicus. Accessory nipples vary in composure and usually are just a rudimentary nipple bud but can include glandular tissue (polymastia). They can be excised if causing irritation.

Accessory breast tissue tends to become more prominent or obvious during pregnancy due to the absence of a duct system leading to symptoms of obstruction (**Fig. 17.1**). Reassurance and an explanation of the cause of the 'lump' is usually all that is required. Surgical excision should be reserved for those truly symptomatic as they are difficult to excise cosmetically and surgery is associated with significant morbidity.[2] As with normal breast tissue, both benign and malignant conditions can develop within accessory breast tissue.

## Breast hypoplasia

This is failure of one or both (rarely) breasts to develop fully and is either congenital or acquired. Genetic causes include Poland's syndrome and ulnar-mammary syndrome. Poland's syndrome is a

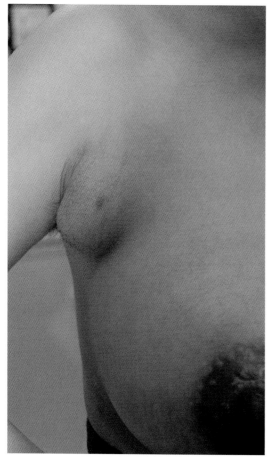

**Figure 17.1** • Accessory breast tissue in the right axilla.

group of conditions associated with the absence of or hypoplasia of the pectoralis major muscle and varying degrees of syndactyly.[3] It is extremely rare and usually only partial in nature. Acquired abnormalities in breast development can be caused by iatrogenic trauma or radiotherapy.

Treatment of hypoplasia depends on the degree of deformity. Mild asymmetry is a common problem which usually only necessitates reassurance. If marked, augmentation of the smaller breast with or without reduction or augmentation of the opposite breast may be required. If possible an anatomical cohesive gel implant should be used but it may be necessary to use an expandable implant first to achieve acceptable skin cover and symmetry. A pedicled or free myocutaneous flap, with or without an implant, can be used to reconstruct any muscle defect and produce symmetry in cases of severe hypoplasia or aplasia. Fat transfer (lipofilling) has

also been described as a technique to correct or aid correction of breast hypoplasia.[4]

Hypoplasia can also be associated with tubular breasts. This deformity can affect one or both breasts and is caused by a constricting ring at the base of the breast, limiting vertical and horizontal growth. The surgical management of this group of conditions is challenging and often unsatisfactory. Tissue expansion combined with radial incisions on the deep aspect of the breast to divide the constricting ring usually improves contour.

Macromastia is the excessive development of the breasts. This tends to occur during puberty (juvenile hypertrophy) or with onset of lactation (gestational). Prepubertal breast enlargement may occur in conjunction with a hormone-secreting tumour. Juvenile hypertrophy results from excessive proliferation of ducts and stromal tissue but no lobule formation. Significant psychological and physical problems can be caused by macromastia and patients with significant breast enlargement will benefit from breast reduction.

# Aberrations of normal breast development and involution

Defining what represents breast disease and what is normal is not a new problem. The ANDI classification[5] was developed to provide a framework to help understanding of the pathogenesis and subsequent management of benign breast disease. Most benign diseases arise from normal physiological processes and range from normality to mild abnormality (aberration) to severe abnormality (disease). The breast passes through three phases related to the levels of circulating hormones and their effects on the ducts, lobule and stroma. The three phases are development, cyclical change and involution (Table 17.1).

## Fibroadenomas

A fibroadenoma is classified as an aberration of normal breast development and is made up of a combination of connective tissue and proliferatory epithelium.[6] Fibroadenomas arise from the hormone-dependent lobule of the terminal duct lobular unit and are influenced by hormonal variances, e.g. increasing in size during pregnancy. The stromal element of these tumours defines their classification and behaviour.

Table 17.1 • Aberrations of normal breast development and involution

| Age (years) | Normal process | Aberration |
|---|---|---|
| <25 | Breast development | |
| | Stromal | Juvenile hypertrophy |
| | Lobular | Fibroadenoma |
| 25–40 | Cyclical activity | Cyclical mastalgia |
| | | Cyclical nodularity (diffuse or focal) |
| 35–55 | Involution | |
| | Lobular | Macrocysts |
| | Stromal | Sclerosing lesions |
| | Ductal | Duct ectasia |

A 'simple' fibroadenoma contains stroma of low cellularity and regular cytology. Phyllodes tumours may arise from fibroadenomas and contain stroma with marked cellularity and atypia. They cannot always be differentiated on core biopsy from simple fibroadenomas.

## Simple fibroadenomas

These are benign, extremely mobile, discrete, rubbery masses that present symptomatically in young women or are an incidental finding during breast imaging. They are a 'frequent' condition and are seen most commonly at the time of greatest lobular development in the late teens and early twenties. They are usually solitary findings but some women develop multiple lesions in one or both breasts. The aetiology is unknown but has been linked to the oral contraceptive and Epstein Barr virus following immunosuppression. They are highly mobile due to encapsulation and pliability of the breast tissue. This can make them appear to be much more superficial on examination than their true position, important to appreciate when embarking on removal under local anaesthetic.

 Fibroadenomas were observed for 2 years in women under 40 years of age: the majority did not change in size (55%), some got smaller or resolved (37%) and a small number increased in size (8%).[7]

In older women the picture is less classical; differentiating breast cancer from a fibroadenoma

is essential. Rapid growth of a fibroadenoma is rare but can occur in either adolescence (juvenile fibroadenoma) or in the perimenopausal age group. Tumours over 5 cm are termed 'giant fibroadenoma' and are more commonly seen in African countries.[8] On macroscopic appearance fibroadenomas are discrete, bosselated, whitish tumours that appear to bulge when cut through. Only rarely does cancer develop within a fibroadenoma but when it does it tends to be non-invasive and lobular in nature.[9]

### Management

Excision is recommended if a fibroadenoma increases significantly in size, if the fibroadenoma is causing significant distortion of the breast profile, where the lesion measures over 4 cm in size, if there is any histological concern about stromal activity or if the patient wishes excision. It is important to take account of the wishes of the patient; these are influenced by the manner in which the facts are presented.

The management of fibroadenomas depends on the patients' age and preference as well as the results of triple assessment. Core biopsy (multiple cores) is now preferred to cytology to confirm the diagnosis of a fibroadenoma. In patients with lesions under 4 cm, where histology confirms the diagnosis, the patient can then be reassured and discharged. In women presenting with multiple clinical and radiological firoadenomata, a core should be undertaken on the largest lesion.

Excision should ideally be undertaken through cosmetically placed incisions. Another option is to remove fibroadenomas with an 8G mammotome.[10] With larger lesions (>5 cm where histology has shown no suggestion that it could be a phyllodes tumour), it is safe to section the tumour in situ and remove it through a small incision to improve cosmetic outcome. Large lesions can also be removed cosmetically through an inframammary incision. Removal of excess skin is rarely required in young women, particularly when removing a large juvenile fibroadenoma. Recurrence of a fibroadenoma can occasionally occur but is rare. When it does so, it may be due to undiagnosed adjacent lesions rather than incomplete excision.

## Tubular and lactating adenomas

A fibroadenoma consists of fibroconnective stroma with glandular structures within. The glandular lining consists of a single or multiple layers of epithelial cells. When the entire lesion consists of glands with very little intervening stroma, this is termed a tubular adenoma. Lactating adenomas are similar to tubular adenomas, but occur in the pregnant or lactating breast and are often multiple. Tubular adenomas are clinically similar to firoadenomas and are managed identically. Mammographically they may demonstrate diffuse punctuate microcalcification within the acini. Lactating adenomas are managed conservatively through breast feeding unless there is clinical concern. They tend to regress following cessation of breast feeding.

## Hamartoma

Hamartomas are not uncommon benign breast lesions composed of variable amounts of adipose, glandular and fibrous tissues. They are usually asymptomatic but may be palpable. Most occur in women over 35. Mammographically they have been described as having a classical appearance (circumscribed area consisting of both soft tissue and lipomatous elements, surrounded by a thin radiolucent zone). Management is similar to that of fibroadenomas.

## Phyllodes tumour and sarcoma

The aetiology of phyllodes (leaf-like) tumours is unknown. They are less common than fibroadenomas (ratio of presentation 1:40[11]) and constitute about 2.5% of all fibroepithelial tumours. The age of onset is 15–20 years later than fibroadenomas. They tend to grow rapidly, producing marked distortion and cutaneous venous engorgement, which can lead to ulceration. The majority are benign in nature and so they are rarely fixed to skin or muscle. When cut during removal they are more brownish in colour than fibroadenomas and can have areas of necrosis within. If a diagnosis of phyllodes tumour is made before operation, then the aim should be to remove it with a clear macroscopic margin.

Differentiating benign from malignant phyllodes can be difficult and involves assessment of the size, ratio of stroma and epithelium, the border of the lesion, stromal cellularity and the number of stromal mitoses, and the presence or absence of necrosis.

Overall, phyllodes tumours recur locally in approximately 20% of patients. Most locally recurrent tumours are histologically similar to the original lesions. Malignant phyllodes tumours recur earlier on average than benign lesions. Regional lymph node metastases are seen rarely in malignant phyllodes tumours, with nodes being affected in approximately 5%. Metastatic lesions, when they

occur, resemble sarcomas. Fewer than 5% of all phyllodes tumours metastasise and approximately 25% of those classified as malignant metastasise depending on the exact criteria used for classification. Treatment of metastatic disease has been discouraging, with no sustained remissions from radiation, hormonal treatment or chemotherapy.

# Nipple discharge

Nipple discharge accounts for 5% of referrals to a breast clinic,[12] with 5% of these caused by in situ or malignant disease.[13] The important features to assess are whether the discharge is from one duct or many, is induced or spontaneous and is affecting one or both breasts. The frequency, colour and consistency of the discharge should also be noted. The aim is to differentiate between physiological causes and ductal pathology. Discharge can be elicited by squeezing around the nipple in 20% of women[14] and is often noted following mammography. If discharge is associated with a lump, then management is directed to the diagnosis of the lump.

Galactorrhoea should only be diagnosed if the discharge is bilateral, copious, off-white in colour and from multiple ducts. Some women continue to produce milk for many months after they have stopped breast-feeding but galactorrhoea usually develops long after cessation of breast-feeding. Prolactin levels should be checked and if raised (>1000 mIU/L) the cause can be secondary to medication or a pituitary tumour. If the serum prolactin is normal, then reassurance and a full explanation of the aetiology are often all that is required. If there are persistent symptoms, the ducts underneath the nipple can be ligated.

Coloured opalescent discharge, from multiple ducts, is common. It may be physiological discharge or it can be from duct ectasia. Serosanguineous and/or bloody discharge from a single duct is more likely to be associated with papillomas, epithelial hyperplasia or carcinoma.

## Investigation

Assessment includes a careful breast examination to identify the presence or absence of a breast mass. Firm pressure applied around the areola can help to identify the site of any dilated duct (pressure over a dilated duct will produce the discharge); this is helpful in defining where an incision should be made for any subsequent surgery. The nipple is squeezed with firm digital pressure and if fluid is expressed, the site and character of the discharge are recorded. Testing of the discharge for haemoglobin determines whether blood is present. Fewer than 10% of patients who have a blood-stained discharge or who have a discharge containing moderate or large amounts of blood have an underlying malignancy. Age is said to be an important predictor of malignancy; in one series, 3% of patients younger than 40, 10% of patients between ages 40 and 60, and 32% of patients older than 60 years who presented with nipple discharge as their only symptom were found to have cancers.[15] The absence of blood in nipple discharge is not an absolute indication that the discharge is unrelated to an underlying malignancy, as demonstrated in a series of 108 patients where the sensitivity of Haemoccult testing was only 50%.[16] Nipple discharge cytology is of little use due to its poor sensitivity.[17,18]

A number of techniques have evolved to determine the aetiology and avoid unnecessary surgery. Ductoscopy, using a microendoscope passed into the offending duct, allows direct visualisation and has the potential for biopsy. There are encouraging reports of its use (see Chapter 3), especially in directing duct excision at surgery[19] and detecting deeper lesions often missed by blind central excision.[20] Ductal lavage is a technique in which the duct is cannulated, irrigated with saline and the subsequent discharge (encouraged with massage) examined cytologically. This technique increases cell yield by 100 times that of simple discharge cytology and in one series showed a sensitivity for cytology obtained by ductal lavage of 64%, with a 100% positive predictive value.[21] Ductography (imaging of the ductal system) can identify intraductal lesions. Although this investigation has only a 60% sensitivity for malignancy, a filling defect or duct cut-off has a high positive predictive value for the presence of either a papilloma or a carcinoma.[22,23] Ductography, however, is a painful procedure and is not widely practised.

At present, the role of ductoscopy appears to be as an adjunct to surgery; by using simple transillumination of the skin overlying the lesion during ductoscopy, limited duct excision is possible. The role of ductal lavage has been questioned due to large variations in its sensitivity and specificity.[24,25] During ductoscopy, visualised lesions can be biopsied and in one report 38 of 46 women with biopsy-proven papillomas were observed for 2 years with no reported

missed cancers.[20] The role of ductoscopy in the assessment of nipple discharge is set to increase as the quality of equipment improves and it becomes more widely available. A benefit of both ductography and ductoscopy is that they allow identification of the site of any lesion in younger women, allowing localisation and excision of the causative lesion while retaining the ability to lactate. A mammogram should be performed as part of the assessment of patients over 35 years of age with a discharge. The sensitivity in this group of patients is low, at 57%.[17] Digital mammography has been shown to have a greater pick-up rate than film mammography in women under 50 or with dense breasts.[26] Ultrasound can sometimes identify papillomas and malignant lesions in the ducts close to the nipple.[27] Papillomas visualised on ultrasound can then be removed using a vacuum-assisted core biopsy device.[28]

If no abnormality is found on clinical or mammographic examination, patients are managed according to whether the discharge is from a single duct or multiple ducts (**Fig. 17.2**). Any patient with spontaneous single-duct discharge should undergo surgery to determine the cause of the discharges if it is:

- bloodstained or contains moderate to large amounts of blood on testing;
- persistent (at least twice per week);
- associated with a mass;
- a new serosanguineous discharge in a postmenopausal woman.

## Aetiology

### Duct ectasia

This is benign dilatation and shortening of the terminal ducts within 3 cm of the nipple. It is a common condition and increases in incidence with age. It should not be confused with periductal mastitis, which occurs in younger women and is secondary to cigarette smoking. Duct ectasia can present as nipple discharge, nipple retraction (giving a slit-like appearance) or a palpable mass. It is usually asymptomatic. The discharge is usually creamy and cheesy in nature. Bilateral multiduct green discharge is physiological and not usually related to duct ectasia.

### Ductal papillomas

There are three main forms: a solitary-duct discrete papilloma, multiple papillomas or juvenile papillomatosis (Swiss cheese disease). Papillomas are characterised by formation of epithelial fronds that

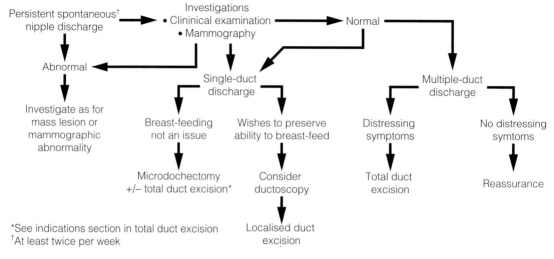

**Figure 17.2** • Investigation of nipple discharge.

have both the luminal epithelial and the outer myo-epithelial cell layers, supported by a fibrovascular stroma. The epithelial component can be subject to a spectrum of morphological changes ranging from metaplasia to hyperplasia, atypical intraductal hyperplasia and in situ carcinoma. A solitary intraductal papilloma, which occurs in a large duct (within 5 cm of the nipple), is the commonest form and is the most likely aetiology of a bloody nipple discharge. They are most frequently seen in the 30–50 age group and can be palpated in one-third of patients. As papillomas have a thin stalk, they have the potential to tort and necrose. Half of women with papillomas have bloody discharge while the other half have a serous discharge.[29]

Multiple intraductal papillomas describe a condition where a woman has many peripheral duct papillomas. It is defined as a minimum of five clearly separate papillomas within a localised segment of breast tissue, usually in a peripheral location. These tend not to present as nipple discharge but as a palpable lump and tend to occur in a younger age than single papillomas. They are only associated with an increased risk of malignancy if they contain areas of atypical hyperplasia. Repeated excision of papillomas in patients with multiple intraductal papillomas can result in significant breast asymmetry. One option in such patients is to excise such lesions with a vacuum-assisted core biopsy device. This provides sufficient material for the pathologist to assess that all excised lesions are benign.

Juvenile papillomatosis is a very rare condition defined as severe ductal papillomatosis occurring in young women <30 years old and usually presents as a painless, mobile mass (similar to fibroadenoma). Treatment is by complete excision. Patients with this condition (and their close family) may be at some increased risk of subsequent breast cancer, especially if the lesion is bilateral and there is significant family history. Close clinical surveillance is indicated.

Ductal carcinoma in situ

One-third of symptomatic in situ cancers present as nipple discharge.[30] Only rarely does an invasive cancer cause nipple discharge in the absence of a clinical mass. In most series, ductal carcinoma in situ (DCIS) is responsible for up to 10% of unilateral single duct nipple discharge.[14] Bloody nipple discharge with or without the presences of Paget's disease constitute one-third of all symptomatic in situ patients. The diagnosis is often made only following surgical excision of the affected duct.

Bloody nipple discharge in pregnancy

A bloody nipple discharge detected either visibly or on testing during pregnancy or lactation is common. In 20% of women who develop nipple discharge during pregnancy, blood is evident on testing. The likely cause is hypervascularity of developing breast tissue; it is benign, resolves spontaneously and requires no specific treatment.[31]

### Nipple adenoma

Nipple adenomas present as a non-discrete, palpable growth of the papilla of the nipple. There may be discoloration and contour change noted. They tend to lead to erosion of the nipple tip and commonly present as a bloody nipple discharge. They are benign in nature and definitive treatment is complete excision. It is caused by ductal hyperplasia of the lactiferous ducts and presents in women of approximately 40–50 years of age.

### Granular cell tumours

This is an uncommon, usually benign neoplasm that originates from Schwann cells of the peripheral nervous system. About 6% of all granular cell tumours involve the breast. The mean age at diagnosis is 40 years. Clinically and on imaging they are difficult to differentiate from a breast carcinoma due to their fibrous consistency, fixation to the pectoral fascia and skin retraction. Granular cell tumours are usually benign but there have been reports of malignant cases. Treatment is a wide local excision, ensuring a clear margin to prevent recurrence. This may include a cuff of muscle.

## Surgery

### Microdochectomy

A single duct can be removed using microdochectomy. This is performed via a radial incision or a circumareolar incision, the latter giving better cosmesis. Expression of the nipple discharge should not be performed until the patient is in theatre and fully draped in order to provide the best chance of identifying the offending duct. This duct is cannulated and either a lacrimal probe placed or methylene blue injected and an incision made. The probe aids identification of the relevant duct and dissection of this from surrounding ducts/breast tissue. A length of at least 2–3 cm should be removed. The excised duct should be opened to ensure a cause for the discharge is present and the distal remnant inspected to ensure that the entire dilated duct has been excised. If the residual duct is dilated, then it should be split, opened and inspected. Microdochectomy should not damage surrounding normal ducts and allows subsequent breast-feeding. If performing a duct excision directed by ductoscopy, then having identified an abnormality in the duct, the light is used to direct the surgical excision. Once the excision has been performed, the nipple should be squeezed gently to ensure that the discharging duct has been excised.

### Total duct excision or division

In women of non-childbearing age, total duct excision is an option for a single-duct discharge. Current evidence suggests that total duct excision is more likely to result in a specific diagnosis and less likely to miss underlying malignancy than microdochectomy.[32] Total duct excision can also be used for multiple-duct discharge if the discharge is copious and affecting quality of life, and is often performed for periductal mastitis. The operation involves dividing all the ducts from the underside of the nipple and removing surrounding breast tissue to a depth of 2 cm behind the nipple–areola complex.[33] A circumareolar incision is used. Patients should be warned that there is a small risk of nipple tip necrosis (<1%), reduced sensation (40%) and nipple inversion associated with this operation. Patients undergoing surgery for periductal mastitis require total removal of all ducts from behind the nipple; leaving remnants of ducts predisposes to recurrence. Because the lesions of periductal mastitis usually contain organisms patients should receive appropriate antibiotic treatment during the operation and for 5 days after surgery. Options for antibiotic therapy include amoxicillin–clavulanate or a combination of erythromycin and metronidazole.

For patients having cosmetic nipple eversion, the procedure can be performed through a limited incision and the ducts divided sufficiently to ensure the nipple everts naturally without the need for sutures.

## Mastalgia

Most women at some point during their lives will suffer from breast pain. The aim for clinicians is to differentiate between true mastalgia (pain originating within the breast) and referred pain. Women with referred pain will describe the pain as unilateral, associated with activity and reproduced by pressure on the chest wall. Non-steroidal anti-inflammatory drugs, either taken orally or applied topically, can relieve such symptoms. True mastalgia is associated with swelling and nodularity of the breasts. It resolves spontaneously in 20–40% of women but can recur.

Due to the hormonal aetiology true breast pain is often worse before and relieved after menstruation. Exacerbating factors include the perimenopausal state (where hormone levels fluctuate) and the use of exogenous hormones (hormone replacement therapy or the oral contraceptive pill).

The cause of mastalgia is unknown but suggestions include excess production of prolactin,[34] excess estrogen,[35] insufficient progesterone,[36] or increased receptor sensitivity in breast tissue caused by a raised ratio of saturated fatty acids to essential fatty acids.[37]

## Assessment

A full history and examination should be performed. In women over 35 years of age, mammography should be performed to exclude an occult malignancy (approximately 5% of women with breast cancer complain of pain,[11] while 2.7% of women presenting with pain as their main problem are diagnosed with breast cancer[38]). If a lump is palpable, then this will dictate further management. Most breast pain and this includes many women with cyclical breast pain, have pain arising in the chest wall. Analgesia, a firm bra worn 24 hours a day and gentle stretching exercise are effective treatments.

The use of a pain chart allows interpretation of the pattern of the pain, gives objective evaluation of treatment and indicates the effect it is having on the patient's life. (Patients with minimal pain are unlikely to fully complete a 3-month chart!)

## Treatment

Reassurance that the symptoms are not related to an underlying malignancy is probably the most effective treatment for mastalgia.[39] Following this, the majority will require no further treatment.

Evening primrose oil (EPO) has been withdrawn because two double-blind, randomised, crossover trials comparing EPO versus placebo showed no benefit for EPO.[40,41] The original work that advocated its use has never been published other than in abstract form.[42] Other agents that have been shown to have some benefit include phytoestrogens (e.g. soya milk)[43] and Agnus castus (a fruit extract).[44]

Reducing fat intake to less than 15% of dietary calories has been shown to improve symptoms in cyclical mastalgia.[45] The patients who responded showed changes in their serum lipid profiles but the study was not blinded so placebo effects cannot be excluded.

In severe pain, prescribed medication can be used but complications need to be explained. Treatment should be either tamoxifen 10 mg daily or danazol. Tamoxifen 20 mg daily was found to be superior to placebo in a double-blind, randomised, controlled

trial and pain relief was maintained in 72% of women 1 year after use.[46] Tamoxifen given in the luteal phase of the menstrual cycle abolished pain in 85% of women. Recurrent pain at 1 year was 25% and the rate of adverse effects was 21%.[47] Tamoxifen 10 mg daily has been compared with danazol 200 mg daily.[48]

Tamoxifen was found to be superior to danazol, with fewer adverse effects: 53% of patients receiving tamoxifen were pain-free at 1 year compared with 37% of patients receiving danazol. Tamoxifen 10 mg daily or danazol can be given during the luteal phase of the cycle with similar improvements in symptoms but with a marked reduction in adverse effects.[47,49]

Tamoxifen is not licensed for use in mastalgia. Toremifene, another selective oestrogen receptor modulator, has also recently demonstrated its effectiveness in treating mastalgia. In a randomised, double-blind trial of 195 women with persistent (lasting longer than 6 months) mastalgia, they assigned patients to toremifene 30 mg daily or a matched placebo for three menstrual cycles. This demonstrated a significant benefit for toremifene but with no significant difference in adverse events between the two groups.[50]

A phase II trial using afimoxifene (4-hydroxytamoxifen) delivered locally to the breast as a transdermal hydroalcoholic gel daily over four cycles has shown statistically significant improvements in signs and symptoms of cyclical mastalgia across patient- and physician-rated scales with excellent tolerability and safety. There is strong evidence that this tamoxifen metabolite is absorbed into the breast tissue but does not have the systemic effects associated with tamoxifen.[51]

Bromocriptine use has diminished due to its high rate of adverse effects (80%).[52] Selective serotonin reuptake inhibitors have shown some benefit in mastalgia as part of premenstrual syndrome;[53] they also have effects on fatty acid profiles.

## Breast cysts

Palpable breast cysts are a common presentation to a breast clinic and affect 7% of women.[11] Microcysts have no significance except their potential to grow. Macrocysts present typically in the fifth decade and are usually multiple in nature. Cysts can be divided into apocrine and non-apocrine depending on the consistency of the fluid found within the cyst. The relevance of this is that apocrine cysts have a higher tendency to recur.[54]

## Imaging

Mammographically breast cysts have characteristic haloes but ultrasound is essential to the management of cystic disease. Not only does it distinguish between solid and cystic lesions but also provides information on the cyst lining and fluid consistency. It is also an adjunct in ensuring accurate differentiation of simple from complex cysts, as well as allowing complete aspiration. A simple cyst shows a smooth outline with no internal echoes and posterior enhancement. Complex (or complicated or atypical) cysts are characterised by internal echoes or thin septations, thickened and/or irregular wall, and absent posterior enhancement. These are rarely malignant and should be reviewed with a follow-up scan several months later. If the cyst wall shows any projections, this may indicate the presence of an intracystic papilloma or carcinoma and core biopsy is indicated.

## Management

Asymptomatic cysts should be left alone. Large or painful cysts should be aspirated to dryness. If the fluid is bloodstained it should be sent for cytology; otherwise it should be discarded. If a palpable mass is still present after aspiration, further imaging and biopsy are indicated. If the cyst recurs, then repeat aspiration can be performed. There is a slightly increased relative risk of developing breast cancer in women with cysts but not significant enough to warrant surveillance.

## Sclerotic/fibrotic lesions

Stromal involution can produce areas of fibrosis. Three different groups of such lesions are described: sclerosing adenosis, radial scars and complex sclerosing lesions (CSLs). Sclerosing adenosis can present with a palpable mass and breast pain. Mammographically it can be associated with microcalcificaton. It differs histologically from radial scars and CSLs in the degree of excessive myoepithelial proliferation seen in addition to the fibrosis. Radial scars and CSLs are considered to be part of the same process but are differentiated on size (radial scar, ≤1 cm; CSL, >1 cm). Radial scars and CSLs are usually asymptomatic and discovered as part of mammographic screening but can present as a palpable mass. Both lesions may serve as a background for the development of atypical epithelial proliferations, including atypical ductal hyperplasia, atypical lobular hyperplasia, lobular carcinoma in situ and DCIS. Even in the absence of atypia there is some suggestion that the presence of such lesions increases the individual's risk of malignancy.[55] All these lesions, though benign in nature, are difficult to distinguish from malignant conditions mammographically, macroscopically and histologically. Percutaneous biopsy of these lesions with a core needle is only reliable when there is no associated atypia, when at least 12 cores are included and where there is concordance with radiological findings.[56] Malignancy cannot be reliably excluded when there is limited sampling, presence of atypia or discordance with the radiology. Then either open excision or vacuum-assisted biopsy is recommended.

## Diabetic mastopathy

This is a form of sclerosis occurring in premenopausal women and occasionally men with long-standing type I diabetes, often associated with other diabetic complications, particularly retinopathy. It can result clinically in one or more hard masses within the breast which are clinically suspicious of malignancy, but on histology the findings are of sclerosing lymphocytic lobulitis or 'diabetic mastopathy'. The disease probably represents an immune reaction to the abnormal accumulation of altered extracellular matrix in the breast, which is a manifestation of the effects of hyperglycaemia on connective tissue. It does not seem to predispose to breast carcinoma or lymphoma and in patients without diabetes has an unknown aetiology.[57]

## Pseudoangiomatous stromal hyperplasia of the breast (PASH)

PASH is a benign myofibroblastic proliferation of non-specialised mammary stroma. It is frequently a microscopic incidental finding in breast biopsies performed for benign or malignant disease. It has been reported to form breast masses and some of these have been reported to be sizeable. Whether PASH is the cause of these masses or an epiphenomenon, for instance extensive PASH is common within a juvenile fibroadenoma, is not clear. The aetiology is not known and assuming that PASH explains the cause of any localised mass is unwise. The histological appearance has caused confusion with mammary angiosarcoma, so immunohistochemical vascular markers are used for distinction.

## Fibromatosis

Fibromatosis or *desmoid tumour* of the breast is an extremely rare entity. Fibromatosis is an infiltrative fibroblastic and myofibroblastic proliferation with significant risk for local recurrence, but no metastatic potential. Fibromatosis is uncommon in the mammary gland and accounts for less than 0.2% of all primary breast lesions. It is usually indistinguishable from malignancy on ultrasound, mammography, physical examination, and on gross evaluation. Fibromatosis is a spectrum of conditions from extremely indolent areas principally of fibrosis to a more proliferative infiltrative lesion that requires excision. Establishing the diagnosis can be difficult on core biopsy and larger vacuum-assisted 8G needle biopsies provide more tissue for the pathologist to assess. Open biopsy may be necessary if a diagnosis is not evident on needle biopsy. Once it is established that the diagnosis is fibromatosis (this may involve sending the biopsy for an expert opinion) then treatment is surgical excision with wide clearance as there is little evidence in benefit of chemotherapy, radiotherapy or antiestrogen therapy. Excision may need to involve removal of underlying chest muscle and ribs. Recurrence can occur if excision is incomplete. Recurrence is often evident because of nerve entrapment which results in local pain.

# Non-ANDI conditions

## Breast infections

Infection is a common problem affecting the breast,[58] and can be divided into lactational, non-lactational and postsurgical. The skin overlying the breast can also become infected either primarily or secondarily because of infection developing in an existing lesion such as a sebaceous cyst or as a consequence of a generalised condition such as hidradenitis suppurativa.

### Lactational infections

Mastitis secondary to breast-feeding occurs in approximately 5% of puerperal women and is most common during the first month or during weaning as the baby's teeth develop. *Staphylococcus aureus* is the usual organism and it enters the duct system through the nipple. There is usually a history of a cracked nipple and/or problems with milk flow. Patients initially present with pain, localised erythema and swelling.

If this progresses, the inflammation can affect large areas of the breast and the patient can become toxic. Promoting milk flow by continuing to breast-feed and the early use of appropriate antibiotics markedly reduces the rate of subsequent abscess formation. Infections developing within the first few weeks may result from organisms transmitted in hospital and may be resistant to commonly used antibiotics. Over half of organisms that cause breast infection produce penicillinase.[59] Co-amoxiclav or flucloxacillin and erythromycin are the antibiotics of preference. Tetracycline, ciprofloxacin and chloramphenicol should not be used to treat infection in breast-feeding women because these drugs enter breast milk and may harm the child.

### Non-lactational infections

Non-lactational infections are grouped into peripheral or periareolar. Those infections in the periareolar area are seen in young women and are often secondary to periductal mastitis (associated with heavy cigarette smoking).[60] How cigarette smoking causes periductal mastitis is unclear. Substances in cigarette smoke may directly or indirectly damage the wall of subareolar ducts. Accumulation of toxic metabolites, such as lipid peroxidase, epoxides, nicotine and cotinine, in the breast ducts has been demonstrated to occur in smokers within 15 minutes of a woman starting to breast-feed.[61] Smoking has also been shown to inhibit growth of Gram-positive bacteria, leading to an overgrowth of Gram-negative bacteria.[62] This may affect the normal bacterial flora and allow overgrowth of pathogenic aerobic and anaerobic Gram-negative bacteria, and would explain the presence of these organisms in the lesions of periductal mastitis. Microvascular changes have also been recorded and may cause local ischaemia. The combination of damage due to toxins, microvascular damage by lipid peroxidases, and altered bacterial flora are almost certainly responsible for the clinical manifestations of periductal mastitis.

Patients present with periareolar inflammation associated with a mass or abscess. The organisms are usually mixed, including anaerobes. Very rarely an infection is related to underlying comedo necrosis in DCIS. For this reason a mammogram should be performed in those patients over 35 years of age after resolution of the inflammation. Periareolar sepsis has a high rate of recurrence.

Peripheral non-lactational breast abscesses are three times more common in premenopausal women than in menopausal or postmenopausal women. The aetiology of these infections is unclear but some are associated with diabetes, rheumatoid arthritis, steroid treatment and trauma.[63] The usual organism responsible is *S. aureus*.

## Postsurgical infection

Infections can present in the acute postsurgical period or after the wound has healed. There is conflicting evidence for the use of prophylactic antibiotics during clean breast surgery.[64] The most common organisms causing infection in the acute period include normal skin flora or organisms derived from the terminal ducts.[65] Most surgeons give antibiotics routinely to patients having implants inserted. Patients having surgery for periductal mastitis are at increased risk of postoperative infection and all these patients should have intraoperative and postoperative antibiotics that cover the range of organisms isolated from this condition. 'Seromas' are frequent and can become infected either during aspiration or as a result of reduced resistance to infection during chemotherapy. Radiotherapy interferes with both the blood and lymphatic flow to the breast and its effect is to reduce resistance to infection in the treated area; when infection occurs, prolonged and high-dose antibiotic therapy is usually required. Delayed infections after breast-conserving surgery or mastectomy are not uncommon (especially after radiotherapy). It is important not to confuse this with so-called 'delayed cellulitis', where the breast becomes painful, red and oedematous. It is unresponsive to antibiotics and has an incidence of 3–5% in patients following radiotherapy for breast-conserving surgery.[66]

If an implant becomes infected, intensive antibiotic therapy is occasionally effective but usually the prosthesis has to be removed. Replacing an infected implant following thorough lavage has been reported to be effective but is rarely performed.[67] It is not uncommon for implants to become infected after a minor surgical intervention (such as dental work) or during chemotherapy given as adjuvant therapy or as treatment for metastatic disease. Prophylactic antibiotics should be considered for patients with implants undergoing major dental work.

## Treatment

The basis of treatment for all breast infections is use of a broad-spectrum antibiotic and draining any collections of pus.

Due to the difficulty of predicting the presence of pus within an inflamed breast, ultrasound with or without aspiration should be performed.[68] The need for open drainage in breast abscesses has been superseded by the use of aspiration.[69–71]

This has allowed management to become outpatient based. Protocols validated within the Edinburgh Breast Unit have demonstrated that few if any breast abscesses require incision and drainage under general anaesthesia.[72] All abscesses should be assessed by ultrasound and if pus is present the surgeon or radiologist aspirates this, usually under ultrasound guidance (**Fig. 17.3**). Patients are reviewed regularly every 2–3 days and any further collections aspirated until no further pus forms. Drainage under local anaesthesia is performed in patients where the overlying skin is thinned or necrotic (**Fig. 17.4**). The incision to drain any breast abscess should be just large enough to allow the pus to drain (usually 1 cm or less), while minimising later scarring. Ultrasound provides a simple method of differentiating an abscess from cellulitis, allows assessment of loculation and permits complete aspiration of all pus. Experience in the Edinburgh Breast Unit

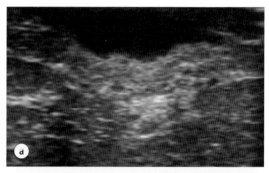
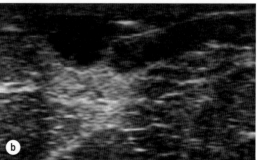

**Figure 17.3** • Aspiration of abscess under ultrasound guidance: **(a)** ultrasound view of a breast abscess; **(b)** the needle can be seen entering the abscess on the right allowing aspiration to be performed.

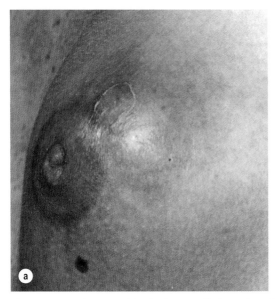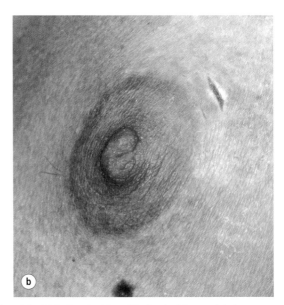

**Figure 17.4** • Abscess of the left breast with thinned overlying skin: **(a)** before incision; **(b)** after incision and drainage through a small stab incision.

of using ultrasound to assist aspiration of breast abscesses is that it is quick and simple to learn and use. When used with local anaesthetic injected into the breast and irrigated into the abscess cavity, aspiration is relatively painless and the local anaesthetic dilutes the pus to allow aspiration. Periareolar non-lactational abscesses can be treated and cured by repeated aspiration. Due to the recurrent nature of this condition, recurrent abscess formation is common and in such patients careful surgical excision of any residual abscess and affected ducts is often required.[34] A mammary duct fistula (an abnormal connection between the infected duct and the skin around the areola) develops in up to one-third of patients after incision and drainage of a periareolar abscess.[73] These require definitive surgical management, with complete excision of the tract (plus the affected ducts under the nipple) and ideally primary closure with antibiotic cover (**Fig. 17.5**). There is a high risk of recurrence in the presence of postoperative wound infection.[74] Laying open the fistula and allowing it to heal by secondary intention is effective but leaves an ugly scar across the nipple.

An important aspect of the management of puerperal breast infections is the continued expression of milk, with the most efficient breast pump being the baby's mouth. Emptying the breast increases the rate of a good outcome in infective mastitis[75] and although bacteria and the antibiotic are present in the milk, this does not appear to harm the child.[76] It

is rarely necessary to suppress lactation but in severe unremitting or repeated infections, agents such as cabergoline are effective at stopping milk flow.

It is essential to remember that inflammatory carcinoma can be difficult to differentiate from breast infection. If the breast does not settle on appropriate management, then fine-needle aspiration and/or core biopsy of any abnormal area should be considered.

## Other infections

### HIV associated

Immunocompromised patients are susceptible to breast infection. This is true of both male and female sufferers.

### Granulomatous mastitis

This is a rare condition, characterised by non-caseating granulomas and microabcesses confined to a breast lobule.[77] Patients present with a hard mass (which is often indistinguishable from a carcinoma) or multiple or recurrent abscesses. The mass can be extremely tender. Young parous women are most frequently affected and there is no association with smoking. The role of organisms in the aetiology of this condition is unclear but one study did isolate corynebacteria from 9 of 12 women with granulomatous lobular mastitis.[78] The most common species isolated was the newly described *Corynebacterium kroppenstedtii*, followed by *Corynebacterium amycolatum* and

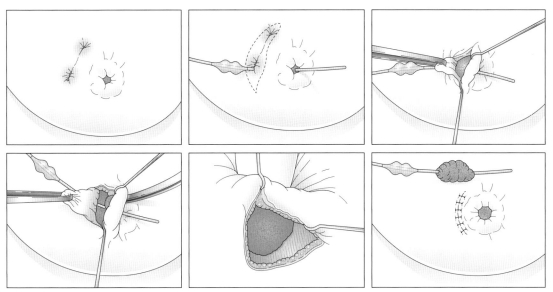

**Figure 17.5 •** Diagrammatic illustration of the steps involved in excision of a mammary duct fistula performed through a circumareolar incision with primary wound closure under antibiotic cover.

*Coryneacterium tuberculostearicum*. These organisms are usually sensitive to penicillin and tetracycline, but treatment with such antibiotics rarely produces resolution of granulomatous lobular mastitis and the role of these organisms is unclear. In patients presenting with a breast mass diagnosed on core biopsy as granulomatous lobular mastitis, excision of the mass should be avoided, as it is often followed by persistent wound discharge and failure of the wound to heal. Steroids have been used with varying reports of their efficacy; we do not use them.[79]

### Hidradenitis suppurativa

Hidradenitis is infection associated with the apocrine glands, affecting axillae, perineum and/or breast areas. It is commoner in smokers and the organisms responsible are similar to those present in periareolar sepsis. Treatment in the acute phase comprises management of any infection/abscesses. Excision of the affected area with skin grafting is effective in approximately 50% of patients and may be the only long-term option for some patients.

## Montgomery's glands

Throughout the areola are blind-ending glands that produce fluid to lubricate the areola during breast-feeding. These glands can block, forming hard nodules on the periphery of the areola. Occasionally these can become infected. Unless symptomatic, the management of these prominent Montgomery's glands is reassurance.

## Lipomas

Due to the fatty nature of the breast it is not surprising that lipomas develop. They tend to present in the fifth decade[11] and have to be distinguished from any sinister cause. Imaging shows a radiolucent lobulated mass. Needle aspiration is often reported inadequate (C1) due to fat only being aspirated. A pseudo-lipoma is a mass that clinically appears to be a simple lipoma but is actually caused by a small cancer that produces compressed fat lobules as the suspensory ligaments of the breast shorten. Liposarcomas occur only very rarely in the breast.[80]

## Fat necrosis

Following trauma to the breast, fat necrosis can occur. Fat necrosis can produce either a mass similar on palpation and imaging to breast carcinoma or a cystic oily collection. Usually patients give a history of direct trauma (or surgery) to the affected breast and examination may reveal bruising. It is important to assess such patients with imaging and not dismiss dimpling and bruising as fat necrosis. Histologically fat necrosis is characterised by anucleate fat cells, surrounded by histiocytic giant cells and foamy macrophages. Severe fat necrosis can follow seat-belt damage and such patients often have a significant defect in the breast with some distortion at the site where the seat-belt has disrupted a significant area of breast fat. Some patients present with bruising but have underlying carcinomas that are only evident following (usual trivial) trauma. The symptoms of fat necrosis tend to settle within a couple of months.

## Mondor's disease

Mondor's disease is spontaneous superficial thrombophlebitis of a breast vein. It is often initially painful and occasionally there may be a history of trauma or surgery to the breast. Clinically, there may be a thickened palpable cord with associated erythema. Its aetiology in the absence of surgery, trauma or infection is unknown but is not thought to be of any significance. It is a self-limiting condition that normally resolves within a couple of weeks. Nonsteroidal anti-inflammatory agents rubbed over the area of tenderness improve pain. Mondor's disease most commonly involves one or more of three venous channels: the thoracoepigastric vein, the lateral thoracic vein and the superior epigastric vein. The upper, inner portion of the breast is never involved.

## Gynaecomastia

True gynaecomastia is caused by hyperplasia of the stromal and ductal tissue of the male breast. It is responsible for considerable embarrassment and worry and is the commonest condition affecting the male breast. Pseudogynaecomastia gives a similar appearance but is due to excess adipose tissue with no increase in stromal or ductal tissue. Both types can present together.[81] Gynaecomastia associated with Kleinfelter syndrome is associated with actual lobule formation and a risk of breast cancer approaching that of the female population.

Gynaecomastia can occur from any age and presents as a concentric painful swelling. It is a common condition, occurring in at least 35% of men at some time. It is benign and usually reversible. An important differential diagnosis is a primary breast cancer.

The aetiology of gynaecomastia is due to a relative hyperestrogenism.[82] This is caused by decreased androgen production, increased estrogen produc-

tion or an increase in peripheral aromatisation. In patients where no endocrine abnormality or drug is found, the cause may be a reduction in androgen receptors and/or a local increase in aromatase activity.[83] Causes can be divided into physiological, pathological, drug induced (medicinal and recreational) and idiopathic.

1. Physiological, or primary, gynaecomastia shows a trimodal pattern, with peaks in the neonatal period, puberty and senescence. It is often self-limiting but will occasionally require treatment.
2. Pathological causes are listed in Box 17.1.
3. Common drugs that produce gynaecomastia include: spironolactone (antiandrogen); histamine $H_2$ antagonists, antipsychotics and methyldopa (gonadotrophin disturbance); digoxin, cannabis and griseofulvin (estrogen receptor competitors); and anabolic steroids (Box 17.2). HIV treatment with highly active anti-retrovirals is also commonly associated.

The degree of gynaecomastia is classified using appearance (Table 17.2). A thorough history will usually elicit the underlying cause. Examination of breast, axilla, testes and abdomen should be performed.

Investigations of gynaecomastia are directed to excluding a primary breast carcinoma or a secondary pathological cause. Biochemical assessment (liver and renal function tests, γ-glutamyltransferase, prolactin,

**Box 17.1** • Pathological causes of gynaecomastia

### Decreased androgens
*Reduced production*
- Chromosomal abnormalities, e.g. Klinefelter's syndrome
- Bilateral cyptorchidism
- Hyperprolactinaemia
- Bilateral torsion
- Viral orchitis
- Renal failure

*Androgen resistance*
- Testicular feminisation

### Increased estrogens
*Increased secretion*
- Testicular tumours
- Carcinoma of the lung

*Increased peripheral aromatisation*
- Liver disease
- Adrenal disease
- Thyrotoxicosis

Box 17.2 • Drugs associated with gynaecomastia

**Hormones**
- Anabolic steroids (body-builders)
- Estrogenic agonists
- Antiandrogens (treatment of prostate cancer), e.g. cyproterone acetate, goserelin

**Recreational drugs**
- Alcohol
- Cannabis
- Heroin

**Cardiovascular drugs**
- Digoxin
- Spironolactone
- Captopril
- Enalapril
- Amiodarone
- Nefedipine
- Verapamil

**Antiulcer drugs**
- Cimetidine
- Ranitidine
- Omeprazole

**Antibiotics**
- Ketoconazole
- Metronidazole
- Minocycline

**Psychoactive agents**
- Tricylic antidepressants
- Diazepam
- Phenothiazines

**Others**
- Domperidone
- Metoclopramide
- Penicillamine
- Phenytoin
- Theophylline

Table 17.2 • Classification of gynaecomastia

| Grade | Clinical appearance |
|-------|---------------------|
| I | Small but visible breast development with little redundant skin |
| IIa | Moderate breast development with no redundant skin |
| IIb | Moderate breast development with redundant skin |
| III | Marked breast development with much redundant skin |

From Simon BE, Hoffman S, Kahn S. Classification and surgical correction of gynecomastia. Plast Reconstr Surg 1973; 51:48–52.[84] With permission from Lippincott, Williams & Wilkins. © American Society of Plastic Surgeons.

α-fetoprotein, β-human chorionic gonadotrophin and total testosterone) is only required in rapidly growing gynaecomastia. Imaging (with mammography and/or ultrasound) plus biopsy (fine-needle aspiration cytology and/or core biopsy) can be performed if the cause of the gynaecomastia is indeterminate, surgery is being considered or cancer is suspected.

## Treatment

Reassurance of the transient and benign nature is often all that is required in the management of physiological gynaecomastia. In drug-related gynaecomastia, withdrawal of the drug or change to an alternative should be considered. For pathological gynaecomastia, the underlying cause needs to be addressed.

For those cases requiring treatment there are two options: medical treatment and surgical excision. Medical management benefits from a high success rate and avoidance of an operation.

 The evidence for the three commonly prescribed drugs (danazol,[85] tamoxifen[86] and clomifene[87]) is based on small non-randomised trials and does not include recurrence rates, optimum dose, length of treatment or associated long-term risks.

In the UK, only danazol is licensed for the treatment of gynaecomastia. A short 6-week course is recommended, with 100 mg b.d. for the first week followed by 100 mg t.d.s. for the second to sixth weeks, response being assessed at the eighth week. Imaging and clinical photography can be used to evaluate success of treatment. Repeat courses may be required. Tamoxifen at a daily dose of 10 mg produces excellent response rates and is favoured in our practice.

Due to the high risk of poor cosmesis associated with gynaecomastia surgery and subsequent risk of litigation, surgery should only be undertaken after medical failure or where the stage of the problem is too large (class IIa/III). Marking the extent of the gynaecomastia prior to surgery is essential. The procedure should be performed via a periareolar incision to reduce scarring. The use of lighted retractors and diathermy aids surgery. A disc of breast tissue should be left behind the nipple combined with an intact pectoral fascia and overlying fat to prevent retraction and fixation to the muscle (saucer deformity). Skin flaps are kept thick to prevent deformity and skin necrosis. Patients should be warned about nipple necrosis, sensory changes and recurrence, as well as cosmetic problems. In extreme cases excess skin is removed, requiring repositioning of the nipple and even free nipple grafts.[88] In young patients, the excess skin will correct itself without need for excision. The use of liposuction alone or combined with limited surgery or mammotomy has been reported to improve cosmetic outcomes. Ultrasound-assisted liposuction allows treatment of more fibrous areas and increases the number of patients suitable for this technique.[89] An approach to management including liposuction is outlined in **Fig. 17.6**.[90]

# Common complications of cosmetic breast surgery

Cosmetic surgical procedures to the breast are increasing in popularity. The frequency of patients presenting with symptoms either secondary or independent to previous operations means an understanding of such procedures and their complications can allow rapid diagnosis and reassurance for the patient. It is *highly* recommended that the operating surgeon assess patients with recognised problems from such surgery. However, it is not uncommon for these patients to be referred to a breast clinic as suspected breast cancer.

Assessment involves a detailed history of the original procedure as well as standard triple assessment. In the augmented patient it is useful to know the type of implant used (size, shape and composition) and its position (subpectoral or submammary). The time since surgery and any surgical complications (e.g. haematoma) should also be noted. Examination will show if any associated mastopexy (breast lift) was performed. In the patient who has undergone a breast reduction it is useful to know an approximate volume reduction and wound healing problems.

Imaging of breasts post-cosmetic surgery brings some technical challenges. Scarring is commonly seen after breast reduction and can make mammographic interpretation difficult. Assessment of the augmented breast should include mammography (using the Ekland technique) and ultrasound. Magnetic resonance imaging (MRI) is useful in assessing areas of concern or if implant rupture is suspected. Due to the obvious risk of puncture any biopsy to an augmented breast should be performed under image guidance.

## Breast augmentation complications

### Capsular contraction

Any foreign tissue placed within a body will produce a reaction or scar. The scarring around an implant produces a capsule, which contracts over time. Due to the relative inertness of silicone and the development of a textured surface around modern implants, such a reaction to a breast implant is usually only a problem after several years. It can be exacerbated by postoperative complications such as haematoma or a subclinical infection. Capsular contraction tends to produce pain, change in shape and hardness of the breast. A grading for capsular contraction is shown in Box 17.3. Treatment depends on severity

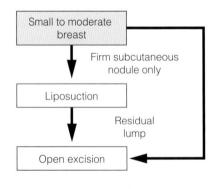
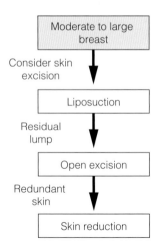

**Figure 17.6** • Algorithm for management of gynaecomastia.

Box 17.3 • Classification of capsular contraction

**Grade I (absent)**

The breast is soft with no palpable capsule and looks natural.

**Grade II (minimal)**

The breast is slightly firm, with a palpable capsule but looks normal.

**Grade III (moderate)**

The breast is firm with an easily palpable capsule and looks abnormal.

**Grade IV (severe)**

The breast is hard, cold, painful and distorted.

of symptoms and patient wishes. Removal plus capsulotomy or capsulectomy for rupture is the standard treatment with or without re-augmentation.

## Rippling/palpable implant edge

Due to the pressure effect of the implant on the breast tissue, some degree of glandular atrophy can occur. This can make the underlying implant more palpable, especially in the thin woman. Round, non-cohesive implants, due to their softness and fluid nature, can have a palpable 'rippling'. This is commonly felt superiorly when placed submammary in a thin woman or if there is marked ptosis. Rippling and sometimes the implant edge can be felt on the medial or lateral edges if there is a large implant or paucity of glandular cover. Treatment is reassurance and explanation or revision, placing the implant in the submuscular plane.

## Capsular rupture

Rupture is most commonly due to implant failure over time but may be caused by trauma or iatrogenic injury. Modern silicone breast implants tend to contain cohesive gel which tends not to have the frequency of rupture seen with liquid silicone implants.

Women with rupture present with pain, change in breast shape and usually a lump. Once identified, treatment is removal of implant plus capsule. Residual silicone can cause a reaction producing hard lumps (siliconomas).

## Breast reduction problems

### Fat necrosis

Scarring and fat necrosis can result from devascularisation of fatty breast tissue or following wound healing problems. This may not be noticed until some time has passed postsurgery. Triple assessment will rule out any malignancy and allow for reassurance.

### Inclusion cyst

An inclusion cyst occurs due to implantation of keratinising squamous epithelium within the dermis when an area of incomplete de-epithelialised skin (usually the pedicle for the nipple) is buried during a breast reduction operation. A discrete lump may be palpable or an impalpable lesion may be discovered at subsequent mammographic screening.

# Assessment of patients with benign breast disease

Commonly encountered questions include the following.

- Is a one-stop clinic the best method of diagnosing breast disease?
- Fine-needle aspiration cytology, core biopsy or both?
- Should benign breast disease become the remit of nurse specialists?

## One-stop clinics

The aim of the one-stop clinic is to provide the patient with all the relevant investigations and diagnosis at the initial visit. This requires the availability of a breast specialist, cytopathologist and breast radiologist to provide immediate interpretation of the examination and investigations. Even with all these available, a definitive diagnosis is not always possible.[91] There are benefits in reducing anxiety in such a service (*especially with benign disease*) but this benefit is only in the short term.[92] Patients like these clinics and they reduce the number of clinic visits and letters, improving administration efficiency. The increased cost of such a service, concerns that immediate reporting may affect accuracy and the possible detrimental psychological aspect for those with cancer[93] need to be considered. It is well recognised that at the time when a patient is given bad news, little else of the consultation is remembered. By concentrating on establishing and delivering a diagnosis at the first visit, it is then possible to have a more useful and constructive second visit when management can be considered. One-stop clinics are likely to continue as patients prefer them, but they may only be feasible in larger units where they are cost-efficient.

## Fine-needle aspiration cytology, core biopsy or both?

Fine-needle aspiration cytology was the mainstay of diagnosis of symptomatic breast lumps for more than 30 years. Its introduction allowed preoperative diagnosis and avoided a large number of open excision biopsies. It has the benefit of being easy to perform, causes little patient discomfort and has a high sensitivity and specificity (in experienced hands[94]). The result can be interpreted quickly, allowing rapid diagnosis. Its major disadvantage is that it does not provide architectural information on the area examined and therefore cannot differentiate in situ and invasive disease. It is possible to grade tumours[95] and provide estrogen receptor status[96] from cytology.

 Core biopsy has taken over as the preoperative technique of choice for diagnosing palpable breast lumps and areas of nodularity.[97] The improved sensitivity and specificity and greater information available (architecture, estrogen receptor and HER-2 status, grade, presence of vascular invasion or calcification) with core biopsy is the reason for this change.

The use of roll cytology, from cores, allows rapid initial diagnosis and adds the benefit of a subsequent histological assessment.[98]

There is increasing evidence that symptomatic lumps should be biopsied under ultrasound guidance.[99] This ensures that the actual lump is visualised with the biopsy needle within it, improving sensitivity. Suitably trained surgeons or breast physicians can undertake these biopsies, thus ensuring that radiologists are not inundated with further work.[100]

## Future management of benign breast disease

The last few years has seen the expansion of breast physicians, nurse specialists and the formation of nurse consultants. Their roles have expanded to help with the increasing breast workload and the lack of breast specialists. There is evidence that such professionals can help in symptomatic clinics, perform follow-up clinics and run symptom-specific clinics (e.g. mastalgia clinics) as long as there is specialist back-up.[101,102] The future roles of both these individuals and breast surgeons are likely to continue to evolve. The breast surgeons of the future may be less involved in diagnosis, and more active surgically.

## Key points

- The majority of patients seen in a breast clinic have benign disease or normal breasts.
- Many conditions occur so commonly against the background of breast development, cyclical activity and involution that they are best considered abberations of this process.
- Following a diagnosis of benign disease reassurance alone is insufficient. An explanation of the cause, possible risks and treatment options is required.
- Persistent (>2 per week) or bloodstained nipple discharge requires a definitive diagnosis which may only be obtained by duct excision.
- Breast pain is common and the majority is related to the chest wall.
- For true cyclical breast pain tamoxifen is effective.
- Breast cysts diagnosed on ultrasound require aspiration only if symptomatic or complex on scan.
- Breast infection requires early antibiotic therapy and rapid referral to hospital if it does not settle rapidly on antibiotics.
- Breast abscesses should be assessed by ultrasound and treated by aspiration or mini-incision and drainage.
- Gynaecomastia is an increasing problem. The cause should be ascertained and surgery only performed after other options have been exhausted.

# References

1. Thrush S, Sayer G, Scott-Coombes D et al. Is the grading of referrals to a specialist breast unit appropriate or effective? Br Med J 2002; 324:1279.

2. Down S, Barr L, Baildam AD et al. Management of accessory breast tissue in the axilla. Br J Surg 2003; 90:1213–14.

3. Nerakha GJ. In: Gallager HS, Leis HP, Synderman RK et al. (eds) The breast. St Louis, MO: Mosby, 1978; pp. 442–51.

4. Pinsolle V, Chichery A, Grolleau JL et al. Autologous fat injection in Poland's syndrome. J Plast Reconstr Aesthet Surg 2008 (Epub ahead of print).

5. Hughes LE, Mansel RE, Webster DJ. Aberrations of normal development and involution (ANDI): a new perspective on pathogenesis and nomenclature of benign breast disorders. Lancet 1987; ii:1316–19.

6. World Health Organisation. Histological typing of breast tumours, 2nd edn. Geneva: WHO, 1981.

7. Dixon JM, Dobie V, Lamb J et al. Assessment of the acceptability of conservative management of fibroadenoma of the breast. Br J Surg 1996; 83:264–5.

8. Hughes LE, Mansel RE, Webster DJT. Benign disorders of the breast. London: Bailliére Tindall, 2001.

9. Ozzello L, Gump FE. The management of patients with carcinomas in fibroadenomatous tumors of the breast. Surg Gynecol Obstet 1985; 116:99–104.

10. Sperber F, Blank A, Metser U et al. Diagnosis and treatment of breast fibroadenomas by ultrasound guided vacuum-assisted biopsy. Arch Surg 2003; 138:796–800.

11. Haagenson CD. Diseases of the breast, 3rd edn. Philidelphia: WB Saunders, 1986.

12. Dixon JM, Mansel RE. ABC of breast diseases: symptoms, assessment and guidelines for referral. Br Med J 1994; 309:722.

13. King EB, Chew KC, Petrakis NL et al. Nipple aspiration cytology for the study of pre-cancer precursors. J Natl Cancer Inst 1983; 71:1115–21.

14. Ambrogetti D, Berni D, Catarzi S et al. The role of ductal galactography in the differential diagnosis of breast carcinoma. Radiol Med 1996; 91:198–201.

15. Selzer MH, Perloff LJ, Kelley RI et al. Significance of age in patients with nipple discharge. Surg Gynecol Obstet 1970; 131:519.

16. Sandison AT. An autopsy of the human breast. National Cancer Institute Monograph No. 8. US Dept of Health, Education and Welfare, 1962, pp. 1–145.

17. Simmons R, Adamovich T, Brennan M et al. Nonsurgical evaluation of pathologic nipple discharge. Ann Surg Oncol 2003; 10:113–16.

18. Groves AM, Carr M, Wadhera V et al. An audit of cytology in the evaluation of nipple discharge: a retrospective study of 10 years' experience. Breast 1996; 5:96.

19. Dooley WS. Routine operative breast endoscopy for bloody nipple discharge. Ann Surg Oncol 2002; 9:920–3.

20. Matsunaga T, Ohta D, Misaka T et al. A utility of ductography and fibreoptic ductoscopy for patients with nipple discharge. Breast Cancer Res Treat 2001; 70:103–8.

21. Shen KW, Wu J, Lu JS et al. Fiberoptic ductoscopy for breast cancer patients with nipple discharge. Surg Endosc 2001; 15:1340–5.

22. King BL, Love SM, Rochman S et al. The Fourth International Symposium on the Intraductal Approach to Breast Cancer, Santa Barbara, California, 10–13 March 2005. Breast Cancer Res 2005; 7(5):198–204.

23. Ambrogetti D, Berni D, Catarzi S et al. The role of ductal galactography in the differential diagnosis of breast carcinoma. Radiol Med (Torino) 1996; 91:198.

24. Khan SA, Baird C, Staradub VL et al. Ductal lavage and ductoscopy: the opportunities and the limitations. Clin Breast Cancer 2002; 3:185–95.

25. Van Zee KJ, Ortega Perez G, Minnard E et al. Preoperative galactography increases the diagnostic yield of major duct excision for nipple discharge. Cancer 1998; 82:1874.

26. Pisano ED, Gatsonis C, Hendrick E et al. The Digital Mammographic Imaging Screening Trial (DMIST) Investigators Group. Diagnostic performance of digital versus film mammography for breast-cancer. N Engl J Med 2005; 353(17):1773–83.

27. Cabioglu N, Hunt KK, Singletary SE et al. Surgical decision making and factors determining a diagnosis of breast cancer in women presenting with nipple discharge. J Am Coll Surg 2003; 196:354–64.

28. Helbich TH, Matzek W, Fuchsjager MH. Stereotactic and ultrasound-guided breast biopsy. Eur Radiol 2004; 14:383–93.

29. Van Zee KJ, Ortega Perez G, Minnard E et al. Preoperative galactography increases the diagnostic yield of major duct excision for nipple discharge. Cancer 1998; 82:1874–80.

30. Rosen PP, Cantrell B, Mullen DL et al. Juvenile papillomatosis (Swiss cheese disease) of the breast. Am J Surg Pathol 1980; 4:3–12.

31. Lafreniere R. Bloody nipple discharge during pregnancy: a rationale for conservative treatment. J Surg Oncol 1990; 43:228–30.

32. Sharma R, Dietz J, Wright H et al. Comparative analysis of minimally invasive microductectomy versus major duct excision in patients with pathologic nipple discharge. Surgery 2005; 138(4):591–6; discussion 596–7.

33. Dixon JM, Kohlhardt SR, Dillon P. Total duct excision. Breast 1998; 7:216–19.

34. Peters F, Pickardt CR, Zimmerman G et al. TSH and thyroid hormones in benign breast disease. Klin Wochenschr 1981; 59:403–7.

35. England PC, Skinner LG, Cotterell KM et al. Serum oestradiol-17β in women with benign and malignant breast disease. Br J Cancer 1974; 30:571–6.

36. Sitruk-Ware R, Sterkers N, Mauvais-Jarvis P. Benign breast disease. 1. Hormonal investigation. Obstet Gynecol 1979; 53:457–60.

37. Gateley CA, Maddox PR, Pritchard GA et al. Plasma fatty acid profiles in benign breast disorders. Br J Surg 1992; 79:407–9.

38. Mansel RE. ABC of breast diseases: breast pain. Br Med J 1994; 309:866–8.

39. Barros AC, Mottola J, Ruiz CA et al. Reassurance in the treatment of mastalgia. Breast J 1999; 5:162–5.

40. Khoo SK, Munro C, Battistutta D. Evening primrose oil and treatment of premenstrual syndrome. Med J Aust 1990; 153:189–92.

41. Blommers J, de Lange-De Klerk ES, Kuik DJ et al. Evening primrose oil and fish oil for severe chronic mastalgia: a randomised, double blind controlled trial. Am J Obstet Gynecol 2002; 187:1389–94.

42. Pashby NH, Mansel RE, Hughes LE et al. A clinical trial of evening primrose oil in mastalgia. Br J Surg 1981; 68:801–24.

43. McFayden IJ, Chetty U, Setchell KDR et al. A randomized double blind crossover trial of soya protein for the treatment of cyclical breast pain. Breast 2000; 9:271–6.

44. Halaska M, Raus K, Beles P et al. Treatment of cyclical mastodynia using an extract of Vitex agnus castus: results of a double blind comparison with a placebo. Ceska Gynecol 1998; 63:388–92.

45. Boyd NF, McGuire V, Shannon P et al. Effect of a low-fat high-carbohydrate diet on symptoms of clinical mastopathy. Lancet 1988; ii:128–32.

46. Fentiman IS, Caleffi M, Brame K et al. Double blind controlled trial of tamoxifen therapy for mastalgia. Lancet 1986; i:287–8.

47. GEMB Group Argentine. Tamoxifen therapy for cyclical mastalgia: dose randomised trial. Breast 1997; 5:212–13.

48. Kontostolis E, Stefanidis K, Navrozoglou I et al. Comparison of tamoxifen with danazol for treatment of cyclical mastalgia. Gynecol Endocrinol 1997; 11:393–7.

49. O'Brien PM, Abukhalil IE. Randomised controlled trial of the management of premenstrual syndrome and premenstrual mastalgia using luteal phase-only danazol. Am J Obstet Gynecol 1999; 180:18–23.

50. Mansel R, Goyal A, Le Nestour E et al. and Afimoxifene (4-OHT) Breast Pain Research Group. A phase II trial of Afimoxifene (4-hydroxytamoxifen gel) for cyclical mastalgia in premenopausal women. Breast Cancer Res Treat 2007; 106(3):389–97.

51. Gong C, Song E, Jia W et al. A double-blind randomized controlled trial of toremifen therapy for mastalgia. Arch Surg 2006; 141(1):43–7.

52. Blichert-Toft M, Anderson AN, Henrikson D et al. Treatment of mastalgia with bromocriptine: a double blind crossover study. Br Med J 1979; 1:273.

53. Eriksson E. Serotonin reuptake inhibitors for the treatment of premenstrual dysphoria. Int Clin Psychopharmacol 1999; 14(Suppl 2):S27–33.

54. Dixon JM, McDonald C, Elton RA et al. Risk of breast cancer in women with palpable breast cysts. Lancet 1999; 353:1742–5.

55. Jacobs TW, Byrne C, Colditz G et al. Radial scars in benign breast-biopsy specimens and the risk of breast cancer. N Engl J Med 1999; 340(6):430–6.

56. Brenner RJ, Jackman RJ, Parker SH et al. Percutaneous core needle biopsy of radial scars of the breast: when is excision necessary? Am J Roentgenol 2002; 179(5):1179–84.

57. Kudva YC, Reynolds CA, O'Brien T et al. Mastopathy and diabetes. Curr Diabetes Rep 2003; 3:56–9.

58. Thrush S, Banerjee S, Sayer G et al. Breast sepsis: a unit's experience. Br J Surg 2002; 89(Suppl 1):75–6.

59. Goodman MA, Benson EA. An evaluation of the current trends in the management of breast abscesses. Med J Aust 1970; 1:1034–9.

60. Schafer P, Furrer C, Merillod B. An association between smoking with recurrent subareolar breast abscess. Int J Epidemiol 1988; 17:810–13.

61. Petrakis NL, Maack CA, Lee RE et al. Mutagenic activity of nipple aspirates of breast fluid. Cancer Res 1980; 40:188–9.

62. Ertel A, Eng R, Smith SM. The differential effect of cigarette smoke on the growth of bacteria found in humans. Chest 1991; 100:628–30.

63. Rogers K. Breast abscess and problems with lactation. In: Smallwood JA, Talor I (eds) Benign breast disease. London: Edward Arnold, 1990; p. 96.

64. Gupta R, Sinnett D, Carpenter R et al. Antibiotic prophylaxis for post-operative wound infection in elective breast surgery. Eur J Surg Oncol 2000; 26:363–6.

65. Collis N, Mirza S, Stanley PR et al. Reduction of potential contamination of breast implants by the use of 'nipple shields'. Br J Plast Surg 1999; 52:445–7.

66. Zippel D, Siegelmann-Danieli N, Ayalon S et al. Delayed breast cellulitis following breast conservation operations. Eur J Surg Oncol 2003; 29:327–30.

67. Nahabedian MY, Tsangaris T, Momen B et al. Infectious complications following breast reconstruction with expanders and implants. Plast Reconstr Surg 2003; 112:467–76.

68. Hayes R, Mitchell M, Nunnerley HB. Acute inflammation of the breast: the role of breast ultrasound in diagnosis and management. Clin Radiol 1991; 44:253–6.

69. Dixon JM. Repeated aspiration of breast abscesses in lactating women. Br Med J 1988; 297:1517–18.

70. O'Hara RJ, Dexter SPL, Fox JN. Conservative management of infective mastitis and breast abscesses after ultrasonographic assessment. Br J Surg 1996; 83:1413–14.

71. Dixon JM. Outpatient treatment of non-lactational breast abscesses. Br J Surg 1992; 79:56–7.

72. Dixon JM (ed.). ABC of breast. London: BMJ Publications, 2000.

73. Bundred NJ, Dixon JM, Chetty U et al. Mammary fistula. Br J Surg 1991; 78:1185.

74. Hanavadi S, Pereira G, Mansel RE. How mammillary fistulas should be managed. Breast J 2005; 11(4):254–6.

75. Thomsen AC, Espersen T, Maigaard S. Course and treatment of milk stasis, non-infectious inflammation of the breast and infectious mastitis in nursing women. Am J Obstet Gynecol 1984; 149:492–5.

76. Anonymous. Puerperal mastitis. Br Med J 1991; 302:1367–71.

77. Howell JD, Barker F, Gazet J-C. Granulomatous lobular mastitis: report of further two cases and comprehensive literature review. Breast 1994; 3:119–23.

78. Paviour S, Musaad S, Roberts S et al. *Corynebacterium* species isolated from patients with mastitis. Clin Infect Dis 2002; 35:1434–40.

79. Taylor GB, Paviour SD, Musaad S et al. A clinico-pathological review of 34 cases of inflammatory breast disease showing an association between corynebacteria infection and granulomatous mastitis. Pathology 2003; 35:109–19.

80. Blanchard DK, Reynolds CA, Grant CS et al. Primary nonphylloides breast sarcomas. Am J Surg 2003; 186.359 61.

81. Daniels IR, Layer GT. How should gynaecomastia be managed? Aust NZ J Surg 2003; 73:213–16.

82. Carlson HE. Gynecomastia. N Engl J Med 1980; 303:795–9.

83. Ismail AA, Barth JH. Endocrinology of gynaecomastia. Ann Clin Biochem 2001; 38:596–607.

84. Simon BE, Hoffman S, Kahn S. Classification and surgical correction of gynecomastia. Plast Reconstr Surg 1973; 51:48–52.

85. Jones DJ, Holt SD, Surtees P et al. A comparison of danazol and placebo in the treatment of adult idiopathic gynecomastia: results of a prospective study in 55 patients. Ann R Coll Surg Engl 1990; 72:296–8.

86. Khan HN, Blamey RW. Endocrine treatment of physiological gynaecomastia. Br Med J 2003; 327:301–2.

87. Plourde PV, Kulin HE, Santner SJ. Clomiphene in the treatment of adolescent gynecomastia. Clinical and endocrine studies. Am J Dis Child 1983; 137:1080–2.

88. Wray RC Jr, Hoopes JE, Davis GM. Correction of extreme gynaecomastia. Br J Plast Surg 1974; 27:39–41.

89. Samdal F, Kleppe G, Amland PF et al. Surgical treatment of gynaecomastia. Five years' experience with liposuction. Scand J Plast Reconstr Surg Hand Surg 1994; 28:123–30.

90. Fruhstorfer BH, Malata CM. A systematic approach to the surgical treatment of gynaecomastia. Br J Plast Surg 2003; 56:237–46.

91. Eltahir A, Jibril JA, Squair J et al. The accuracy of 'one stop' diagnosis for 1110 patients presenting to a symptomatic breast clinic. J R Coll Surg Edinb 1999; 44:226–30.

92. Dey P, Bundred N, Gibbs A et al. Costs and benefits of a one stop clinic compared with a dedicated breast clinic: randomised controlled trial. Br Med J 2002; 324:507–10.

93. Harcourt D, Ambler N, Rumsey N et al. Evaluation of a one-stop breast clinic: a randomised controlled trial. Breast 1998; 7:314–19.

94. Dixon JM, Lamb J, Anderson TJ. Fine needle aspiration of the breast: importance of the operator. Lancet 1983; ii:564.

95. Robinson IA, McKee G, Nicholson A et al. Prognostic value of cytological grading of fine-needle aspirates from breast carcinomas. Lancet 1994; 343:947–9.

96. Zoppi JA, Rotundo AV, Sundblad AS. Correlation of immunocytochemical and immunohistochemical determination of estrogen and progesterone receptors in breast cancer. Acta Cytol 2002; 46:337–40.

97. Britton PD. Fine needle aspiration or core biopsy? Breast 1999; 8:1–4.

98. Albert US, Duda V, Hadji P et al. Imprint cytology of core needle biopsy specimens of breast lesions. A rapid approach to detecting malignancies, with comparison of cytologic and histopathologic analyses of 173 cases. Acta Cytol 2000; 44:57–62.

99. Hatada T, Ishii H, Ichii S et al. Diagnostic value of ultrasound-guided fine needle aspiration biopsy, core needle biopsy, and evaluation of combined use in the diagnosis of breast lumps. J Am Coll Surg 2000; 190:299–303.

100. Whitehouse PA, Baber Y, Brown G et al. The use of ultrasound by breast surgeons in outpatients: an accurate extension of clinical diagnosis. Eur J Surg Oncol 2001; 27:611–16.

101. Garvican L, Grimsey E, Littlejohns P et al. Satisfaction with clinical nurse specialists in a breast care clinic: questionnaire survey. Br Med J 1998; 316:976–7.

102. Earnshaw JJ, Stephenson Y. First two years of a follow-up breast clinic led by a nurse practitioner. J R Soc Med 1997; 90:258–9.

# 18

# Litigation in breast surgery

Tim Davidson
Tom Bates

## Introduction

Litigation in breast disease has accelerated at an alarming rate. In the USA, the value of malpractice claims for delay in the diagnosis of breast cancer is now second only to that for neurological damage to neonates.[1,2] Poor cosmetic outcome is also a frequent cause for litigation and heightened public awareness has increased patients' expectations of recompense for real or perceived injury.

Doctors have been made increasingly aware of the need to warn patients of the risks involved with any procedure, be it diagnostic or therapeutic, to involve patients in decision-making, and to seek fully informed consent. Patient information leaflets, involvement of breast-care nurses and more detailed consent forms signed by the operating surgeon are now standard practice but have done little to stem the tide of litigation as expectations continue to rise.

## Basic principles

The legal process differs between countries and although the present account is based on civil law in England and Wales, the general principles in use elsewhere are similar.[3] For a claimant to succeed in law, she must satisfy the court (in the UK a judge, or in some countries a jury) that there was a failure or breach of duty of care (*liability*) and that as a foreseeable result she suffered an injury (*causation*). For the case to succeed, the court must find in favour of the claimant with regard to both liability and causation. Negligence cases are heard in civil court and the judge determines on the balance of probabilities whether the defendant is liable. This is entirely different from a criminal court determining guilt or innocence where the level of proof is beyond all reasonable doubt (which many equate to a degree of confidence >95%). If the court finds in favour of the claimant, the court awards financial recompense to redress, as far as money is able, the injury that she has suffered.

## The award of damages

The sole remedy available to the successful claimant is an award of damages – a sum of money intended to restore the claimant to the position she would have been in but for the negligent act. Explanation and apology to the claimant or her family, desirable though they may be, are not within the power of civil law, nor are recommendations for retraining, suspension or deregistration of doctors who find themselves as defendants.

The award comprises two components, general and special damages. General damages compensate for pain, suffering and loss of amenity, and are based upon judicial guidelines that are upgraded regularly to allow for inflation. Special damages are specific to the individual claimant and include past losses, which can be identified with some accuracy, and future losses, which can only be estimated. It is the future loss of earnings and the costs of providing care for the claimant and/or dependants that generate very high claims. A young woman with children and a high income will attract a high value award if she (or her surviving family) can demonstrate that her premature death resulted from lack of care.

In English law the magnitude or perceived culpability of the negligent act has no bearing on the sum awarded. This contrasts with the position in the USA, where cases that proceed to trial (the minority) rely on jury decisions which often incorporate an element of punitive or exemplary damages, a sum the jury considers warranted by the wrongfulness of the defendant's act. The extent to which this affects the size of the award can be seen by comparing the average value of claims concluded by settlement ($282 000) with that secured by jury verdict ($870 000).[2]

## Breach of duty

### Duty of care

Any doctor – GP, radiologist, surgeon or pathologist – owes each individual patient a duty of care. This is rarely an issue. In the NHS the doctor acts as a servant of the hospital trust or community health authority which is covered by the NHS Litigation Authority which administers a scheme that acts as a mutual insurer for participating trusts (Clinical Negligence Scheme for Trusts).[4] When acting in a private capacity, the doctor is covered by a professional defence organisation of his or her choice.

### The Bolam test

A doctor is not negligent if he or she acts in accordance with a practice accepted at the time as proper by a responsible body of medical opinion. The Bolam test arises from the case of a patient who received electroconvulsive therapy and sustained fractures.[5] Negligence was alleged because the patient was not given muscle relaxants and was inadequately restrained. Some doctors would have used muscle relaxants and restraints, others not. The doctor was not found negligent because he acted in accordance with a practice accepted at the time, even though other doctors may have advocated a different practice.

The Bolam test requires a higher degree of skill from a specialist in his or her own field than from a

GP. If a patient is referred to a breast surgeon and the standard of care falls below that which the patient could reasonably have expected from a breast specialist, there has been a breach of the duty of care. The Bolitho modification of Bolam adds the requirement that for the practice or opinion formed to be acceptable, it must be based on logical argument; an irrational practice cannot be argued as acceptable in court simply because a body of medical opinion agrees with its use.[6]

### Guidelines

National and local guidelines of good clinical practice are now in use throughout the NHS and breast practice has been in the vanguard, with guidelines covering patient referral, diagnosis, treatment and organisational arrangements within breast units.[7–9] Breaches of guidelines are not indicative of, or equivalent to, negligent practice and guidelines are constantly being amended in the light of scientific knowledge, healthcare resources, government targets, etc. Consideration must always be given to the time at which the alleged breach of duty took place and for a guideline to be relevant it must have been in the public domain at the time.

Clinical practice that complies with guidelines is inevitably much easier to defend against allegations of negligence. A diagnostic excision biopsy exceeding 20 g, the current NHS Breast Screening Programme (BSP) guideline, does not equate to negligent practice; however, a patient claiming excessive deformity after such a procedure is unlikely to succeed in litigation if her biopsy specimen weighed under 20 g. There is ongoing debate regarding the medico-legal implications of surgical guidelines.[10] Carrick et al.[11] reported that whereas 41% of surgeons surveyed believed that guidelines would protect them against litigation, 37% believed that they would increase their exposure to claims.

### Consent

Great emphasis is now placed on warning patients of the risks of any proposed management. Consent obtained by a junior doctor without the knowledge and skill to undertake the intended procedure or to discuss the possible complications and alternatives is no longer considered acceptable. The degree of disclosure is primarily a matter of clinical judgement, but catastrophic complications (such as loss of a flap in breast reconstruction) must be included even if their occurrence is rare.[3] Where a procedure (such as breast reduction) is being undertaken primarily for cosmetic reasons, the surgeon is advised to include even minor potential consequences in the documentation of informed consent.

## Causation

The second hurdle to be overcome by the claimant is to prove that the negligent act caused an injury which was forseeable. Causation may be obvious where there is a poor cosmetic outcome from breast reduction, but may be difficult to prove where there has been a delay in the diagnosis of breast cancer.

### Did the delay necessitate more radical treatment?

Where the patient has had a mastectomy on the basis of tumour size, it is often plausible to suggest that earlier diagnosis would have made breast conservative surgery an option. For multifocal tumours, it can be argued that mastectomy would have been needed from the outset. When the patient has received chemotherapy it is sometimes argued that this would not have been necessary if the diagnosis had been made sooner when, for example, the axillary nodes would probably have been negative. However, this line of argument is open to counterattack on the basis that failure to give chemotherapy would have omitted a treatment likely to have made a difference to prognosis.

### Did the delay in diagnosis reduce the chance of cure?

This is a controversial area since there is public expectation, promoted over the years by health campaigners, that earlier diagnosis offers better chance of a cure. Where expert opinion is divided, the court often prefers the evidence in favour of delay having caused a reduced survival time.

### The burden (level) of proof

In civil litigation the court determines the facts, which means that the judge makes a decision *on the balance of probabilities*. This means that the successful claimant will normally recover damages in full, although in one case where the claimant was held to have lost an 80% chance of cure, a deputy high court judge directed that damages should be calculated accordingly.[12,13]

The all-or-none nature in awarding damages is arguably the most troubling aspect for experts involved in clinical negligence. For example, if the court finds that as a result of negligence a woman has suffered a reduction in her chance of survival from 60% to 40%, she will be awarded the full amount to compensate her (or her family) as though the loss had definitely occurred on the basis that *on balance* she is now more likely to die. If the court finds, however, that her chance of survival is reduced from 90% to 60%, it may award her nothing on the basis that *on balance* her chance of survival remains unchanged.

In the case of *Hotson* v. *East Berkshire Area Health Authority* (1987), the House of Lords formulated the current UK position on causation. The defendant was in breach of duty in failing to diagnose a fracture of a femoral epiphysis following a fall. The child developed avascular necrosis with significant disability. The evidence was that the child had a 75% risk of developing this complication due to the accident and the trial judge and the Court of Appeal held that he was entitled to 25% of his damages for the 25% loss of a chance that prompt treatment might have prevented the complication. However, the House of Lords overturned the decision and held that on balance of probabilities he was going to develop it even in the absence of negligence or, put another way, he had failed to establish that he was within the 25% who would not develop it.

The inherent unfairness was again recognised in the case of *Gregg* v. *Scott* (2002), a claim for failure to diagnose an axillary lump as non-Hodgkin's lymphoma. The Court of Appeal held that the delay had reduced his chance of survival, although this had always been less than 50%, from 42% to 25% survival at 10 years. The case was appealed to the House of Lords who dismissed the claimant's appeal for loss of a chance and upheld the traditional approach. So the burden of proof in deciding causation, for the time being at least, remains unchanged.

## Delay in the diagnosis of breast cancer

Delay in diagnosis may occur as a result of failure to refer the patient from primary care, false-negative mammography, failure to perform triple assessment, misinterpretation of fine-needle aspiration cytology (FNAC) or the misfiling of a positive test result. There are three phases, where the major responsibility often rests with the patient herself, with the referring GP or with the breast specialist in the clinic.[14,15]

## Phase 1: patient delay

When a woman first becomes aware of a breast cancer, she may delay seeking advice for fear of the diagnosis or the treatment. She may be over-optimistic about the likely diagnosis or she may deny the possibility that she has cancer. Delay is longer on average in disadvantaged populations and at the extremes of age, but the absence of a palpable lump may also falsely reassure a woman that her symptoms are not serious.

## Phase 2: delay in primary care

The GP who sees many cases of symptomatic breast disease each year but only one or two breast cancers is in an increasingly difficult position and GPs are increasingly facing litigation for delays in referral. Relying on a negative mammogram without an expert clinical examination or needle biopsy to complete a triple assessment may increase the risk of false reassurance. The GP is therefore faced with referring most women with breast symptoms for a specialist opinion and referral guidelines have been in use since 1995.[16,17]

## Phase 3: after specialist referral

Breast units throughout the UK submit audit data on compliance with 2-week *target referrals* for suspected cancer and these data are now in the public domain.[18] However, the prioritisation of referral letters is counter-productive if non-urgent cases have to wait longer, with about 25% of breast cancers still to be found in non-urgent referrals. NHS '31/62' cancer targets (allowing 31 days from urgent referral to diagnosis and 62 days to commencing treatment) will identify units where delays in this phase breach national guidelines.

The role of triple assessment, and the circumstances in which it fails, are critical to this phase. The specialist centre is also faced with the problem that women under 35 form the majority of the diagnostic workload (66%) but the fewest number of breast cancers (3%).[19]

## The North American experience

Two studies commissioned by the Physician Insurers Association of America (PIAA)[1,2] showed delay in the diagnosis of breast cancer to be the commonest cause of clinical litigation in the USA, and a striking feature of both studies was young age: women under 50 accounted for 69% of claimants and received 84% of the damages paid, whereas only 25% of cancers occur in women under 50.[20]

The most common reasons cited for the delay were (in descending order):

- physical findings failed to impress;
- failure to follow up the patient;
- negative mammogram report or misreading of the mammogram;
- failure to perform a biopsy.

False-negative or equivocal mammography, whether symptomatic or screening, was cited in 80% of cases and, not surprisingly, radiologists were the most frequent defendants. Radiologists are particularly at risk when the patient refers herself, since triple assessment may be incomplete because of lack of a clinical examination.

In 487 cases where liability was admitted, the mean delay was 14 months. The mean payout for all delays was $301 000, with higher damages for longer delays and to younger patients.[2] There are now statistical models for predicting the size of damages,[21] particularly when the patient has young children and the economic consequences of a reduced lifespan are more relevant.

# Diagnosis of breast cancer

Triple assessment is the foundation upon which clinicians diagnose breast lumps. However, the extent to which the accuracy of these tests is reduced in younger women is not well appreciated (**Fig. 18.1**). It has been suggested that perfection of diagnosis will require removal of every solid mass,[22] but this would represent a retrograde step. The practice of defensive medicine, in place of conventional wisdom, will certainly be encouraged by a litigious public and diagnostic tests whose sensitivity falls below 95%.

## Physical examination

About 70% of all breast cancers are palpable, but with tumours 0.6–1 cm diameter this figure falls

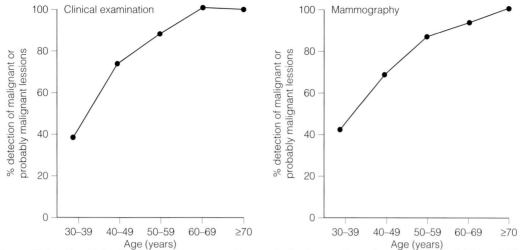

**Figure 18.1** • Sensitivity of clinical and mammographic examination by age. Reproduced from Dixon JM, Mansel RE. Symptoms, assessment and guidelines for referral. In: Dixon JM (ed.) ABC of breast diseases, 2nd edn. London: BMJ Books, 2000; p. 6. With permission from Wiley Publishing Ltd.

to 50%.[23] The larger the breast and the greater the density of breast tissue, the more difficult physical examination becomes. Cyclical changes in breast parenchyma may require repeat examination at different phases of the menstrual cycle. Coexisting benign lumps, scars and distortion from previous surgery, the ridge of tissue above the inframammary fold and the underlying ribs all add to the uncertainty of clinical examination. Changes during pregnancy and lactation may be a pitfall for the obstetrician who wishes to reassure an anxious patient. Other difficulties include: inflammatory cancers masquerading as infection; the presence of implants with an associated fibrous capsule; and the effect of hormone replacement therapy (HRT), which increases the density of breast parenchyma both clinically and radiologically.

The sensitivity of clinical examination in women aged 30–39 can be as low as 25%.[24] A sensitivity of 90% can only be expected in older women, when the atrophic nature of the breast parenchyma and the low incidence of benign disease combine to make clinical diagnosis a relatively simple task. The low sensitivity of clinical examination, coupled with the low incidence of breast cancer and the considerable numbers of young women attending breast clinics, must largely explain why failure of physical findings to impress the clinician was one of the most common reasons for delay in diagnosis in the PIAA study.[2]

## Mammography

False-negative mammography is one of the principal reasons for delay in diagnosis of breast cancer,[1,2,25,26] since it gives the clinician and patient false reassurance. Age is an important factor in false-negative reporting (Fig. 18.1) since the radiographic density in young women makes tumour detection more difficult.

The Health Insurance Plan Project estimated that the mean time by which the diagnosis of breast cancer can be advanced by screening (lead time) is 1.7 years;[27] other estimates vary from 0.4 to 3.0 years.[28] It is therefore probable that up to 25% of interval cancers were in fact present at the time of the initial mammogram.[29] Interval cancers are more often node positive but this may be due to length bias, with cancers detected between screens more aggressive than prevalent cancers detected at the initial screen. The number of cancers missed by the initial screen is inversely proportional to age: 36% of cancers in women aged 40 compared with just 9% in those aged 75.[20]

## Ultrasound

The use of ultrasound to augment mammography has expanded since the mid-1990s (see Chapter 1). It is now an integral part of breast imaging to perform ultrasound in a patient of any age with a lump, especially when an abnormality is not detectable on clinical or mammographic examination. There is a trend for ultrasound-guided core biopsy to replace FNAC, although both techniques are currently acceptable. The expertise required for ultrasound examination and the use of guided core biopsy have placed breast imaging outside the competency of the general radiologist. The breast surgeon using ultrasound in the clinic may be similarly compromised unless training in the technique can be verified.

## Fine-needle aspiration cytology

For many years FNAC has allowed cost-effective tissue diagnosis of a palpable lump without the need for open biopsy. How much reliance can one place in FNAC? Dixon et al.[24] reported that the sensitivity of FNAC could be increased from 66% to 99% by restricting the biopsy to one aspirator. In comparison, the sensitivity of FNAC in women under 36 was as low as 78%,[22] though Dixon et al.[24] found that accuracy was not related to age if inadequate samples were excluded from the calculations.

In a review of 112 reports of FNAC of breast masses by Layfield et al.,[30] the overall accuracy was over 95% but concern was raised over the range of false-negative and false-positive reporting (1–35% and up to 18% respectively) and of unsatisfactory specimens (1–68%). Despite the introduction of FNAC, delay in diagnosis of greater than 50 days still occurred, and 85% of such delays were in women under 55[31] and with smaller tumours.[32] In small tumours, a sampling error is probably more common than misinterpretation of the cytology and ultrasound-guided core biopsy is advisable.

## Efficacy of triple assessment

If it is assumed that breast cancer detection by clinical examination, imaging and FNAC are independent of each other, it is possible to calculate the theoretical rate at which all three tests will give a false-negative result. The false-negative rates of the three investigations have been multiplied and expressed as a percentage in Table 18.1. It is probable that the sensitivities of these tests are not totally independent of each other, and therefore the predicted rate that all three tests will be false negative for an individual is a conservative estimate. For a woman under 35 with breast cancer, there may be a 12% chance that all three tests will give a false-negative result. If generally accepted optimal sensitivities are taken, the chance that all three tests will produce a false-negative result falls to approximately 1 in 1000 patients with these data skewed towards the older age groups; the likely overall rate of false-negative triple assessment in the clinic is between 1.4%[33] and 4%.[32]

## Cancer control window

The theory that early detection of a tumour will lead to cure depends on the concept that at the time of earlier treatment the tumour has not metastasised. The period of time between the earliest possible detection of the cancer and the time at which the tumour metastasises has been described as the cancer control window.[34] If the tumour has already metastasised by the time it reaches the threshold size for detection, there is no window and only effective systemic therapy might cure the patient.

Table 18.1 • False-negative rates of triple assessment for women under 35 compared with the generally quoted results[19,20,31]

| | False-negative rate | |
| --- | --- | --- |
| | Women <35 years | Optimal |
| Clinical examination | 0.75 | 0.12 |
| Mammography | 0.75 | 0.12 |
| Fine-needle cytology | 0.22 | 0.05 |
| All three false negative | 12.3% | 0.072% |

## Tumour doubling time

The usual threshold diameter for detection of a breast cancer by physical examination is 1 cm; such a tumour consists of $10^9$ cells and is the result of 30 doublings. It is possible for mammography to detect tumours as small as 2 mm, which equates to a tumour of $10^7$ cells and about 23 doublings.

Assuming a constant doubling time, early detection of breast cancer is a misnomer, since at least two-thirds of the biological life of the tumour will have been completed at the time of detection.[35] In medico-legal terms, if the alleged delay in diagnosis was 14 months for a cancer with a doubling time of 90 days, such a delay would equate to the number of cells increasing by one order of magnitude (i.e. from $10^9$ to $10^{10}$ cells). This represents a major increase in tumour load but is a very short period in the lifespan of the tumour and it is difficult to be sure that this period of delay would have a significant effect. In civil law, however, the court wants to know whether such an effect is more likely than not to alter the patient's prognosis or treatment. It is generally held by the claimant and her legal advice that delay in treatment is the cause of metastasis rather than the inherent biology of the tumour itself.

Lymph node status is the most important prognostic indicator at the time of surgical excision. Tubiana and Koscielny[36] suggested that breast cancer represents a continuum from slow-growing tumours with late axillary involvement and distant dissemination to the most aggressive, rapidly growing and early metastasising subtype. Assuming the growth rate of the nodal metastasis approximates to that of the primary tumour, it is possible to estimate the theoretical time at which the tumour must have metastasised, and not infrequently this would have occurred before the threshold size for detection of the primary tumour.[35]

As with other cancers, it is generally accepted that breast cancer begins as a single cell or a small group of cells that exhibit an exponential growth pattern. The time taken for a tumour to double in *volume* is known as the doubling time. Doubling times for breast cancers have been estimated by measuring the size of mastectomy scar recurrences[37] and also by serial mammographic evaluation.[38]

Pearlman[37] categorised patients as having fast- (<25 days), intermediate- (26–75 days) and slow-growing (>76 days) tumours based on measurement of tumour doubling time; 5-year survival rates were 5%, 62% and 100% respectively. Although lymph node metastases are more commonly found in fast-growing tumours, it would be wrong to assume that the survival of patients was entirely a consequence of tumour doubling time. Galante et al.[38] emphasised the importance of the metastatic potential of the tumour, suggesting that within fast-, intermediate- and slow-growing tumours there may be subsets with high and low metastasising potential.

# Vignettes on breach of duty

The following vignettes illustrate areas of breach of duty that have arisen in medico-legal breast cases and the comments following each vignette raise issues which would be discussed in conference with counsel.

## Vignette 1: Radiological delay in diagnosis

A woman aged 54 years attended for the second round of breast screening and was found to have an opacity on mammography that proved malignant. She asked to see the previous films taken 3 years earlier. When these were produced it was evident to her experts that the cancer had been present 3 years previously.

### Comments

- One-quarter of screen-detected cancers are apparent with hindsight 3 years earlier on mammograms and, very occasionally, 6 years earlier.
- Such a 'missed diagnosis' may be obvious to a radiologist with knowledge of the outcome but if the mammograms are interspersed with normal films, as in the screening situation, more often than not they will be passed as normal. However, when the expert radiologist's opinion is that any competent breast radiologist working to an acceptable standard should have reported the abnormality, liability has to be admitted.
- Radiologists in the NHS BSP who have a high detection rate (sensitivity) for breast cancer may also have a high recall rate (low specificity). Conversely, radiologists with a lower detection rate may recall fewer patients unnecessarily.
- The net result of the increasing medico-legal threat to breast radiologists has been an increase in recall and biopsy rates.[39]

## Vignette 2: False-positive cytology, lymphoedema and alteration of records

A 60-year-old patient was referred to a breast clinic with a clinically suspicious breast lump. Mammography was suspicious (R4) and FNAC was malignant (C5). The patient underwent wide local excision and axillary clearance for what subsequently proved to be a histologically benign condition. She complained of a poor cosmetic outcome and a painful swollen arm which she had not been warned about. The nursing records stated 'patient was warned of the risk of lymphoedema'.

### Comments

- A false-positive cytology result is a rare but potentially devastating event. From a medico-legal standpoint, an external expert review of the cytology should be the first step. If experts are agreed that the cytologist acted reasonably in reporting the slides as malignant, attention will then focus on the surgeon.
- The surgeon has to be aware that a false-positive cytology can occur and for this reason most surgeons will not carry out mastectomy without histological confirmation from a core biopsy. Histology is mandatory in the absence of a fully concordant malignant triple assessment and should have been obtained in this case. Axillary clearance for a benign condition is a potentially significant injury and it is unfortunate that this patient developed lymphoedema.
- The tense of the warning suggested to the judge that this was a retrospective note. Judges place most credence on handwritten contemporaneous records and alterations to the notes are often quite obvious. Any addition to the notes must be clearly identified as such by signing and dating the record and any temptation to alter the record after the event must be firmly resisted.

## Vignette 3: Failure of preoperative assessment and postoperative management

A 65-year-old woman presented with a small but obvious carcinoma in the tail of the breast. The surgeon performed FNAC, which showed malignant

cells (C5), and he carried out wide local excision of the tumour without preliminary breast imaging and without performing axillary staging. The tumour was grade 2 but the resection margins and the presence of vascular invasion were not reported. The patient was started on tamoxifen but was not referred for consideration of radiotherapy.

### Comments

- The management of this patient falls short of an acceptable standard in a number of respects (breach of duty), but until such time as she develops evidence of recurrence, which may never occur, any harm (causation) remains potential.
- A preoperative mammogram might have shown widespread microcalcification or multifocal tumour and in this situation conservative surgery would not have been appropriate. There might also have been an undetected cancer in the contralateral breast.
- To fail to report the margin status and managing a patient with conservative surgery without consideration of radiotherapy is unacceptable.
- It is clear that this case was not discussed at a multidisciplinary meeting.
- Axillary node status should have been assessed and has been recommended in UK guidelines since 1995.[7,9]

## Vignette 4: Pneumothorax following FNAC

A dental nurse aged 32 presented with a lump in the tail of the breast. An ultrasound examination was negative and an experienced clinical assistant in the breast clinic carried out FNAC. Unfortunately, he pierced the pleura and caused a pneumothorax that required hospitalisation and pleural drainage. The patient was not warned of the risk and complained of persistent chest pain over a period of many months.

### Comments

- Did the clinician fail in his duty of care by advancing the needle too far or by failing to warn the patient? The literature suggests a risk of around 1 in 10 000.[40–42] It is not rare to strike a rib with the needle at FNAC. Piercing the pleura may be more common because a trivial pneumothorax may go undetected.

- In several cases the court has found pneumothorax to be a rare but recognised complication that can occur without breach of duty, although a recent case ruled this injury to be negligent, which was an unexpected judgement.[42] There is often a reluctance on the part of trusts to defend or appeal low-value cases under £10 000 (as would be the case for damages here).
- In defending a claim of negligence, it is important to be able to show that the clinician was experienced in the technique.[42] Were this to be a trainee, it would be necessary to establish that he or she had been properly supervised.
- Pneumothorax has been reported following needle localisation by a radiologist and following aspiration of axillary seroma, performing FNAC and/or core biopsy. Using image guidance should theoretically reduce the risk.

## Vignette 5: False-negative FNAC, trainees in the diagnostic setting and lobular carcinoma

A 38-year-old patient was referred to a breast clinic with a breast lump. Mammography was negative and a specialist registrar found an indefinite lump of which he was not suspicious. He carried out FNAC but failed to achieve an adequate specimen (C1). At follow-up 6 weeks later a repeat FNAC showed an adequate benign sample (C2). She was discharged from the clinic but re-presented 6 months later with an invasive lobular carcinoma at the same site.

### Comments

- Trainees must be adequately supervised and only permitted to see patients by themselves when their trainer is satisfied that they are competent and understand local protocols. The 1995 British Association of Surgical Oncology (BASO) guidelines required that a trainee should also have been attending the breast clinic for at least 2 months,[7] though this requirement has been omitted from subsequent revisions of the guidelines.[8,9] Trainees should not be brought in to fill an unforeseen hiatus in the breast clinic and adherence to diagnostic protocols is essential.
- There is a learning curve in achieving adequate samples with FNAC and it is likely that this will be achieved more quickly with immediate reporting of cytology with instant feedback on

sample adequacy. The rate of inadequate FNAC samples should be monitored for each clinician.
- Clinicians should be aware that lobular cancers are prone to false-negative mammography. There is also an increased rate of inadequate cytology (C1) and of difficulty with false-negative interpretation (C2).
- The diagnosis of breast cancer in young women is difficult and in the situation where a patient complains of a lump but on clinical examination or mammography nothing is obvious, ultrasound is advisable with guided biopsy if a lesion is seen.

# Delay in diagnosis: causation issues

In a case of delay in diagnosis, it is often relatively straightforward to establish whether there has been a breach of duty of care. The next hurdle to be overcome by the claimant is to satisfy the court, on the balance of probabilities, that this delay caused her harm. The public and the judiciary have the expectation that early diagnosis carries a better outlook. It is not surprising therefore that counter-arguments of lead-time bias and predeterminism of tumour biology tend to fall on deaf ears.

Having established a breach of duty of care, the issue of causation may include the allegation that less treatment would have been required, e.g. mastectomy or chest wall radiotherapy would not have been necessary. It may also be argued that psychological damage has ensued. However, the main issue centres around whether the claimant has suffered a reduced expectation of life or if, for instance, by the time the matter comes to court she has died, whereas she would have lived longer. Expert opinion is often divided and if the experts cannot agree then the court makes a judgement. Whenever an estimation is given as to reduction in survival, allowance should be made for lead-time bias.

Richards et al.,[43] after a systematic review, concluded that there is an average reduction in 5-year survival of 7% with a delay of 3–6 months and 12% with a delay of more than 6 months. Dische et al.[44] extrapolated a 1.8% decrease in survival from Richards et al.'s data for each 1-month delay up to 6 months. In the same issue of the *Lancet*, Sainsbury et al.[45] reported no such effect but produced the apparently contradictory finding that patients with the shortest delay had the worst prognosis. This latter finding has been previously reported by Afzelius et al.[46]

The survival in patients with the best-prognosis tumours (small, special type, grade I, node negative) is not different from that of the normal population, and clearly a formula attributing a reduction in survival for each month of delay would be inappropriate in such tumours. However, if one accepts this, then for some tumours with a worse prognosis there must be a greater loss of survival.[44] It would nevertheless seem intuitive that the most aggressive tumours with rapid metastatic potential are likely to be incurable from early in their natural history, suggesting diagnostic delays in such cancers are less likely to have an impact.

## Vignettes on causation

The following real vignettes illustrate some of the causation issues that arise once liability has been established. Delay in diagnosis remains an area of considerable uncertainty and the comments reflect our experience of differing arguments presented to the court.

### Vignette 6: 12-month delay in diagnosis of node-positive carcinoma

A 32-year-old woman was referred to a breast clinic with a lump in the breast. Ultrasound showed an indeterminate opacity 1.0 cm in diameter consistent with a fibroadenoma but no sample was taken by FNAC or core biopsy. She was discharged from the clinic but returned a year later with a clinical carcinoma at the same site. This measured 2.1 cm on both ultrasound and histology and was grade 3; one of four nodes was positive. Liability for delay in diagnosis was admitted in failing to carry out a biopsy at the first visit.

## Comments

* The Nottingham Prognostic Index (NPI)[47–50] and adjuvantonline are often used to determine the difference in outcome by calculating the change of value of the index over the period of delay.
* Both NPI and adjuvantonline rely on the following assumptions about the individual case.

Assumption 1: the tumour grade remains constant – this is usually agreed by both sides.

Assumption 2: in this particular case a record of tumour size at the first visit was available, but if no clinical measurement was recorded and there was no imaging, an approximate tumour size has to be derived from a putative tumour volume, itself derived by working back from the tumour volume at diagnosis using tumour doubling times. This calculation assumes (i) that tumour growth is exponential, (ii) that in calculating tumour diameter the tumour approximates a sphere (or an ellipsoid), and (iii) that the doubling time chosen is appropriate for the tumour in question. Tumour size itself is a weak determinant of prognosis but the derived earlier tumour size is further used to calculate the likely nodal status.

Assumption 3: the nodal status at the time of the breach of duty is usually unknown, but is often disputed by the experts. Axillary node status is invariably presumed to have been negative by the claimant, and this claim is supported by tables for tumour grade and tumour size which show the probability of positive nodes. Only in grade 2 and 3 tumours greater than 2.5 cm does the probability of positive nodes rise above 50% (Table 18.2). Therefore, *on balance* it may

Table 18.2 • Nottingham Prognostic Index groups

| Group | Index value | 10-year survival (%) |
| --- | --- | --- |
| Excellent (EPG) | 2.0–2.4 | 96 |
| Good (GPG) | 2.41–3.4 | 93 |
| Moderate I (MPGI) | 3.41–4.4 | 82 |
| Moderate II (MPGII) | 4.41–5.4 | 75 |
| Poor (PPG) | 5.41–6.4 | 53 |
| Very poor (VPG) | ≥6.41 | 39 |

From the Nottingham Primary Breast Cancer Series. Data relate to patients with primary operable breast cancer, treated from 1990 to 1996.[48]

be argued that the nodes would have been negative at the earlier time when the tumour was smaller and the diagnosis missed.

## Vignette 7: 2-year delay in diagnosis of node-negative grade 1 carcinoma

A 40-year-old woman presented with a lump in the breast and a triple assessment was carried out. The tumour measured 1.5 cm on ultrasound and mammography, and FNAC was reported as benign (C2). She was discharged but 2 years later returned with a carcinoma 3 cm in diameter on histology. The tumour was grade 1 and four nodes sampled were clear. Review of the original cytology indicated that this had been under-reported and an expert opinion graded the slides unequivocally malignant (C5). Liability was admitted. The patient was treated by breast conservation and postoperative radiotherapy.

### Comments

- The standard of care must be judged by the standard reasonably expected of a cytologist working at the same level. It is inappropriate to ask a world expert in the field to judge the opinion of a doctor from a district general hospital.
- Although the tumour doubled in size over the 2-year period of delay, it remained within the good prognosis group. The treatment would have been the same with an earlier diagnosis and therefore the case did not succeed on causation.

## Vignette 8: 3-year delay in diagnosis of a carcinoma missed on screening

A woman of 50 responded to an invitation for screening and was recalled for magnification views of a localised area of microcalcification. There was a soft-tissue opacity and the appearance was judged benign on further views and ultrasound. She was returned to routine screening but 3 years later the screening films showed an obvious carcinoma at the same site. This was a 2.0 cm grade

2 infiltrating carcinoma with an extensive in situ component; four of 10 nodes were positive. An opinion from a breast-screening radiologist rated the original films as suspicious of ductal carcinoma in situ (R4) and stated that the focus of microcalcification should have been biopsied by any competent breast radiologist.

### Comments

- Delay due to radiological misinterpretation tends to be a matter of years rather than months. Screening by 3-yearly mammography probably reduces breast cancer deaths by up to 25%, and it is likely that a delay in diagnosis of 3 years will affect survival in a proportion of cases.
- The potential loss of survival in this case would be considerable since the original lesion would, on the balance of probabilities, have been an area of high-grade ductal carcinoma in situ with a near-normal expectation of life if it had been adequately treated at age 50. At age 53 the patient now has a relatively poor prognosis but on balance is still more likely to survive 10 years (Table 18.2).

## Vignette 9: 14-month delay in the breast clinic and failure to recommend chemotherapy

A 30-year-old woman was referred with a lump in the breast and was seen by a succession of specialist registrars. An initial ultrasound showed a 1-cm opacity consistent with a fibroadenoma but the FNAC was reported as mildly atypical (C3) and the pathologist advised 'consider biopsy to confirm'. However, the registrar took no action because the pathologist always seemed to produce equivocal reports. A 6-month follow-up appointment was given. The GP did not wait for this appointment but referred the patient again to the consultant, who immediately diagnosed breast cancer. The tumour was 4 cm, grade 3 and heavily node positive. The patient was treated by wide local excision, axillary clearance and radiotherapy. She was not given chemotherapy or hormone treatment until she developed bone secondaries 16 months later. Liability was admitted for the delay in diagnosis and the failure to give chemotherapy at the time of diagnosis.

## Comments

- Ignoring advice to consider a biopsy because 'he always says that' suggests an unacceptable failure of communication between clinician and cytologist.
- Arranging a 6-month follow-up for a breast lump that is presumed benign is illogical.
- The place of a trainee giving an independent opinion in a breast clinic is an ongoing area of contention.
- The judge took evidence from five expert witnesses. It was agreed that when first seen the tumour would have been grade 3, 1 cm in diameter and node negative. The tumour had increased in size to 4 cm in the 14 months of delay and opinion was divided as to whether this was ever potentially curable. The experts for the claimant were far more optimistic than those for the defence but in the event the judge preferred the latter.[51]
- The judge considered that, on balance, the breach of duty 'caused her to die 18 months before, sadly, she would have died anyway'.
- Unfortunately, the damages amounted to less than the defence had already paid into court. Civil litigation rules resulted in the family winning the case but receiving none of the settlement.

# Poor cosmetic outcome

Litigation arising from poor cosmetic outcome after surgery for breast cancer was uncommon in the past. This situation changed with the trend towards breast conservation surgery (see Chapter 4) and where surgical options have not been fully discussed.

The mastectomy rate in the UK remains close to 40%, and where mastectomy is required the increasing demand for reconstruction is reflected in national guidelines.[52] Litigation has risen in line with patients' expectations, and an unsatisfactory cosmetic outcome is now the second commonest reason for legal action against breast surgeons, although the typical size of claim is considerably less than for alleged delay in diagnosis.

Comprehensive clinical notes should record evidence of discussions with the patient regarding either immediate or later breast reconstruction. It is to the clinician's benefit to record that alternative treatment options and potential complications of surgery have been discussed. The presence of the breast-care nurse to augment and further document the surgeon's advice is advisable and her written record, usually kept separately from the clinical notes, can make all the difference when allegations of inadequate preoperative information are part of a claim for breach of duty on the part of the reconstructive surgeon.

Preoperative markings should be made on the ward by the operating surgeon, explained to and agreed with the patient without pressure of time, and a record kept of this operative planning. Hasty skin marking in the anaesthetic room or on a patient already anaesthetised are not compatible with a reasonable standard of care.

A request for immediate reconstruction can present difficulties offering the most appropriate reconstruction and yet not breach guidelines for commencing treatment. This tension has presented medico-legally where patients offered a more basic form of reconstruction such as a subpectoral implant in order to expedite mastectomy may, once the cancer has been dealt with, feel that the advice fell below a reasonable standard. The breast surgeon must make available to the patient the appropriate range of reconstructive options.

Should a patient pursue litigation for her cosmetic outcome, the Bolam principle[5] would apply in determining breach of duty, i.e. the practice would be compared with that held to be reasonable by a similar body of professionals, in this case breast surgeons trained to undertake breast reconstruction. When a poor cosmetic outcome is due to a recognised complication rather than poor judgement and provided the patient has been warned of the risk, she does not have a case against the surgeon.

Reduction mammoplasty, breast augmentation and surgery for gynaecomastia remain high-risk areas for patient dissatisfaction and should never be undertaken on an occasional basis. Evidence of appropriate discussions about potential problems needs to be adequately recorded in the notes and correspondence, together with the use of appropriate information leaflets and clinical photographs to explain the proposed procedure. Consent forms should record both the confirmation of signed informed consent as well as documenting that the literature has been received and understood.

Concerns that plastic surgeons might present expert opinions in court demanding a higher standard of reconstructive skill (such as free flap reconstruction) and suggesting that the breast surgeon had not met his duty of care remain as yet unfounded. An audit of the surgeon's operative results is not currently expected by the court, nor are there prescribed minimum numbers of procedures to comply with good practice. At present there is no certificate of competency in training in breast reconstruction within the UK, but current reconstructive guidelines[52] outline the requirements for good practice.

## Vignette 10: Poor cosmetic outcome after reconstruction by a breast surgeon

A 52-year old patient with multifocal cancer was advised to have a mastectomy by a breast surgeon and after discussion with the breast-care nurse she requested immediate reconstruction. He offered her a tissue expander, which was inserted at the time of mastectomy, but it was not possible to achieve symmetry with the large contralateral breast. Contralateral breast reduction was carried out, with a poor cosmetic outcome. She was subsequently referred to a plastic surgeon for revision surgery and then sued her first surgeon.

### Comments

- With cosmetic and reconstructive surgery, the damage is self-evident, i.e. causation is less of an issue than breach of duty. With delay in diagnosis the converse is often the case.
- Patient expectation of a good cosmetic outcome is arguably less demanding for postmastectomy reconstruction than for purely cosmetic surgery of the breast. Nevertheless, there is growing demand for a wider choice and more sophisticated reconstruction techniques.
- The first question that must be addressed is the adequacy of training in reconstructive surgery. If the level of training was appropriate, the second question is whether the standard of advice and operative skill met that which the patient could reasonably have expected. Unless the answer to both questions is in the affirmative, the surgeon is liable.
- Most breast surgeons undertaking reconstruction in the UK have attended training courses on the use of the latissimus dorsi flap and their experience with this robust flap has on the whole proved satisfactory. Some breast surgeons undertake pedicled transverse rectus

abdominis muscle reconstruction, but free tissue transfer is beyond the capability and theatre time constraints of most breast surgeons.

## The Woolf report

In a review of the UK civil justice system, Lord Woolf singled out clinical negligence cases[53] because the difficulty in proving both liability and causation accounts for much of the excessive cost and the high proportion of cases which fail. The root of the problem, however, lies less in the complexity of the law than in the climate of defensiveness. Patients feel let down when treatment goes wrong, sometimes because of unrealistic expectations, and doctors feel they are under attack from aggrieved patients and react defensively. The patients' disappointment is then heightened by what they perceive to be a refusal to acknowledge fault and an attempt to cover up.

In cases valued at less than £12 500, the median figure for the costs of litigation was 137% of the value of the claim. The general rule is that 'costs follow the event' – so the unsuccessful party is responsible for the costs of both sides. Privately financed claimants or lawyers acting on a no-win, no-fee basis are therefore reluctant to pursue actions where the chances of success are small. However, if the claimant is supported by legal aid and loses the case, costs are not recoverable by the defendant. Over 90% of claims in the UK are legally aided because of the high costs of litigation; most often the defendant is the NHS Trust, hence expenses incurred by both the claimant and defendant are funded from the public purse. This explains the pressure to settle low-value claims even if defensible and a reluctance to appeal a doubtful judgement.

The recommendations of the Woolf report are intended to improve the resolution of disputes between patients and doctors, and reduce delay and cost while treating both parties fairly. The NHS Ombudsman's role has been extended, but has no jurisdiction over financial compensation. Lord Woolf's recommendations include:

- A pre-litigation protocol where claimants should notify defendants with a written intention to sue 3 months before action. If liability is disputed, defendants should provide a reasoned answer.
- The special lists on the Queen's Bench to include a list of judges familiar with clinical negligence cases and training of trial judges in medical issues.

# Chapter 18

- Standard tables to quantify clinical negligence claims.
- Fast-track options for claims under £10 000 so that these can be litigated on a modest budget with a single expert acceptable to both parties appointed by the court.
- Medical experts are now required to address their report to the court and not to the instructing party.[54] 'The expert witness has a duty … to provide objective unbiased opinion to the court on matters within his expertise, never assuming the role of an advocate.'

## Risk management

Failure of communication and poor rapport often prompt patients into taking legal action. A woman who feels that her complaints have been taken seriously and investigated thoroughly is less likely to sue. In cases where the doctor–patient relationship breaks down, referral to another specialist may be the best course of action.

The recommendations of the PIAA study[2] cover the most common pitfalls:

- Always perform an adequate examination and document findings, especially when the referring GP's findings were unimpressive.
- Do not abandon the diagnostic pursuit because the clinical findings are unimpressive.
- If a mass is detected, investigations must rule out malignancy.
- Obtain a tissue diagnosis in a palpable mass with a negative mammogram.
- Repeat the study if a mammogram is of poor technical quality, and arrange additional views or ultrasound if mammography is equivocal.
- Compare the results of the present imaging with previous studies.
- With localisation biopsy, ensure the correct lesion is localised in both open and needle procedures; specimen radiography should always be done.

Many of these recommendations will best be achieved by establishing and adhering to a multidisciplinary approach in the care of breast patients, and this is arguably the most robust safeguard of good practice in both diagnostic and treatment aspects of breast surgery.

### Key points

- Delay in diagnosis remains the biggest cause of litigation by breast patients.
- Missed diagnosis of breast cancer is commonest, and the settlements highest, in premenopausal women.
- False reassurance from a negative mammogram is a common factor.
- Triple assessment should be reviewed in the breast multidisciplinary meeting.
- Disordant triple assessment always needs to be addressed.
- Clinical practice that complies with guidelines is easier to defend.

# References

1. Physician Insurers Association of America. Breast cancer study. Rockville, MD: PIAA, 1990.

2. Physician Insurers Association of America. Breast cancer study. Rockville, MD: PIAA, 1995; pp. 1–27.

3. Branthwaite M. Law for doctors: principles and practicalities. London: Royal Society of Medicine Press, 2000.

4 NHS Litigation Authority. Available at http://www.nhsla.com

5. Bolam v. Friern Hospital Management Committee [1957] 2 All ER 118; [1957] 1 WLR 582.

6. Bolitho v. City & Hackney Health Authority [1997] 4 All ER 771; [1997] 3 WLR 1151.

7. Breast Surgeons Group of the British Association of Surgical Oncology. Guidelines for surgeons in the management of symptomatic breast disease in the United Kingdom. Eur J Surg Oncol 1995; 21(Suppl A):1–13.

8. Breast Surgeons Group of the British Association of Surgical Oncology. Guidelines for surgeons in the management of symptomatic breast disease in the United Kingdom (1998 revision). Eur J Surg Oncol 1998; 24:464–76.

9. The Association of Breast Surgery at BASO. Guidelines for the management of symptomatic breast disease. Eur J Surg Oncol 2005; 31:S1–21.

10. Hurwitz B. Clinical guidelines and the law. Br Med J 1995; 311:1517–18.

11. Carrick SE, Bonevski B, Redman S et al. Surgeons' opinions about the NMRC clinical practice guidelines for the management of early breast cancer. Med J Aust 1998; 169:300–5.

12. Brahams D. Loss of chance of survival. Lancet 1996; 348:1604.

13. Judge v. Huntington Health Authority [1995] 6 Med LR 223.

14. Andrews BT, Bates T. Delay in the diagnosis of breast cancer: medico-legal implications. Breast 2000; 9:223–7.

15. Tennvall J, Moller T, Attwell R. Delaying factors in primary treatment of breast cancer. Acta Chir Scand 1990; 156:591–6.

16. Austoker J, Mansel R, Baum M et al. Guidelines for referral of patients with breast problems. Sheffield: NHS Breast Screening Programme, 1995.

17. Davidson T. Delay in diagnosing breast cancer: medicolegal implications. Trends Urol Gynaecol Sexual Health 1998; 3:11–12.

18 Dr Foster guide to hospitals and consultants. Available at http://www.hospital.drfoster.co.uk

19. Salih A, Webb MW, Bates T. Does open-access mammography and ultrasound delay the diagnosis of breast cancer? Breast 1999; 8:129–32.

20. Lannin DR, Harris RP, Swanson FH et al. Difficulties in diagnosis of carcinoma of the breast in patients less than fifty years of age. Surg Gynecol Obstet 1993; 177:457–62.

21. Zylstra S, Bors-Koefoed R, Mondor M et al. A statistical model for predicting the outcome in breast cancer malpractice lawsuits. Obstet Gynecol 1994; 84:392–8.

22. Yelland A, Graham MD, Trott PA et al. Diagnosing breast carcinoma in young women. Br Med J 1991; 302:618–20.

23. Woodman CBJ, Threlfall AG, Boggis CRM et al. Is the three year breast screening interval too long? Occurrence of interval cancers in NHS Breast Screening Programme's north western region. Br Med J 1995; 310:224–6.

24. Dixon JM, Anderson TJ, Lamb J et al. Fine needle aspiration cytology, in relationship to clinical examination and mammography in the diagnosis of a solid breast mass. Br J Surg 1984; 71:593–6.

25. Mitnick JS, Vazquez MF, Plesser KP et al. Breast cancer malpractice litigation in New York State. Radiology 1993; 189:673–6.

26. Joensuu H, Asola R, Holli K et al. Delayed diagnosis and large size of breast cancer after a false negative mammogram. Eur J Cancer 1994; 30A:1299–302.

27. Walter SD, Day NE. Estimation of the duration of a pre-clinical disease state using screening data. Am J Epidemiol 1983; 118:865–6.

28. Fox H, Moskowitz M, Saenger L et al. Benefit/risk analysis of aggressive mammographic screening. Radiology 1978; 128:359–65.

29. Daly CA, Apthorp L, Field S. Second round cancers: how many were visible on the first round of the UK National Breast Screening Programme, three years earlier? Clin Radiol 1998; 53:25–8.

30. Layfield LJ, Glasgow BJ, Cramer H. Fine needle aspiration in the management of breast masses. Pathol Ann 1989; 24:23–62.

31. Bates AT, Bates T, Hastrich DJ et al. Delay in the diagnosis of breast cancer: the effect of the introduction of fine needle aspiration cytology to a breast clinic. Eur J Surg Oncol 1992; 18:433–7.

32. Jenner DC, Middleton A, Webb WM et al. Inhospital delay in the diagnosis of breast cancer. Br J Surg 2000; 87:914–19.

33. Barber MD, Jack W, Dixon JM. Diagnostic delay in breast cancer. Br J Surg 2004; 91(1):49–53.

34. Spratt JS, Spratt SW. Medical and legal implications of screening and follow-up procedures for breast cancer. Cancer 1990; 66:1351–62.

35. Plotkin D, Blankenberg F. Breast cancer: biology and malpractice. Am J Clin Oncol 1991; 14:254–66.

36. Tubiana M, Koscielny S. Cell kinetics, growth rate and the natural history of breast cancer. The

Heuson Memorial Lecture. Eur J Clin Oncol 1988; 24:9–14.

37. Pearlman AW. Breast cancer: influence of growth rate on prognosis and treatment evaluation. A study based on mastectomy scar recurrences. Cancer 1976; 38:1826–33.

38. Galante E, Gallus G, Guzzon A et al. Growth rate of primary breast cancer and prognosis: observations on a 3- to 7-year follow up in 180 breast cancers. Br J Cancer 1986; 54:833–6.

39. Elmore JG, Taplin SH, Barlow WE et al. Does litigation influence medical practice? The influence of community radiologists' medical malpractice perceptions and experience on screening mammography. Radiology 2005; 236(1):37–46.

40. Christie R, Bates T. The risk of pneumothorax as a complication of diagnostic fine needle aspiration or therapeutic needling of the breast: should the patient be warned? Breast 1999; 8:98–9.

41. Gately CA, Maddox PR, Mansel RE. Pneumothorax: a complication of fine needle aspiration of the breast. Br Med J 1991; 303:627–8.

42. Bates T, Davidson T, Mansel R. Litigation for pneumothorax as a complication of fine-needle aspiration of the breast. Br J Surg 2002; 89:134–7.

43. Richards MA, Westcombe AM, Love SB et al. Influence of delay on survival in patients with breast cancer: a systematic review. Lancet 1999; 353:1119–26.

44. Dische S, Bentzen G, Bond S. The influence of delay in diagnosis of breast cancer upon outlook. Clin Risk 2000; 6:4–6.

45. Sainsbury R, Johnston C, Haward B. Effect on survival of delays in referral of patients with breast-cancer symptoms: a retrospective analysis. Lancet 1999; 353:1132–5.

46. Afzelius P, Zedeler K, Sommer H et al. Patients' and doctors' delay in primary breast cancer. Acta Oncol 1994; 33:345–51.

47. Galea MH, Blamey RW, Elston CW et al. The Nottingham Prognostic Index in primary breast cancer. Br Cancer Res Treat 1992; 22:207–19.

48. Thompson AM, Pinder SE. Prognostic factors. In: Dixon JM (ed.) The ABC of breast diseases, 3rd edn. Oxford: Blackwell Publishing, 2006; pp. 77–80.

49. Blamey RW, Ellis IO, Pinder SE et al. Survival of invasive breast cancer according to the Nottingham Prognostic Index in cases diagnosed in 1990–1999. Eur J Cancer 2007; 43(10):1548–55.

50. Blamey RW, Pinder SE, Ball GR et al. Reading the prognosis of the individual with breast cancer. Eur J Cancer 2007; 43(10):1545–7.

51. Taylor v. West Kent Health Authority [1997] 8 Med LR 251–7.

52. Association of Breast Surgery at BASO, BAPRAS and the Training Interface Group in Breast Surgery. Oncoplastic breast surgery – A guide to good practice. Eur J Surg Oncol 2007; 33:S1–23.

53. Woolf HK. Medical negligence. In: Access to justice: final report to the Lord Chancellor on the civil justice system in England and Wales. London: HMSO, 1996; pp. 169–96.

54 Civil Procedure Rules. Available at http://www.justice.gov.uk/civil/procrules

# Index

Note: Page numbers in *italics* refer to figures and page numbers in **bold** refer to tables.